Phlebotomy Technician Specialist

THOMSON

DELMAR LEARNING

Australia • Brazil • Canada • Mexico • Singapore • Spain • United Kingdom • United States

Phlebotomy Technician Specialist

Certification Exam Review

Kathryn A. Kalanick, CMA, NCPT, CPI

THOMSON

DELMAR LEARNING

Australia • Brazil • Canada • Mexico • Singapore • Spain • United Kingdom • United States

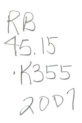

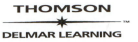
THOMSON

DELMAR LEARNING

Phlebotomy Technician Specialist: Certification Exam Review

by Kathryn A. Kalanick

Vice President, Health Care Business Unit:
William Brottmiller

Director of Learning Solutions:
Matthew Kane

Acquisitions Editor:
Sherry Dickinson

Senior Product Manager:
Darcy M. Scelsi

Editorial Assistant:
Angela Doolin

Marketing Director:
Jennifer McAvey

Marketing Channel Manager:
Chris Manion

Marketing Coordinator:
Andrea Eobstel

Technology Director:
Laurie Davis

Technology Project Manager:
Jamilynne Myers

Production Director:
Carolyn Miller

Production Manager:
Barbara A. Bullock

Art Director:
Jack Pendleton

Content Project Manager:
Stacey Lamodi

Library of Congress Cataloging-in-Publication Data

Kalanick, Kathryn A.
   Phlebotomy technician specialist : certification exam review / Kathryn A. Kalanick.
      p. ; cm.
   Includes bibliographical references and index.
   ISBN 1-4180-0140-6 (alk. paper)
   1. Phlebotomy—Examinations, questions, etc. 2. Medical technologists—Certification—Study guides. I. Title.
   [DNLM: 1. Phlebotomy—United States—Examination Questions. 2. Allied Health Personnel—United States—Examination Questions. 3. Certification—United States—Examination Questions. QY 18.2 K14p 2007]
   RB45.15.K355 2007
   616.07'561—dc22

                                    2006027332

NOTICE TO THE READER

DEDICATION

This book is dedicated to every student who has touched
my life: You have inspired me to reach
and achieve more than I ever
dreamed possible.

Contents

Preface

It is no longer adequate simply to be trained as a layperson in the field of medicine. Every discipline requires a standardized formal education and either licensure or certification. Certification by profession is no longer the exception; it is the rule. In today's society of specialists, certification sets a standard of demonstrated competency. Certification is evidence that an individual has mastered the skills required to perform in a specific technical area, in this case phlebotomy.

The purpose of certification is twofold: First, it establishes that the individual has met the required competencies with the skills to perform as a credentialed phlebotomist. Second, upon successful completion of the certification exam, the phlebotomist is given credentials and/or a title. Certified phlebotomists are authorized to use the appropriate initials after their names. Certification exams are generally given on a national or state level, in conjunction with an educational program, and are affiliated with the program's approval or the school's accrediting organization.

The goal of this examination review book is to provide both the new phlebotomy graduate and other allied health professionals meeting the certification exam requirements a comprehensive review guide for concentrated study of phlebotomy content and procedures. In addition to the standard phlebotomy concepts, the latest trends and safety measures, as outlined by Occupational Safety and Health Administration (OSHA), have been included as well as the standards set forth by Clinical and Laboratory Standards Institute (CLSI).

The features that distinguish this review book from others on the market are its comprehensive review, critical thinking activities, and the ability to generate multiple practice exams. The review book has been designed around Thomson Delmar Learning's top two phlebotomy textbooks: *Phlebotomy Technician Specialist: A Practical Guide to Phlebotomy* (Kalanick) and *The Complete Textbook of Phlebotomy* (Hoeltke). It encompasses the knowledge base and testing areas, by percentage, of the top phlebotomy certification agencies; so, regardless of which national certification exam you select or are required to take, you can be assured that the content has been addressed.

Agencies that administer certification examinations in phlebotomy are:

- American Association of Allied Health Professionals, Inc. (AAAHP)
- American Medical Technologists (AMT)
- American Society for Phlebotomy Technicians (ASPT)
- American Society of Clinical Pathologists (ASCP)
- National Center for Competency Testing (NCPT)
- National Phlebotomy Association: Certified Phlebotomy Technician (CPT)
- National Accrediting Agency for Laboratory Personnel Phlebotomy Examination (CLPlb)

The book is divided into two sections. Section I addresses examination preparation, providing the applicant with study techniques for successfully preparing and passing written examinations. Section II is divided into six modules. Each module includes a thorough review of the topics and concludes with multiple-choice questions, presented in the same or similar format to the actual certification exams, and critical thinking activities to help the reader begin to apply the concepts learned.

ORGANIZATION

During the development of the content and exams for this review book, each phlebotomy certification agency's suggested content review material and the percentage of each testing section were taken into consideration. The material was cross-referenced and analyzed to provide the reader with an approximation of each agency's examination. Although the exams vary slightly from agency to agency and not every phlebotomy certification examination has the exact number of questions on the same topic, the review book provides a broad enough content and question base to cover the information regardless of which examination the applicant is studying for.

Module 4: Review of Medical Terminology and Anatomy and Physiology
30 Questions = 6%
Module 5: The Health Care System
20 Questions = 5%
Module 6: Specimen Collection, Processing, and Handling
300 Questions = 63%
Module 7: Point-of-Care Testing, Other Laboratory Tests, and Nonblood Specimens
50 Questions = 10%

Module 8: Legal, Ethical, and Professional Communications, and Clerical Skills and Duties
50 Questions = 10%

Module 9: Regulatory Agencies, Safety Standards, and Infection Control
30 Questions = 6%

RATIONALE FOR THE BOOK'S ORGANIZATION

As an allied health professional and educator for over 25 years, a certified medical assistant, a nationally certified phlebotomist, and a certified postsecondary instructor, and having maintained continuous personal certification through examination, both written and practical, and continuing education in all three disciplines, I understand the value of a well written and user-friendly review book. As a practitioner and educator, I have extensive experience working with thousands of medical assistants and phlebotomists in classrooms, laboratories, clinics, and hospitals.

Working with students and graduates in preparation for certification examinations in a variety of disciplines over the course of my career has provided me with insight into the specifics of what it takes to prepare for this tremendous achievement. It is my goal with this review book to provide the certification applicant with a comprehensive review of the most testable topics, provide critical thinking opportunities, and create a testing format in which applicants can take multiple practice exams to improve their overall knowledge and comfort level prior to taking a national certification exam. Through practice tests, applicants are given the means to achieve these goals by improving their comprehension and retention of material.

The CD that accompanies the book allows applicants to take a pretest to assess their current level of understanding.

This allows them to see areas of weakness and focus their study on those areas. The CD also allows applicants multiple opportunities to take practice exams. They can use the CD to structure practice exams either to focus on a specific area or to simulate an entire certification exam, practicing on questions from all topic areas. The practice exams can be restructured each time to accommodate each applicant's specific needs. For example, if the applicant is consistently struggling through one particular topic area, an exam can be tailored to address just that topic area. When the applicant feels comfortable with one topic area, additional topics can be added. This process can be restructured time and time again. After completion of this review process, the applicant will have the self-confidence to take and pass the certification exam.

ACKNOWLEDGMENTS

The dedication, perseverance, and commitment of everyone who reviewed the manuscript, along with their suggestions and advice, are greatly appreciated. Each individual has made a substantial contribution to the overall format, content, and correctness of the text. Thank you.

I would also like to thank my daughter, Andrea King, NCMA, for her research and suggestions and for the countless hours she spent typing test questions. A note of gratitude is significantly due to Diane Caudill, CMA, NCPT, CPI, for her input and suggestions in developing the critical thinking exercises.

A special word of thanks goes to Maureen Rosener, acquisitions editor. I have thoroughly enjoyed the many projects we have worked on together. And Darcy Scelsi, senior product manager, your facilitation of this project and your assistance are deeply appreciated. Thanks go to my husband: Your encouragement and support are forever cherished.

SECTION I

Exam Preparation

MODULE **1**

The Examinations

INTRODUCTION

The purpose of this manual is to assist you, the student, in preparing for exams you are likely to encounter in your training, as well as the AMT, ASCP, or NCA phlebotomy certification exam. The manual is arranged according to the content of these exams and is divided into two sections. Section I is comprised of three modules and provides general information about studying, test taking, and the organization and format of the certification exams. Module 1 addresses exam question formats, and Modules 2 and 3 address basic study and test-taking strategies to familiarize you with the mechanics of the testing process and to help overcome test anxiety. A pre-test can be created using the CD located in the back of the book. Taking a pre-test will assess your basic knowledge base. Its purpose is to identify any knowledge weaknesses you may have and to direct you to the appropriate modules for further study. Practice tests are designed to further assess test performance, identify knowledge weakness, and provide guidance on continued study.

To study while you are taking classes, it is recommended that you do the following:

1. Read Section I.
2. Review the appropriate modules or sections of modules corresponding to the required texts being studied or the classes or topics within the classes you are taking.
3. As you prepare for in-class exams, review Modules 2 and 3 in Section I; employ any or all of the study or test-taking suggestions that will be of use.
4. Use the outlines in the modules you are studying as a tool to prepare for the test. Augment the outlines with other information emphasized by the instructor or texts being used.

To prepare for a certification exam, it is recommended that you follow a process of organized study as follows:

1. If you have used this text during the course of your phlebotomy training, most or all of the chapters will be familiar to you.
2. Read Section I.
3. Take a pre-test generated from the CD located in the back of the book. Score the test and calculate the score.
4. Depending on which topic areas have the lowest score—turn to the appropriate section of the manual and study the outline using the appropriate suggestions discussed in Module 2 Section I.
5. Attend to the weaker of the remaining two sections as described above.
6. Eventually, you may wish to browse through all the modules, studying specific areas in detail as warranted.
7. A post-test can be generated from the CD located in the back of the book. It is suggested that you take a post-test prior to taking an actual certification exam.

EXAM QUESTION FORMAT

All certification exams consist of A-type multiple-choice questions. The following describes the significant features of the A-type multiple-choice question.

Components of a Multiple-Choice Question

A multiple-choice question is commonly called an item; it has two parts: a stem and a list of response options. The stem is that part of an item that poses a question, problem, or incomplete statement. The stem can have either positive or negative polarity. A stem that is positively polarized arranges the question in the context of what is true; for example, "Which of the following procedures requires informed consent?" A stem that is negatively polarized arranges the question in the context of what is false; for example, "All of the following procedures require informed consent except:". Likewise, the stem can be either a complete sentence or an incomplete sentence. Complete stems are statements or questions that contain a complete thought and can be answered before reviewing the response options. A response option is paired with the stem that either answers the question or is strongly associated with it. Incomplete stems present a portion of a statement or incomplete thought that must be paired with a response option to complete a sentence or thought.

The response options represent the possible answers to an item posed by the stem. There must be at least three options to be considered a multiple-choice question, however, most items contain four or five options. Options are usually identified by a letter (lower- or uppercase) or a number. One of the options represents the best response; whereas, the others, called distracters, represent less desirable responses and are considered incorrect. Options can be presented in four grammatical arrangements: a sentence, a completion of a stem, an incomplete sentence, or a single word.

Positive Polarity. This is the most common multiple-choice question arrangement. It consists of a stem and four or five lettered options (one best answer and three or four distracters). The candidate is required to select the one best answer. For example:

Which of the following is a function of the skeletal system?
a. absorption of nutrients
b. homeostasis
c. sensation
d. framework for support
e. elimination of waste

Negative Polarity. A format commonly found in each exam presents a stem that generally calls for what is false. Stems having negative polarity generally include the term **"EXCEPT"** capitalized and bold-faced. The question, therefore, calls for the exception. For example:

Each of the following is a function of the skeletal system **EXCEPT**
a. framework for support
b. blood cell production
c. protection of internal organs
d. sensation
e. site of attachment of muscles

In both examples, D is the correct response; whereas, A, B, C, and E are distracters.

Adapted from Cody, J.D. & Kelley-Amey C. (2006). *Medical Assisting Exam Review,* 2e. New York: Thomson Delmar Learning.

MODULE 2

Study Techniques

STUDY METHODS

Successfully preparing and passing a written test, whether it is a test given in a phlebotomy course, or a certification examination, requires the ability to learn and recall information. Therefore, the intent of this module is to provide some guidance for developing test preparation and study skills.

Note-Taking

Note-taking is an important component of effective learning. It is the means by which one records and organizes information for later review and study. Although taking notes is typically performed during a lecture to capture the information provided by an instructor or speaker, note-taking techniques can similarly be used while studying written material as a means of recording and organizing its important concepts. The development of note-taking skills, therefore, will serve you well in your education and certification test preparation. Regardless of the method used, the critical aspect of effective note-taking is keeping the information organized so that subordinate points are placed in close proximity to the concepts they support or illuminate so that these relationships are visibly apparent. The major portions of this text, for example, are organized in an outline format to do just that. This organized way to record or present information clarifies the interrelationships within the information as a whole, as well as the detail necessary to sustain these relationships. This permits the student or examinee to not only learn the details of a given subject, but to understand how these details are related to one another to create a unified subject. The three most common methods of taking notes include the outline format, mind-mapping format, and Cornell format. These methods are discussed below.

Outline format (see Figure 2-1). This format, preferred by the author and extensively used throughout this text, organizes information using headings, subheadings, and subordinate points. A systematic labeling system using Roman numerals (I, II, III . . .), Arabic numerals (1, 2, 3 . . .), and lowercase and uppercase letters keeps the headings and subordinate information organized so that the important note-taking features described above are maintained.

```
I.   Nervous System
     A.  Function
     B.  Organization
         1.  Central Nervous System
         2.  Peripheral Nervous System
             a.  Afferent (Sensory) Nervous System
             b.  Efferent (Motor) Nervous System
                 (1) Somatic Nervous System
                 (2) Autonomic Nervous System
                     (a) Sympathetic Nervous System
                     (b) Parasympathetic Nervous
                         System
                         i)  Promotes digestion and
                             elimination functions.
                         ii) Restores normal resting
                             function after episodes of
                             stress.
II.  Sensory System
     A.  Function
     B.  Organization
```

Figure 2-1

Outline format.

Mind-mapping (see Figure 2-2). A more creative variation of the outline format, mind-mapping is often preferred by students who think and process information outside the linear constraints of strict outlining. The note-taker typically begins by recording the main topic or idea at the center of the page. From the central main idea, the student records the subordinate or supporting information as an extension or branch of the main idea. Information subordinate to these branchings is recorded as further extensions much like the limbs and branches of a tree. Like outlining, mind-mapping organizes information so that the details of a subject clearly demonstrate its unifying features.

Cornell format (see Figure 2-3). This note-taking method is used by drawing a vertical line from the top to the bottom of the note-page approximately two inches from the left edge. Written notes are recorded to the right of the line, perhaps using either the outline or mind-mapping format, or any format the student chooses. The

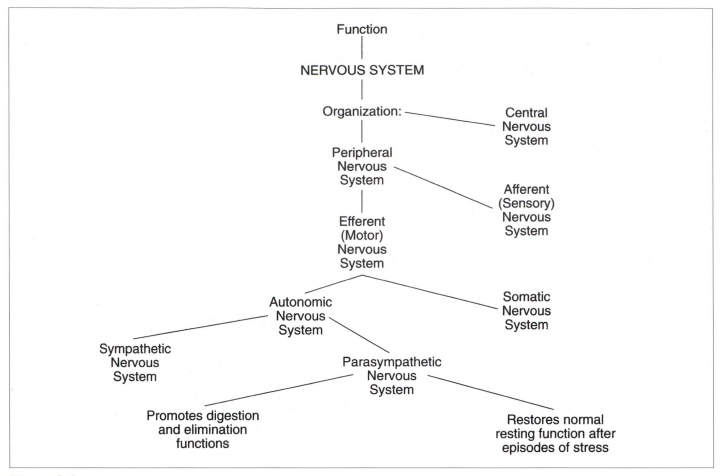

Figure 2-2

Mind-mapping format.

space to the left of the vertical line is used to record any information the student chooses to enhance organization, topic integration, and the like. This may include highlighting key terms or main ideas, as well as references to written sources such as texts and periodicals. Additionally, this space may be used to record other information while the student studies the notes, such as questions, examples, supporting concepts, information from other sources that clarify the notes, etc.

Effective note-taking, especially the methods discussed above, forces students to organize the information as it is heard or read. This permits greater concentration on the subject matter and enhances the cognitive processes vital to comprehension and memory. The following points discuss additional guidelines to consider when taking notes.

- Record your name, the date, and the page number on each page of your notes.
- Attempt to prepare your notes in your own words rather than in the speaker's or author's
- Record only the information that makes the concepts understandable, not everything you hear or read.
- Ask the lecturer to clarify anything said or written on the board that you do not understand.

- Instead of recording all information shown on overheads and slides, request copies, or offer to make copies for your notes if appropriate.
- Avoid using a recording device unless it clearly improves your note-taking or learning. It is a courtesy to speakers to seek permission to record their lectures.
- Record your notes clearly enough the first time to avoid recopying them later. Your time is better spent studying your notes rather than rewriting them.
- Avoid using the notes of others. It is useful, however, to compare your notes with others to identify any important concepts that you may have missed or misinterpreted.
- Use shorthand techniques, standardized or ones of your own design, for frequently occurring words such as *the, and, by, with, of,* etc. The use of medical shorthand, abbreviations, and acronyms can be valuable in quickly and accurately recording information.
- Concepts repeated or written on the board are usually important and should be included in your notes.
- Participate by asking questions and contributing ideas, especially if they clarify your notes.

See p. 22 of text	NERVOUS SYSTEM Function:
	Organization:
Brain/spinal cord	Central Nervous System
	Peripheral Nervous System
Sends sensory information to brain.	Afferent (Sensory) Nervous System
Sends signals to organs and body.	Efferent (Motor) Nervous System Somatic Nervous System
Confusing (?)	
	Autonomic Nervous System Sympathic Nervous System
Clarify	Parasympathetic Nervous System: Promotes digestion and elimination functions.
	Restores normal resting function after episodes of stress.
Read next week	SENSORY SYSTEM
	Function:
	Organization:

Figure 2-3

Cornell format.

- If a lecturer has a tendency to skip around, leave plenty of space in your notes for additions.
- If important information is repeated that has been recorded earlier, use connecting arrows instead of recording the information again.
- Use pencil or erasable ink when recording notes so that errors can be easily and neatly corrected.
- Record references to authors, texts, and other sources in the margins of your notes.

Time Management

Lack of time is the most common excuse for poor test performance. More often than not, it is not a lack of time but a lack of time management. Just getting started and beginning the study process tends to be more difficult than studying itself; however, delaying your study activities will only interfere with your ability to effectively prepare for an exam. This is especially crucial with regard to certification exams since they may be offered only two or three times a year. The following are some basic tips for organizing your study time:

- Study difficult or boring subjects first. Students generally find the administrative component the least interesting, and anatomy and physiology the most difficult; perhaps these are good places to start.
- Avoid cramming by spacing out your study time. Attempt to devote a specific time each day or week for study.

- Study during the time of day when you function best. Some are naturally morning people, others are night people; keep this in mind when scheduling your study time.
- Study material organized on three-by-five-inch index cards (or a cassette recorder) during waiting periods. When you are waiting for the bus or in line at the theater, keep material on hand to study while you wait.
- Negotiate an agreement with significant others concerning your study time.
- Do not permit others to interfere with your study time: learn to say "NO."
- Attempt to accomplish one more thing in the time allotted.
- In the event of time constraints, perfection cannot be a high priority.

Developing Discipline

Effective study requires discipline. One method you can exercise to develop greater discipline is described as follows:

Study as long as you are interested, but no longer. Once you have become uninterested or bored, make the commitment to stop; however, read one more page or solve one more problem; then stop, even if your interest is renewed. During the next study session, take the same approach, but this time complete two study units before stopping. In the following study session, complete three study units before quitting, and so on. Using this technique helps you to develop greater discipline in the effective use of study time.

An additional method is the common "To Do" list. In planning your test preparation activities and study time, itemize all of the things you need to do to prepare for the exam. Organize this list by prioritizing each activity into one of three categories: A, B, and C. The A category represents tasks that are the most important and must be completed first. Category B items have intermediate importance and will ultimately fall into the A category as A tasks are completed. Category C items have the least importance and are routinely completed as time permits. As a rule of thumb, you should spend 80 percent of your time attending to the top 20 percent of your objectives; that is, category A items. Likewise, you should spend the other 20 percent of your time on the remaining 80 percent of your objectives; that is, category B and C items.

SQ3R Method

SQ3R is a five-step guide to assist in the study of any subject. SQ3R is shorthand for SQRRR—an acronym that means Survey, Question, Read, Recite, and Review. This method is useful because it organizes the study process into manageable steps to facilitate learning. The following is a brief description of each step:

Survey. To survey the material you are studying, scan the table of contents, paragraph headings, illustrations, examples, summaries, and sample questions to get a sense of the basic content of the material and its organization.

Question. Based on the content just surveyed, formulate in your mind questions that might be answered within the material. Or, read any review or discussion questions at the end of each chapter as a stimulus for pinpointing important concepts and information in the chapter. Write down the questions on paper or in the margins of the text, referring to them as needed.

Read. Read the material and focus your energies on understanding the subject matter while attempting to answer the questions created in the previous step.

Recite. Attempt to recite aloud the material you recall from the reading. Review the questions posed earlier to stimulate recall.

Review. Review the material to identify information gaps and to clarify poorly understood concepts. Repeat the process until you are satisfied with your performance.

This can be an especially effective technique as it allows for the creation of associations and relationships within the material as a means of improving understanding and recall. The chapters of this manual are organized in a manner suitable to the SQ3R methodology.

Study Groups

Studying in groups can enhance the learning process by making the study process more enjoyable and more energetic. By studying in a group arrangement, students are permitted to exchange ideas and impressions thereby confirming or questioning each other's understanding. Group study requires more participative activity and is much less passive than independent study. It is recommended, however, that you limit your study group to three to five members; larger groups often lead to excessive socializing. Group study requires greater logistical commitment than does studying alone, so it is important that group members agree to, and adhere to, the study group's objectives. The following are some suggestions concerning study groups:

1. Formulate and agree on the study group's purpose and ultimate objective. The group must agree on what it wishes to accomplish. In studying for a course test or certification exam, the group's ultimate objective would naturally be to pass the test. Whatever the case, members may have different goals. One member may wish to concentrate on a single portion of the exam, whereas others may wish to concentrate on other areas. To be effective, however, the group must agree on the goals it wishes to pursue and attempt to align each member's agenda to the group's overall study plan. If there is wide disparity, perhaps it is best to form smaller study groups or seek other group members with parallel needs.

2. Schedule the study sessions and establish an agenda for each. Agree on meeting times and places as well as a tentative agenda for each meeting. It is important to maintain a certain level of flexibility as subsequent meeting agendas may be affected by what occurred in the preceding study session; adjust the schedule accordingly to meet each member's needs while focusing on the study group's goals.

3. Test each other through questions. Questioning is an effective way of assessing what you know and remember. There are a variety of ways of approaching this step; one way would be to ask selected members specific questions soliciting the assistance of others as needed. Another technique would be to ask open-ended questions of the group in general to stimulate discussion and to explore new ways of looking at different concepts.

4. Practice teaching each other. One of the most effective ways to learn something is to have to teach it. Within a group, each member has a favorite topic or commands a certain level of expertise in a particular subject area. By taking advantage of this, members can choose an area and give a lecture or some form of presentation to help other members organize or learn that subject. Another approach is to have members who are weak in a given subject give a presentation on

that subject. Discussing techniques each uses to help remember certain facts or concepts is valuable as well.

5. Conduct open-ended discussions. It may be very useful, as well as helpful to clarify one's own understanding, to discuss and debate selected issues, especially if these issues are controversial. Legal and ethical issues are particularly suitable to this forum.

6. Rely on each other for support. If you have a particular skill that others lack, such as dosage calculations, attempt to make yourself available to tutor one of your group members. Help each other out; not only in study but in other areas as well, such as day care and transportation.

Cramming

Cramming, although pedagogically unsound, is sometimes necessary. When confronted with the need to cram, students are often tempted to learn everything lightly; however, this approach allows for marginal recall. First, it is better to focus on your weakest areas. Taking the practice tests will permit you to identify your weakest subject areas. It is recommended that you spend 25 percent of your time learning the material and the remaining 75 percent drilling yourself on that material. Second, use outlines, flash cards, or a cassette recorder as resources for your study drills. Reading material repeatedly is an inefficient means of studying; instead, recite the material aloud to imprint the information in your memory. Last, avoid studying the day before the exam to allow your batteries to recharge. Relax and avoid any pretest anxiety.

Memory Techniques

A considerable number of questions on phlebotomy tests and on certification exams are knowledge-based questions requiring the recall of facts and information. The vast majority of your study time, therefore, will probably be devoted to memorizing facts, terminology, principles, concepts, and theories. There are a number of devices that have been developed to assist you in memorizing and recalling information. Some of these devices are described below.

Repetition. Memorization is imprinting information in the brain through repetitive processes for later recall. The more senses employed in this process, the more effective the recall. Repetition techniques reinforce learning, retention, and recall, however, this form of learning is rote in nature, having little impact on comprehension. Selected repetition techniques are described as follows:

- Index cards are an excellent tool for memorizing information through repetition. They can be used to learn terminology, steps in a procedure, or any information of a factual nature.

- Cassette recorders are effective tools as well. Suppose, for example, you want to remember the five basic functions of the skeletal system as outlined in the anatomy and physiology chapter:

Anatomy and Physiology
A. Skeletal system functions
1. Framework for support
2. Protection of internal organs
3. Blood cell production
4. Attachment for muscles
5. Calcium and phosphorous storage and release

You might record the following statement: "The five functions of the skeletal system are . . ." Now pause long enough to list them in your mind. Then record the functions by stating them out loud. Continue doing this with the outlines as appropriate. Play back the recording, attempting to recite the answers before they are given. Continue this process as needed to memorize the material.

Pegword System. The pegword system was introduced in England by John Sanbrook in 1879. It is a powerful method of memorizing items on a list. The items on a list are associated with a series of numbered objects shown below:

One: Bun
Two: Shoe
Three: Tree
Four: Door
Five: Hive
Six: Sticks
Seven: Heaven
Eight: Gate
Nine: Wine
Ten: Hen

For example, suppose you want to remember the following list:
1. car
2. knife
3. stethoscope
4. apple
5. girl
6. window
7. box
8. book
9. pencil
10. shirt

Now read back over the list and attempt to memorize them for a moment. Next, without peeking, attempt to write down as many items as you can remember. Most people rarely recall all of them. Now visualize the matchup of the items in the list with the numbered objects shown above as follows:

One: A *car* sitting in a *bun.*
Two: A *knife* sticking out of a *shoe.*
Three: A *stethoscope* hanging from a *tree.*
Four: An *apple* wedged in a *door.*
Five: A *girl* holding a bee*hive.*
Six: A *window* surrounded by *sticks.*
Seven: A *box* floating in *heaven.*

Eight: A *book* balanced on a *gate*.
Nine: A *pencil* floating in *wine*.
Ten: A *shirt* worn by a *hen*.

Visualize these paired images for a moment attempting to memorize them. Now, without peeking, write down, in order, the items from the list. If done properly, you should have been able to remember all of them. Not only can you list the items in order with this technique, but you can identify, out of order, each item by number. The key is to create a mental image of the items to be remembered. Because this technique allows you to organize the information in your memory, research has demonstrated an increase in recall ability by a factor of two to four. The nice thing about this method is that the imagery need not make any sense; according to experts, the more absurd the association, the stronger the recall.

Rhyming. Rhyming, an ancient technique, can be a useful device to improve memory. Examples include eight times eight fell on the floor, picked it up with sixty-four ($8 \times 8 = 64$); in fourteen hundred ninety-two, Columbus sailed the ocean blue; thirty days hath September, April, June, and November, all the rest are thirty-one, but for February the excepted one. A clever variation to this technique can be used to prevent confusing carpals (hand-bones) with tarsals (footbones): Hands steer a car(pals), feet step on tar(sals).

Alpha Prompts. Associating information with letters of the alphabet can be helpful. Reciting the names of the fifty states, for example, is easier when listed alphabetically. The ABCs of basic life support is a common example: A-airway, B-breathing, and C-circulation. The classic signs for diabetes mellitus are the three Ps: polyuria, polydipsia, and polyphagia.

Acrostics. Acrostics are devices such as acronyms and related arrangements that aid information recall. An acronym is a mnemonic device that uses the first letter of a series of words. Examples include: ROY G. BIV to remember the colors of the visible light spectrum—Red, Orange, Yellow, Green, Blue, Indigo, and Violet; HOMES to remember the names of the Great Lakes—Huron, Ontario, Michigan, Erie, and Superior. Another acrostic arrangement uses the first letter of the words in a phrase or saying to provide a memory cue. Examples include: *Kings Play Cards On Fairly Good Satin* to remember the taxonomic organization of organisms—Kingdom, Phylum, Class, Order, Family, Genus, and Species; *All Dieters Eat Kilocalories* to remember the fat-soluble vitamins A, D, E, and K.

Comprehension, Application, and Analysis

Methods of exercising and testing the comprehension, application, and analysis of information are best conducted during group study sessions described earlier. The majority of techniques discussed thus far apply to knowledge questions: those that require recall of facts and information. Comprehension questions, on the other hand, not only require information recall but require understanding of the information as well as its significance. Comprehension is demonstrated when one can summarize, paraphrase, interpret, or translate the information, as well as determine the implications, consequences, or effects of the information. A technique useful in developing comprehension that is appropriate to group study is to examine how and why an issue or concept of discussion is important or relevant. For example, when learning that trauma can lead to shock, it is important to know why this occurs. When injury occurs, the autonomic nervous system responds by constricting blood vessels, creating inadequate peripheral blood flow and causing insufficient return of blood to the heart for subsequent transport of oxygen to body cells and tissues. Application questions not only require remembering and comprehending information, but also require the ability to take the underlying theories or principles supporting the information and apply them to other situations or scenarios. Application questions force the student to use the information, not just remember and understand it. A useful exercise is to attempt to associate new information to what is already known. For example, when reviewing the principles of asepsis, attempt to recall the last time you performed such a procedure and relate the principles and theories that support your actions step-by-step. Another useful exercise employs identifying principles or theories common to more than one situation. For example, the principle of capillary action is common to many medical procedures and interventions.

Analysis questions require the ability to recall, understand, and apply information as well as the ability to dissect and evaluate its arrangement, structure, and organization. Analysis allows you to differentiate among the various theoretical and principal components of a concept to identify any underlying interrelationships and significance. For example, when studying disease processes, it is learned that there are myriad causes for hepatitis. Analytical skills can be exercised by attempting to identify the various reasons hepatitis occurs, given different clinical pictures.

SUMMARY

To perform well on a course exam or a certification exam requires greater than minimal commitment to organized study. Your task, therefore, is to develop a study plan that identifies the subject areas to be studied, as well as the time commitment needed for each. Once you have organized your study plan and a timetable, you must then exercise discipline and adhere to the plan. There are no clear shortcuts, so make the commitment to study for the exam no matter how difficult, and follow the advice of Winston Churchill: "Never! Never! Never! Never give up!"

Adapted from Cody, J.D. & Kelley-Amey C. (2006). *Medical Assisting Exam Review*, 2e. New York: Thomson Delmar Learning.

MODULE 3

Test-Taking Stratagems

By themselves, test-taking stratagems are poor substitutes for lack of knowledge; however, phlebotomy programs that require a wide variety of coursework, as well as broad-based tests like most certification exams make it difficult to know all of the material well. Employing a test-taking principle here and a technique there, improves the probability of increasing one's test score, especially for those who are predisposed to test anxiety. Test-taking is a skill distinct from recalling, understanding, applying, and analyzing information; therefore, learning how to take a test is an integral component of the test-taking challenge. Whether you are preparing for a certification exam or a test in a phlebotomy course, the following are some suggestions and advice on successfully taking tests.

Tips on Multiple-Choice Questions

As discussed in Module 1 Section I, the AMT, ASCP, and NCA exams consist of multiple-choice questions. These questions consist of a stem and four or five lettered response options; that is, three or four distracters and "one best answer." Consider the following suggestions when answering this question type.

- Read the question carefully before jumping to the response options.
- Identify whether the question is asking for the true response (positive polarity) or the false response (exception—negative polarity).
- Do not read into the question information that is not provided. Likewise, do not dismiss information that is provided.
- Attempt to answer the question in your mind prior to reviewing the options.
- If the answer you have determined is not among the response options, choose the best available option or attempt to identify the correct option by eliminating the distracters.
- Always stick with your initial response unless you have made an obvious error and you are certain of the correct response.
- If the options cover a wide range of quantities and you do not know the correct option, choose one in the middle of the range.

- After eliminating as many distracters as you can, and the remaining options are similar except for a word or two, choose the one that has the greatest complexity or wordiness.
- In sentence completion questions, eliminate the grammatically incorrect options.
- Do not choose an option that is partially true or partially false.
- Heed terms that are underlined, *italicized*, CAPITALIZED, or in **bold type**.
- Options associated with patient-relation questions that imply all is well, deny patient feelings, change the subject raised by patients, encourage cheerfulness, or renounce professional responsibility usually represent distracters; avoid choosing them.
- If a question totally confounds you, mark it with a "?" and skip it. If time permits return to the question and do the following:
  - Choose one of two options that are similar, except for a word or two.
  - Choose one of two options that sound or look similar.
  - If two quantities are approximately equal, choose one.
  - Choose the option that appears to have the greatest detail, complexity, or wordiness.
  - Two or more options that are plausible where no one is clearly better than the others are usually distracters; eliminate them.
  - Choose the option that uses the same terms or language found in the stem.
  - If two options are opposites, choose one.
  - Choose one of the central options avoiding the first or last option.
- If none of the above suggestions help you narrow down the possibilities, answer all the questions marked "?" with the same letter. This will increase the statistical chances of choosing the correct response option.
- If very little time remains, quickly mark the unanswered questions with the same letter as described above.

True-False Questions

Although simple true-false questions will not be found in any of the certification exams, they may be used in a phlebotomy course. Simply stated, a true-false question is usually a statement regarding a concept, fact, or state of affairs; the student is to determine whether the statement, as it is written, is either true or false. If a test consists of a variety of question types to include true-false questions, and depending on the complexity of the test and time allotted to complete it, it is advisable to answer true-false questions quickly as they generally are awarded the least number of points; this should make intuitive sense since guessing will provide a 50 percent probability of being right. If, on the other hand, a test is composed of entirely true-false questions, answer each one carefully. There are two other points to bear in mind: 1) if any part of a true-false statement is false, the whole statement must be considered false, and 2) absolute qualifiers such as always; never, all, and none generally make the statement false.

True-false-substitution questions are an interesting variation of the simple true-false type that may be used as a testing instrument in a phlebotomy course. A statement is made with one or more words underlined. If the statement is true, the student simply marks it true; however, if the statement is false, the student must substitute the underlined word(s) with a word or phrase that will make the statement true. This question type is more difficult and offers a smaller probability of guessing correctly than does the simple true-false question:

_____ The neuron is the functional physiologic unit of the kidney.

> This statement as it is presented is false, the neuron is not the functional unit of the kidney, it is a nerve cell. If the underlined word were replaced with the word *nephron* in the space provided, the statement would then be true.

Fill-in-the-Blank and Essay Questions

Fill-in-the-blank items are equally common question types in phlebotomy courses. It consists of a sentence containing a blank space for insertion of a word or phrase to correctly complete the sentence. Preparing for fill-in-the-blank questions often demands overlearning because of the specificity required in answering such a question correctly.

Essay questions are considered among most students to be the most difficult testing format. Fortunately, this format is not found on any of the certification exams; however, essay questions are common in phlebotomy courses. Unlike a multiple-choice question where the question and answer are clearly stated, and the student merely recognizes and selects the correct option, essay questions require the student to verbalize an answer without reference to any source other than one's own

memory and comprehension. Students clearly realize that studying for an essay test is a whole different matter when compared to a multiple-choice test. As an evaluation instrument, essay questions are designed to test the student's knowledge, comprehension, application, and analysis of the subject matter as described in Module 2 Section I. Often, essay questions also allow the instructor to evaluate a student's writing or communication skills. According to education psychologists, having knowledge and understanding of a subject is a skill distinct from the ability to explain this knowledge and understanding. This is often frustrating to students who, having the proper knowledge of a concept, experience great difficulty in explaining the concept to another. This text was designed not only for the purpose of helping candidates prepare for certification exams, but to be used as a study aid to help students prepare for phlebotomy course exams as well. The following advice, therefore, is provided to assist students in answering essay-type questions:

- Become familiar with the meaning of key words commonly found in essay questions (see Figure 3-1).
- Mentally, or on your paper, prepare a mind-map or brief outline to organize your thoughts. Writing your outline on paper may earn some points even if you don't have time to prepare a formal answer.
- Leave plenty of space between the points and sub-points of your outline for later inclusions.
- Think about the question further while you refer to your outline; include additional points that come to mind in the spaces left in your outline.
- Once you are satisfied with the organization of your thoughts on paper, prepare the written response to the question while referring to the outline to keep your writing organized.
- Write neatly and legibly.
- Avoid writing any introductory information, and get directly to the point. Although this is an essay question, it is not an essay. Avoid filler sentences that add useless information to your answer.
- Time permitting, review your writing for errors and clarity.

Attitude

Test scores are not a measure of self-worth; however, we often associate our sense of worthiness with our performance on an exam. Thoughts such as "If I don't pass this test, I'm a failure" are mental traps not rooted in truth. Failing a test is failing a test, nothing more. It is in no way descriptive of your value as a person or as a health care professional. Believing that test performance is a reflection of your virtue places unreasonable pressure on your performance. Not passing the certification test only means that your certification status has been delayed. Maintaining a positive attitude is, therefore, important. If you have studied hard, reaffirm this mentally and believe

• Analyze	Identifying the parts of a concept, explaining each along with their interrelationship.
• Compare	Explain the similarities among two or more things. Contrasting may be implied.
• Contrast/Distinguish	Explain the differences among two or more things. Comparisons may be implied.
• Criticize/Evaluate	Formulate an evaluation or judgment regarding the merits of the issue in question.
• Define	Provide a meaning for a term or concept. Do not rely on examples only.
• Describe	Identify the characteristics, traits, or qualities, or formulate a mental picture of the issue in question.
• Discuss	Examine or explain the importance or relevance of the issue in question.
• Enumerate	List the issues in question.
• Illustrate	Provide examples of the issue in question.
• Interpret	Provide an explanation of an issue's meaning according to one's or another's understanding.
• Outline	List the important features, concepts, or parts of the issue in question.
• Prove	Provide valid reasons and evidence to support the issue in question.
• State	Directly identify the issue in question.
• Summarize	Provide a brief account or explanation of the important points of the issue in question.
• Trace	Identify the sequence, progress, or order of the issue in question.

Figure 3-1

Essay questions key words.

that you will do well. If, on the other hand, you did not study as hard as you should have or wanted to, accept that as beyond your control for now and attend to the task of doing the best you can. If things do not go well this time, you know what needs to be done in preparation for the next exam. Talk to yourself in positive terms. Avoid rationalizing past or future test performance by placing the blame on secondary variables. Thoughts such as, "I didn't have enough time," or "I should have . . . ," only compound the stress of test-taking. Take control by affirming your value, self-worth, and dedication to meeting the test challenge head on. Repeat to yourself "I can and I will pass this exam."

Exagiophobia

Exagiophobia (Cody, 1991) is a term used to describe the abnormal fear of tests; it is derived from the Greek *exagion* meaning a weighing, as in a test or trial, and the Greek *phobos* meaning fear. Exagiophobia or test anxiety, is a common occurrence and sometimes can be manifested to phobic proportions. Fear creates unwanted tension, unclear thinking, and ultimately prevents success on exams by predisposing your mind to failure. Desensitizing yourself to the fear response can be an effective means of overcoming and controlling your fear of the test situation. A common method psychologists use to help clients overcome anxieties and phobias is through phobic desensitization. The patient is taught to relax while gradually re-entering the phobic situation. This is done first through imagination and later in reality, all the while keeping the anxiety and fear response to a minimum. This method is effective when relaxation becomes associated with the anxiety or fear response. To attempt phobic desensitization, practice the following steps:

Develop and practice a method of relaxation. Any method that works for you will do fine; for example,

1. get comfortable and loosen any tight clothing
2. contract your toe muscles and count to ten
3. relax your toes and enjoy the release of tension
4. do the same with your feet muscles and continue on up your body to the facial muscles
5. close your eyes taking a deep breath for as long as it takes to naturally count to five
6. hold your breath for approximately five more seconds
7. exhale slowly to a count of five.

Practice a desensitization routine. Once you have developed a relaxation technique that works for you, practice desensitizing yourself to the fear response. You can do this by imagining a testing situation as vividly as you can. If you become anxious or uneasy, clear your mind and proceed through the relaxation process. Once relaxed, attempt to visualize a testing situation for 30 seconds without any feelings of anxiety. Again, if you become uncomfortable, exercise the relaxation technique you have chosen. Periodically continue this exercise until you can imagine a testing situation for 3 minutes or longer without any feelings of uneasiness. Once this is accomplished, take the practice test using your relaxation technique as warranted.

It has been the author's experience that the vast majority of examinees spend no more than 85 percent of the available time to complete either exam, so take your time and use whatever methods seem appropriate to gain control of the test situation. A few minutes periodically devoted to phobic desensitization will probably not cause you to go over time.

Beginning Your Phlebotomy Technician Education

As you embark on your training as a phlebotomist, it is recommended that you refer to this review guide as you study and prepare for phlebotomy course exams and ultimately a certification exam. As you read your course texts and classroom notes, refer to the appropriate modules in this text to help you understand and highlight important concepts and principles. Information in this guide that clarifies your reading or notes should be recorded in the margins or spaces of your text or in your notes to promote comprehension and recall abilities. If this guide was not available early in your training, but near the end, review your class notes and corresponding modules in this guide as described above. This may include your course texts as well. Therefore, be willing to do what is necessary, according to your own preferences and idiosyncrasies, to nurture comprehension and recall abilities.

Months Before the Certification Exam

The earlier you start preparing for the exam the better. It is recommended that you begin your preparatory activities no later than two months prior to the exam date. Spend the first month studying the material you are weakest in; devote half of the remaining time to the next weakest area, and the latter half of the remaining time briefly going over your strongest area. Be sure to exercise test-taking strategies by completing some practice tests. Attempt to plan and adhere to a study schedule identifying microgoals along the way. Week one for example,

may have as a goal the memorization of all medical terms that are not readily recognizable to you. You might prepare for this activity by constructing flash cards to help memorize these word parts.

The Day Before the Exam

The day before the exam, follow your normal routine. Take time to assemble the materials you will need for the exam by placing them in a readily accessible location. Avoid any study activity and attempt to get a good night's rest. Set your alarm to allow you to get to the test facility at least 30 minutes before the exam.

Exam Day

Once you begin the test, progress from the simple to the complex; turn to the section that you feel most confident about. Employ any of the test-taking strategies mentioned previously as needed. Answer the easy questions first, skipping over the more difficult ones until later. Move on to the next section having the next level of difficulty, and leave the most difficult section for last. There should be enough time to go over the entire exam to answer the questions you skipped over. Once all items have been answered, go over the answer sheet to ensure that all the circles are filled in properly and extraneous marks erased.

SUMMARY

Test-taking skills are an important component of the examination challenge. By becoming familiar with the test format and various discriminatory techniques, you can avoid unnecessary distractions and neutralize any potentially negative effects the test arrangement may have on your score. As you prepare for and take practice tests, attempt to use whatever techniques seem appropriate. The reasons for taking practice tests are threefold: Developing familiarity with the exam format, exercising test-taking techniques, and identifying knowledge weaknesses. It is up to you, so take control and succeed. Good luck to you!

Adapted from Cody, J.D. & Kelley-Amey C. (2006). *Medical Assisting Exam Review,* 2e. New York: Thomson Delmar Learning.

SECTION II

Exam Review

MODULE 4

Review of Medical Terminology and Anatomy and Physiology

I. MEDICAL TERMINOLOGY

A. The language of medicine
1. Medical terms are derived from the Latin and Greek languages. Terms can be broken down into word roots, suffixes, and prefixes by combining forms.
2. Example:
   a. OTORHINOLARYNGOLOGY
      ot/o—Ear
      rhin/o—Nose
      laryng/o—Larynx
      logy—The study of
      Otorhinolaryngology is the study of the ear, nose, and larynx.

B. Word roots
1. The word root is the basis of all medical terms. It establishes the meaning of the term. The root generally pertains to a tissue, organ, or body system, or it may indicate color.
2. Examples:
   a. CARDIOLOGY
      cardi—Word root meaning heart
      Cardiology is the study of the heart.
   b. CYANOSIS
      cyan—Root word meaning blue
      Cyanosis is a bluish discoloration of the skin.

C. Combining vowels
1. Combining vowels are used to appropriately join word parts and for ease of pronunciation.
2. Typically the letters "o" and "i" are used as combining vowels.
3. Table 4-1 lists some common combining vowels.
4. Rules:
   a. A combining vowel is used between two root words.

b. If a root word is followed by a suffix, a combining vowel is used only if the suffix begins with a consonant.
   (1) Example: In CARDIOLOGY, the combining vowel "o" is used between the root "cardi" and the suffix "logy."
c. If a suffix begins with a vowel, no combining vowel is necessary.
   (1) Example: In CARDITIS, the root is "card" and the suffix is "itis."
d. There are some exceptions to this rule.
   (1) Example: GASTROENTERITIS

D. Prefixes
1. Prefixes are added at the beginning of a word to change the meaning. Prefixes are often used to indicate an amount, location, or time.
2. Example:
   a. ENDOCARDIUM
      endo—Prefix meaning within
      card—Root word meaning heart
      um—Suffix meaning structure or tissue
      Endocardium means the inner lining of the heart.
3. A prefix never stands alone.
4. Many prefixes are paired with a prefix with the opposite meaning.
5. Example:
   a. "Post-" means after and "pre-" means before.
6. Table 4-2 lists commonly used prefixes.

E. Suffixes
1. Suffixes are added to the end of a term to add to or change its meaning. Suffixes are commonly used to indicate a procedure, condition, disorder, or disease.

Table 4-1
Commonly Used Combining Vowels

abdomin/o	abdomen	**gastr/o**	stomach, belly
abrupt/o	broken away from	**glyc/o**	glucose, sugar
abscess/o	going away, collection of pus	**hem/o**	blood, relating to the blood
aer/o	air, gas	**hemat/o**	blood, relating to the blood
agglutin/o	clumping, stick together	**hemangi/o**	blood vessel
aneurysm/o	aneurysm	**hepat/o**	liver
angin/o	choking, strangling	**immun/o**	immune
aort/o	aorta	**jugul/o**	throat
appendic/o	appendix	**lip/o**	fat, lipid
arteri/o	artery	**lymph/o**	lymph, lymphatic tissue
articul/o	joint	**micr/o**	small
arthr/o	joint	**morph/o**	shape, form
asphyxi/o	absence of a pulse	**my/o**	muscle
aspirat/o	to breathe in	**myel/o**	bone marrow
ather/o	plaque, fatty substance	**myocardi/o**	myocardium, heart muscle
atri/o	atrium	**nephro/o**	kidney
attenuat/o	diluted, weakened	**nerv/o**	nerve, nerve tissue
bacill/o	little stick or rod	**neur/o, neur/i**	pertaining to the nerves, nervous tissue
bacteri/o	bacteria, rod or staff		
bilirubin/o	bilirubin	**nucle/o**	nucleus
brachi/o	arm	**nucleol/o**	little nucleus, nucleolus
bronc/i,	bronchial tube, windpipe	**occlud/o**	shut, close up
broncho/o	bronchial tube, windpipe	**occult/o**	hidden, concealed
calc/o	calcium	**onc/o**	tumor
carcin/o	cancerous	**oste/o**	bone
cardi/o	heart	**path/o**	disease, suffering
caud/o	tail	**phleb/o**	vein
cauter/o	burn, burning	**plasm/o**	something molded or formed
cephal/o	relating to a head	**pulm/o**	lung
cerebell/o	cerebellum	**pulmon/o**	lung
cerebr/o	brain, cerebrum	**py/o**	pus
cholesterol/o	cholesterol	**ren/o**	kidney
coagulat/o	congeal, curdle, fix together	**resuscit/o**	revive
cocc/i, cocc/o,	berry-shaped bacterium	**retr/o**	behind, backward
constrict/o	draw tightly together	**scler/o**	sclera, white of eye
contagi/o	unclean, infection	**sphincter/o**	tight band
contaminat/o	pollute, render unclean by contact	**staphyl/o**	cluster, bunch of grapes
corpuscul/o	little body	**strept/o**	twisted chain
crani/o	skull	**syring/o**	tube
cry/o	cold	**systol/o**	contraction
cyst/o	urinary bladder, cyst, sac of fluid	**thorac/o**	chest
cyt/o	cell	**thromb/o**	clot
derm/o	skin	**tox/o, toxic/o**	poison
diastol/o	standing apart, expansion	**trache/o**	trachea, windpipe
dilat/o	spread out, expand	**tunic/o**	covering, cloak, sheath
ecchym/o	pouring out of juice	**tympan/o**	tympanic membrane, eardrum
electr/o	electric, electricity		
encephal/o	brain	**varic/o**	swollen or dilated vein
endocrin/o	secrete within	**vascul/o**	little vessel
eosin/o	red, rosy, dawn-colored	**ven/o**	vein
erythem/o	flushed, redness	**ventr/o**	in front, belly side of body
erythr/o	red	**ventricul/o**	ventricle of brain or heart
fibrin/o	fibrin, fibers, threads of a clot	**venul/o**	venule, small vein

Table 4-2

Prefixes

a-, an-	away from, negative, no, not without	**inter-**	between, among
ab-	away from	**intra-, intro-**	within, into, inside
ac-, ad-, af-	toward, to	**mal-**	bad, poor, evil
as-, at-	toward, to	**med-, mes-**	middle
al-	like, similar	**mega-**	large, great
ante-	before, forward	**meta-**	change, transformation, subsequent to, behind, hindmost, after, or next
anti-	against, counter		
bi-	twice, double, two	**multi-**	many, much
brachy-	short	**neo-**	new, strange
brady-	slow	**nitro-**	nitrogen
cent-	hundred	**non-**	no
circum-	around, about	**nuli-**	none
co-, com-, con-	together, with	**ortho-**	straight, normal, correct
contra-	against, counter, opposite	**os-**	mouth, bone
cort-	covering	**pan-**	all, entire, every
cyst-	bag, bladder	**para-**	apart from, beside, near, abnormal
de-	from, not, down, lack of	**per-**	excessive, through
demi-	half	**peri-**	around, surrounding
di-	twice, twofold, double	**poly-**	many
dia-	through, between, apart, complete	**post-**	after, behind
dis-	negative, apart, absence	**pre-**	before, in front of
dys-	difficult, painful, bad	**pro-**	before, in behalf of
ecto-	out, outside	**re-**	back, again
em-	in	**retro-**	behind, backward, back of
en-	in, into, within	**semi-**	half
endo-	within, in, inside	**sub-**	under, less, below
epi-	upon, above, on, upper	**super-**	above, excessive, higher than
eu-	well, easy, good	**sym-**	with, together
ex-, exo-	out of, outside, away from	**syn-**	union, association
extra-	on the outside, beyond, outside	**tachy-**	fast, rapid
fore-	before, in front of	**tetra-**	four
hem-	relating to the blood	**trans-**	across, through
hemi-	half	**tri-**	three
hydra-	relating to water	**ultra-**	beyond, excess
hyper-	over, above, increased, excessive	**um-**	structure or tissue
hypo-	under, decreased, deficient, below	**un-**	not
in-	in, into, not, without	**uni-**	one
infra-	beneath, below, inferior to	**venter-**	the abdomen

2. Example:
   a. CARDIALGIA
      cardi—Root meaning heart
      algia—Suffix meaning pain
      Cardialgia means pain in the heart.
3. Suffixes cannot stand alone.
4. Table 4-3 lists some commonly used suffixes.

F. Abbreviations
   1. Abbreviations are used frequently to shorten medical terms, laboratory tests, and medical phrases. Some abbreviations can have more than one meaning.

2. Examples:
   a. Ca—Calcium
   b. CA—Cancer
3. Be sure to use abbreviations correctly—*When in doubt, spell it out.* Many institutions have approved abbreviations lists to reduce errors within the institution. Abbreviations should be used with caution.
4. Table 4-4 lists some commonly used abbreviations.

Table 4-3

Suffixes

Suffix	Meaning	Suffix	Meaning
-able	capable of, able to	-ile	capable of (being) able to, pertaining to
-ac	pertaining to	-ism	state of, condition
-ago	attack, diseased state or condition	-istis, -itis	inflammation
-agra	excessive pain, seizure, attack of severe pain	-ium	structure, tissue
-aise	comfort, ease	-kinesis	motion
-al	pertaining to	-lith	stone, calculus
-algesic	painful	-lithiasis	presence of stones
-algia	pain	-lysis	setting free, break down, separation, destruction
-ar	pertaining to	-lyst	agent that causes lysis or loosening
-arche	beginning	-lytic	reduce, destroy
-ary	pertaining to	-mania	obsessive, preoccupation
-ase	enzyme	-megaly	large, great, extreme, enlargement
-blast	embryonic, immature	-meter	measure
-cele	tumor, cyst, hernia	-necrosis	death of tissue
-centesis	surgical puncture to remove fluid	-oid	like, resembling
-cidal	pertaining to death	-ologist	specialist
-cide	causing death	-ology	the science or study of
-clasis	break	-oma	tumor, neoplasm
-clast	break down	-osis	disease, an abnormal condition
-clysis	irrigation, washing	-ostomosis	surgically creating a mouth or opening cutting, surgical incision
-crasia	a mixture or blending	-ostomy	create a new surgical opening
-crit	separate	-otomy	cut into
-cytic	pertaining to a cell	-ous	pertaining to
-cytosis	condition of cells	-paresis	partial or incomplete paralysis
-dema	swelling (fluid)	-pathic	pertaining to, affected by disease
-desis	bind, tie together, surgical fixation of bone or joint	-penia	lack, deficiency, too few
-duct	opening	-pexy	surgical fixation, to put in place
-dynia	pain	-phage	one that eats, a cell that destroys
-eal	pertaining to	-phagia	eating, swallowing
-ectasia	stretching	-phasia	speak or speech
-ectasis	stretching, dilation, enlargement	-pheresis	removal
-ectomy	surgical removal, cutting out, excision	-phoresis	carrying, transmission
-emesis	vomiting	-phoria	to bear, carry, feeling, mental state
-emia	blood, blood condition	-phylactic	protective, preventive
-esis	state or abnormal condition	-phylaxis	protection
-esthesia	sensation, feeling	-physis	to grow
-exia, -exis	condition	-plasia	formation, development, growth
-ferent	carrying	-plasm	formative material of cells
-form	form, figure, shape	-plasty	surgical repair
-fuge	to drive away	-plegia	stroke, paralysis, palsy
-gene	production, origin, formation	-plegic	paralysis, one affected with paralysis
-genesis	growth	-pnea	breathing
-genic	producing, forming	-poiesis	formation
-genous	producing	-porosis	passage, porous condition
-grade	go	-praxia	action, condition concerning the performance of movements
-gram	tracing, picture, record	-ptosis	drooping, sagging, prolapse, dropping down
-graph	instrument for recording, picture	-ptysis	spitting
-graphy	process of recording a picture or record	-rrhage,	burst forth
-ia	state or condition	-rrhagia	bursting forth
-iac	pertaining to	-rrhaphy	suturing, stiching
-iasis	condition, pathologic state, abnormal condition	-rrhea	flow, discharge
-ible	able to be, capable of being	-rrhexis	rupture
-ic	pertaining to	-sarcoma	tumor, cancer
-ific	making, producing	-scope	instrument for visual examination
-iform	shaped or formed like, resembling	-scopic	pertaining to visual examination
-igo	attack, diseased condition		

(continued)

Table 4-3

Suffixes (continued)

-scopy	see, visual examination	**-tome**	instrument to cut
-stalsis	contraction	**-tomy**	cutting, incision
-statis	stopping, controlling	**-tripsy**	crushing stone
-stenosis	narrowing, tightening, stricture of a duct or canal	**-tropic**	having an affinity for, turning toward
		-uresis	urination
-stomosis,		**-uria**	urination, urine
-stomy	furnish with a mouth or outlet, new opening	**-us**	thing
-tic	pertaining to	**-version**	to turn

Table 4-4

Common Medical Abbreviations

abd	abdomen	**CAT**	computed axial tomography
AB	abnormal	**cath**	catheter, catheterize
ABG	arterial blood gas	**CBC**	complete blood count
AC, a.c.	before meals	**CC**	chief complaint
ACLS	advanced cardiac life support	**CCU**	coronary care unit
ACTH	adrenocorticotropic hormone	**CDC**	Centers for Disease Control
ADH	antidiuretic hormone	**Ch, chol**	cholesterol
ad lib	as desired	**CHF**	congestive heart failure
adm	admission	**CK**	creatinine kinase
AIDS	acquired immune deficiency syndrome	**cm**	centimeter
AKA	also known as	**CML**	chronic myelocytic leukemia
alb	albumin	**CNS**	central nervous system
alk	alkaline	**c/o**	complains of
ALL	acute lymphocytic leukemia	**CO₂**	carbon dioxide
ALT	liver test	**contra**	against
alt hor	alternate hours	**COPD**	chronic obstructive pulmonary disease
alt noct	alternate nights	**CPK**	creatinine phosphokinase
AM, a.m.	morning	**CPR**	cardiopulmonary resuscitation
AMA	against medical advice; American Medical Association	**creat**	creatinine
		C & S	culture and sensitivity
AMI	acute myocardial infarction	**CSF**	cerebrospinal fluid
AML	acute myelocytic leukemia	**CT**	computed tomography
AMS	amylase	**CVA**	cardiovascular accident, cerebrovascular accident
amt	amount		
ANS	autonomic nervous system	**CXR**	chest x-ray film
ant	anterior	**d**	day
A&P	anterior and posterior	**Diag, Dx**	diagnosis
aq	aqueous	**DIC**	diffuse intravascular coagulation
ASA	aspirin	**diff**	differential
ASAP	as soon as possible	**disch**	discharge
AST	aspartate aminotransferase (also know as SGOT serum glutamic oxaloacetic)	**DNA**	deoxyribonucleic acid
		DNR	do not resuscitate
		DOA	dead on arrival
BID, bid, b.i.d.	twice a day	**DOB**	date of birth
bil	bilateral	**Dx**	diagnosis
Bld	blood	**EBV**	Epstein-Barr virus
B/P, BP	blood pressure	**ECG**	electrocardiogram, electrocardiograph
BUN	blood urea nitrogen	**ECHO**	echocardiogram
Bx	biopsy	**E. coli**	Escherichia coli
C	Celsius; centigrade	**EEG**	electroencephalogram
c	without	**EENT**	eye, ear, nose, and throat
Ca	calcium	**EIA**	enzyme immunosorbent assay
CA	cancer	**EKG**	electrocardiogram; electrocardiograph
CAD	coronary artery disease		

(continued)

Table 4-4
Common Medical Abbreviations (continued)

ELISA	enzyme-linked immunoassay, enzyme-linked immunosorbent assay		**KVO**	keep vein open
eos, eosins	eosinophils		**L**	liter
ER	emergency room		**lab**	laboratory
ESR	erythrocyte sedimentation rate		**lac**	laceration
et	and		**lat**	lateral
ETOA	ethyl alcohol		**lb**	pound
ex	excision		**LD**	lactic dehydrogenase
exam	examination		**LDL**	low-density lipoprotein
exp	expiration		**lg**	large
F	Fahrenheit		**liq**	liquid
FAS	fetal alcohol syndrome		**LLQ**	left lower quadrant
FBS	fasting blood sugar		**LMP**	last menstrual period
FH	family history		**LOC**	level/loss of consciousness
FOB	fecal occult blood		**LTC**	long-term care
FTT	failure to thrive		**LUQ**	left upper quadrant
F/U	follow-up		**lymphs**	lymphocytes
FUO	fever of unknown origin		**lytes**	electrolytes
FX, Fx	fracture		**m**	minim
g	gram		**mcg**	microgram
GI	gastrointestinal		**MCH**	mean corpuscular hemoglobin
gm	gram		**MCHC**	mean corpuscular hemoglobin concentration
gr	grain		**MCV**	mean corpuscular volume
GSW	gunshot wound		**mEq**	milliequivalent
GTT	glucose tolerance test		**mg**	milligram
gtt	drops		**MI**	myocardial infarction
GU	genitourinary		**mL**	milliliter
GYN, Gyn	gynecology		**mm**	millimeter
H, hr	hour		**mono**	monocytes
H₂O	water		**MRI**	magnetic resonance imaging
H&H	hemoglobin and hematocrit		**Na**	sodium
Hb, hgb	hemoglobin		**NaCl**	sodium chloride
HbF	fetal hemoglobin		**NEG, neg**	negative
HBV	hepatitis B virus		**NG**	nasogastric
hct	hematocrit		**NKA**	no known allergies
HA	headache		**No**	number
HDL	high-density lipoprotein		**noct**	night
HIV	human immunodeficiency virus		**NPO**	nothing by mouth
H&P	history and physical		**N/S**	normal saline
ht	height; hematocrit		**O₂**	oxygen
Hx	history		**OB**	obstetrics
ICU	intensive care unit		**OB-GYN**	obstetrics and gynecology
Ig	immunoglobulin		**OCC**	occasional
IgA	immunoglobulin A		**OD**	overdose
IgD	immunoglobulin D		**O&P**	ova and parasites
IgG	immunoglobulin G		**OR**	operating room
IgM	immunoglobulin M		**oz**	ounce
IM	infectious mononucleosis, intramuscular		**p**	after; phosphorus; pulse
inf	inferior; infusion		**Pap**	Papanicolaou
I&O	intake and output		**Path**	pathology
irrig	irrigation		**pc**	after meals
isol	isolation		**PCO₂**	pressure of carbon dioxide in the blood
IV	intravenous, intravenously		**PCV**	packed cell volume
IVP	intravenous pyelogram		**PE**	physical examination
K	potassium		**Peds**	pediatrics
kg	kilogram		**pH**	acidity; hydrogen ion concentration
KO	keep open		**PI**	present illness

(continued)

Table 4-4

Common Medical Abbreviations (continued)

PKU	phenylketonuria	**SLE**	St. Louis encephalitis; systemic lupus erythematosus
PLTS	platelets		
PM, p.m.	evening or afternoon	**SSMA**	sequential multiple analysis
PMNS	polymorphonuclear leukocytes	**SMAC**	sequential multiple analysis computer
PNS	peripheral nervous system	**SOAP**	symptoms, observations, assessments, plan
PO, p.o.	by mouth; orally; postoperative		
Polys	polymorphonuclear leukocytes	**SOB**	shortness of breath
pos	positive	**sp gr**	specific gravity
post-op	postoperatively	**SR**	sedimentation rate
PP	postpartum; postprandial (after meals)	**staph**	staphylococcus
PPT	partial prothrombin time	**stat**	immediately
preop	preoperative	**STD**	sexually transmitted disease
prep	prepare	**strep**	streptococcus
prn	as needed	**subcu**	subcutaneous
prog	prognosis	**Sx**	symptoms
pro time	prothrombin time	**T**	temperature
psych	psychiatry	**T₃**	thiiodothyronine (thyroid hormone)
pt	patient; pint		
PTT	partial thromboplastin time;	**T₄**	thyroxine (thyroid hormone)
PT	prothrombin time	**TB**	tuberculosis
PVD	peripheral vascular disease	**T&C**	type and cross match
Px	prognosis	**temp**	temperature
q	every	**TIA**	transient ischemic attack
qh, q.h.	every hour	**TIBC**	total iron binding capacity
q2h, q.2h.	every 2 hours	**TID, t.i.d.**	times interval difference, three times a day
qm	every morning		
qns	quantity not sufficient	**TKO**	to keep open
qoh	every other hour	**TPN**	total parenteral nutrition
qt	quart; quiet	**TPR**	temperature, pulse, respiration
q.q	each	**Trig**	triglycerides
quad	quadrant	**TSH**	thyroid-stimulating hormone
RBC	red blood cell; red blood count	**Tx**	traction; treatment
RBCV	red blood cell volume	**UA**	urinalysis
Rh neg	Rhesus factor negative	**UK**	unknown
Rh pos	Rhesus factor positive	**URI**	upper respiratory infection
RIA	radioimmunoassay	**UTI**	urinary tract infection
RLQ	right lower quadrant	**UV**	ultraviolet
RNA	ribonucleic acid	**VCUG**	voiding cystourethrogram
R/O	rule out	**VD**	venereal disease
RPR	rapid plasma reagin	**VDRL**	Venereal Disease Research Laboratories
RR	recovery room; respiratory rate	**VP**	venipuncture; venous pressure
rt	right; routine	**VS**	vital signs
RT	radiation therapy; respiratory therapy	**W**	water
RUQ	right upper quadrant	**WBC**	white blood cell; white blood count
Rx	prescription; take; therapy;	**wd**	wound
s	without	**WNL**	within normal limits
SCA	sickle cell anemia	**w/o**	without
SCPK	serum creatinine phosphokinase	**wt**	weight
SCT	sickle cell trait	**x**	multiplied by, times
sed rate	sedimentation rate	**XR**	x-ray
seg	segmented neutrophils	**y/o**	year(s) old
semi	half	**YOB**	year of birth
SIDS	sudden infant death syndrome	**yr**	year

II. ANATOMY AND PHYSIOLOGY

A. Introduction
   1. Anatomy is the study of the structure of an organ and the relationship of that organ to other parts of the body. The term "anatomy" is derived from two Greek words: ana, meaning apart, and temuein, to cut.
   2. Physiology is the study of the function of living organisms and their structures.
B. Anatomic terminology (See Figure 4-1.)
   1. Body positions
      a. When a person is standing in the anatomical position, the body is standing erect with the arms at the sides and palms turned forward and with the head and feet also facing forward.
      b. When a person is in the supine position, the body is lying face up.
      c. When a person is in the prone position, the body is lying face down.
   2. Directional terms
      a. Anterior (ventral)—In front of; abdominal side of the body
      b. Posterior (dorsal)—Behind or at the back of; opposite to anterior
      c. Superior—Above, upper of two parts, toward the vertex
      d. Inferior—Beneath, lower, indicating a structure below another

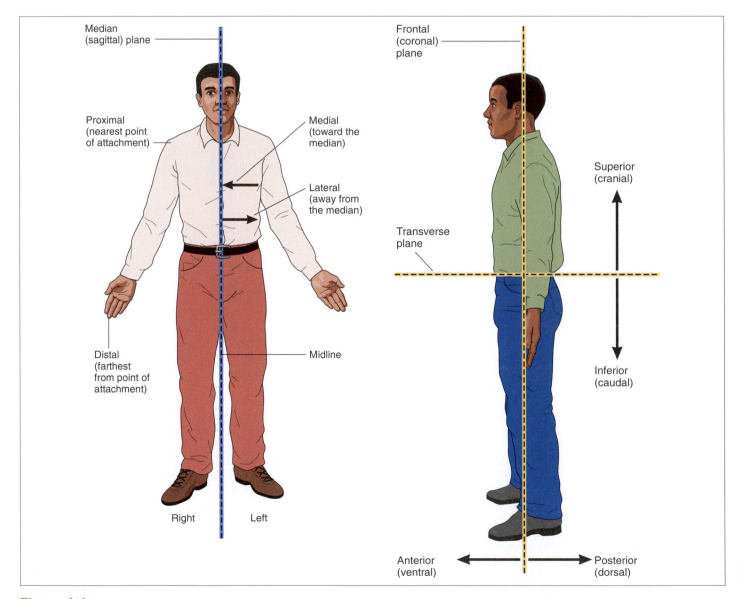

Figure 4-1

Directional Terms.

e. Medial—Toward the midline of the body

f. Lateral—Toward the side of the body

g. Proximal—Nearest the point of attachment, center of the body, or point of reference

h. Distal—Farthest from the point of origin of a structure, opposite of proximal

i. Superficial—Pertaining to or situated near the surface

j. Deep—Pertaining to or situated below the surface

k. Cranial—Toward the head; superior

l. Caudal—Toward the tail; inferior

m. Supine—The position of lying on the back with the face upward

n. Prone—The position that is horizontal with the face downward

3. Anatomical planes (See Figure 4-2.)

   a. A plane is an imaginary line dividing the body.

     (1) Sagittal—Longitudinal imaginary line dividing the body into unequal right and left parts

     (2) Midsagittal—Imaginary longitudinal line dividing the body into equal right and left halves

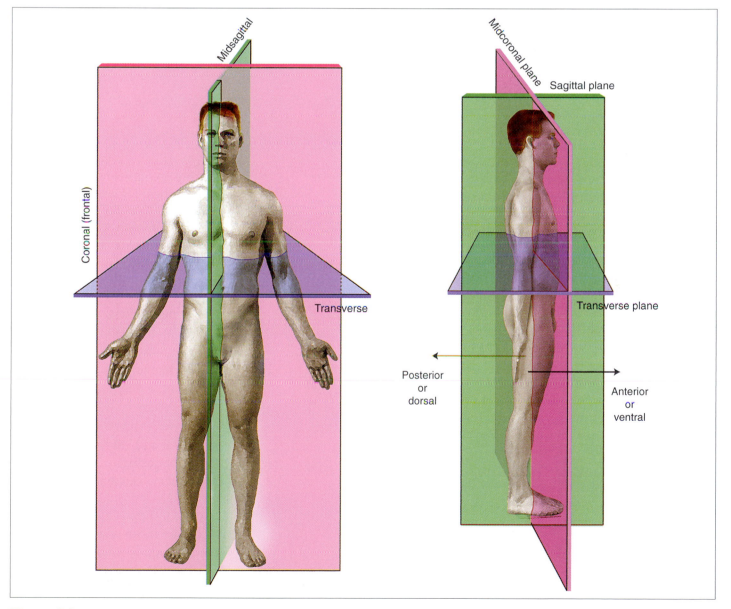

Figure 4-2

Body Planes.

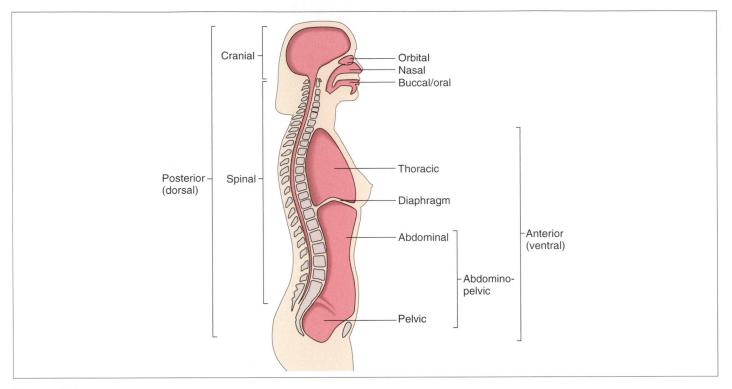

Figure 4-3

Body Cavities.

(3) Frontal—Plane parallel to the long axis of the body and at right angles to the midsagittal plane

(4) Transverse—Plane that divides the body into top and bottom halves

4. Body cavities—Body cavities are hollow spaces that house internal organs. (See Figure 4-3.) The body is made up of two major cavities: the dorsal cavity and the ventral cavity.

(a) Dorsal—Posterior cavity of the body, which houses the brain and spinal column

(1) Cranial—Cavity within the dorsal cavity that houses the brain

(2) Spinal—Cavity within the dorsal cavity that houses the spinal cord

(b) Ventral—Anterior cavity of the body, which is made up of the thoracic and abdominopelvic cavities

(1) Thoracic—Chest cavity

(a) The mediastinum is the region of the thoracic cavity containing the heart and blood vessels between the sternum and vertebral column and between the lungs.

(b) This cavity also contains the lungs.

(2) Abdominopelvic—Usually referred to as the abdominal cavity (containing the stomach, liver, gallbladder, pancreas, spleen, small intestines, appendix, and

part of the large intestine) or the pelvic cavity (containing the urinary bladder, the reproductive organs, the rectum, and the remainder of the large intestine).

(a) The diaphragm separates the abdominal cavity from the pelvic cavity.

(b) Nine regions of the abdominopelvic cavity (See Figure 4-4.)

(i) Upper regions:

Right and left hypochondriac

Epigastric

(ii) Middle regions:

Right and left lumbar

Umbilical

(iii) Lower regions:

Right and left iliac/inguinal

Hypogastric

(c) Abdominal quadrants (See Figure 4-5.)

(i) Right upper quadrant (RUQ)

(ii) Right lower quadrant (RLQ)

(iii) Left upper quadrant (LUQ)

(iv) Left lower quadrant (LLQ)

C. Body functions

1. The body is in the continual process of maintaining equilibrium to ensure survival.

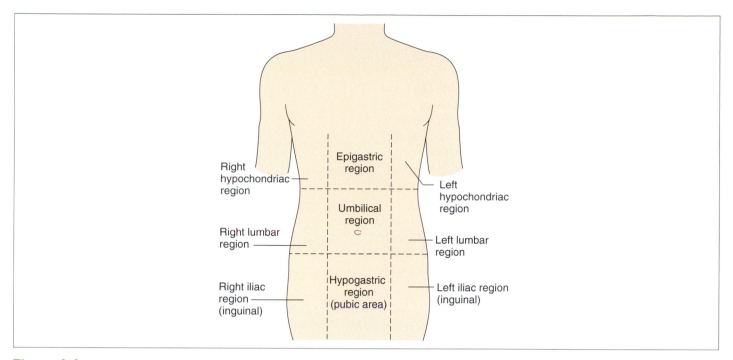

Figure 4-4

Abdominal Regions.

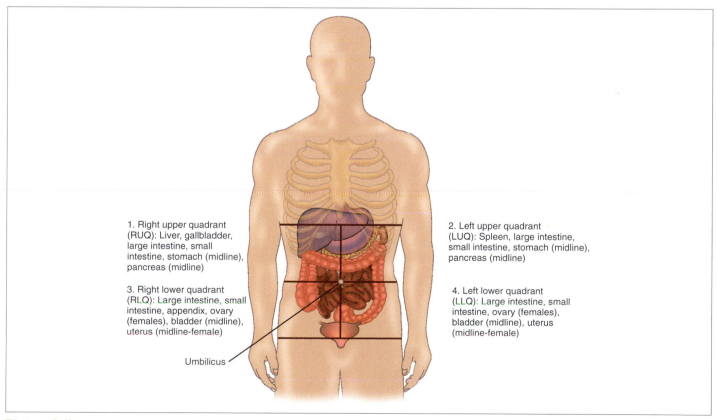

1. Right upper quadrant (RUQ): Liver, gallbladder, large intestine, small intestine, stomach (midline), pancreas (midline)

3. Right lower quadrant (RLQ): Large intestine, small intestine, appendix, ovary (females), bladder (midline), uterus (midline-female)

2. Left upper quadrant (LUQ): Spleen, large intestine, small intestine, stomach (midline), pancreas (midline)

4. Left lower quadrant (LLQ): Large intestine, small intestine, ovary (females), bladder (midline), uterus (midline-female)

Umbilicus

Figure 4-5

Abdominal Quadrants.

a. Homeostasis is the maintenance of the internal environment of the body, which enables all the cells of the body to obtain nutrients and oxygen.

b. Metabolism is the physical and chemical reactions taking place on a cellular level, resulting in the growth, repair, energy release, and use of food by the body's cells. Metabolism consists of two processes:

   (1) Anabolism—The building up of complex materials from simpler materials such as food and oxygen

   (2) Catabolism—The breaking down and changing of complex substances, such as food molecules, into simpler ones, such as carbon dioxide and water with release of energy

D. Structural units of the body

  1. Cells

    a. The cell is the basic unit of structure and function for all life and is responsible for all activities of the body.

    b. The cell is the smallest living unit in the body.

    c. The human body is comprised of a trillion microscopic cells.

    d. The micrometer (formerly known as the micron) is the unit of measurement used to determine cell size.

     (1) Examples:

      (a) A red blood cell (RBC) is 7.5 microns.

      (b) An ovum is 1,000 microns.

    e. Cells come in a variety of shapes and sizes and each has its own unique function.

    f. Cells share a basic structure. (See Figure 4-6.)

     (1) Cytoplasm—Protoplasm outside the nucleus of a cell

     (2) Cell membrane—Structure that encloses the cell

     (3) Nucleus—Core, or center, of a cell containing large quantities of DNA

     (4) Organelles—Microscopic, specialized structures within the cell having a special function or property

     (5) Centrioles—Two cylindrical organelles found near the nucleus in a tiny body called the centrosome; perpendicular to each other

     (6) Endoplasmic reticulum—Transport system of the cell; can be smooth or rough

     (7) Golgi apparatus—Membranous network that resembles a stack of pancakes; stores and packages secretions

     (8) Lysosomes—Cytoplasmic organelle containing digestive enzymes

     (9) Mitochondria—Organelle that supplies energy to the cell

    (10) Ribosome—Submicroscopic particle attached to endoplasmic reticulum; site of protein synthesis in cytoplasm of cell

  2. Tissues

    a. Tissues are made of similar cells working together to perform a specific function.

    b. There are four types of tissues: epithelial, connective, muscle, and nerve.

     (1) Epithelial tissue covers surfaces and protects structures.

      (a) It is found in both the internal and external structures.

      (b) Specialized epithelial tissue produces secretions such as digestive juices, hormones, and perspiration.

      (c) This type of tissue is named according to size, shape, structure, and function.

     (2) Connective tissue is the most abundant and widely distributed; it is found almost everywhere in the body.

      (a) The functions of connective tissue vary depending on structure and appearance.

      (b) This type of tissue forms a supporting framework.

      (c) Examples:

       (i) Blood and lymph tissue

       (ii) Cartilage

       (iii) Supportive bone tissue

     (3) Muscle tissue provides the body with movement by shortening or contracting. There are three types of muscle tissue.

      (a) Skeletal—Striated and voluntary; attaches to bones and allows for movement

      (b) Smooth—Nonstriated and involuntary; responsible for pushing blood through veins and arteries

      (c) Cardiac—Striated and involuntary; found only in the heart, causes the contractions of the heart

     (4) Nerve tissue is composed of specialized cells that are able to send and receive information. These tissues are found in the brain, spinal cord, and the nerves themselves.

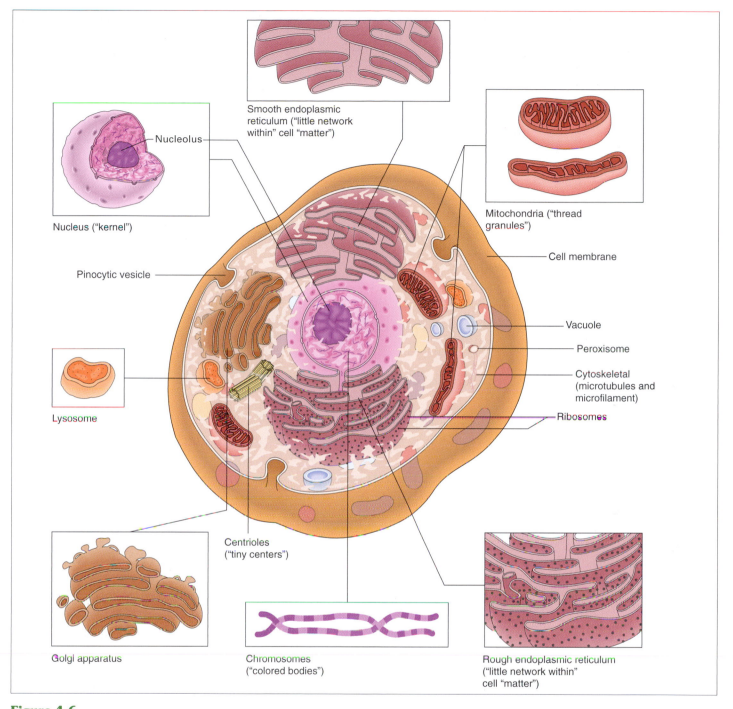

Nucleolus

Nucleus ("kernel")

Smooth endoplasmic reticulum ("little network within" cell "matter")

Mitochondria ("thread granules")

Cell membrane

Pinocytic vesicle

Vacuole

Peroxisome

Cytoskeletal (microtubules and microfilament)

Lysosome

Ribosomes

Centrioles ("tiny centers")

Golgi apparatus

Chromosomes ("colored bodies")

Rough endoplasmic reticulum ("little network within" cell "matter")

Figure 4-6

Structure of a Cell.

3. Organs
   a. Organs are composed of numerous tissues grouped together to perform a specific function.
      (1) Example:
          The heart
   b. Organs cannot function independently. They function together to create specific body systems.

E. The skeletal system
   1. Functions:
      a. Shapes and supports the body.
      b. Protects vital organs.
      c. Assists in movement.
      d. Stores minerals.
      e. Manufactures blood cells, a process called hematopoiesis.

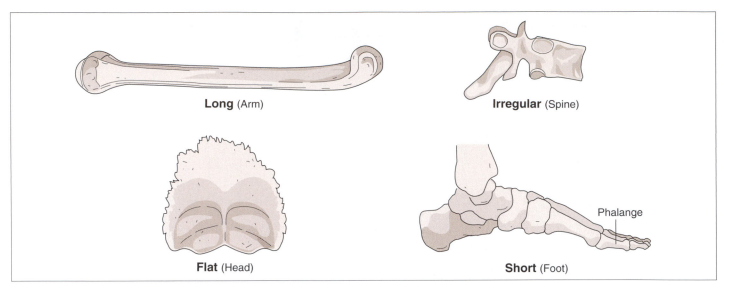

Long (Arm)

Irregular (Spine)

Flat (Head)

Short (Foot)

Phalange

Figure 4-7

Shapes of Bones.

2. There are 206 bones in the adult body.

3. Classification of bones by shape (See Figure 4-7.)

   a. Long bones—Femur, tibia, fibula, humerus, radius, and ulna

   b. Flat bones—Skull, scapula, and ribs

   c. Irregular bones—Vertebrae

   d. Short bones—Carpal and tarsals

4. Bones are connected by ligaments, and cartilage protects connections at joints throughout the body. Joints allow for movement.

5. Structure of bone (See Figure 4-8.)

   a. Bones are made up of hard dense tissue that is covered by a membrane called periosteum, which contains blood vessels and allows for the exchange of nutrients and waste products.

   b. The outer layer of bone is called compact bone. Compact bone is heavier and rigid compared to the inner layer of bone.

   c. The inner layer of bone, called spongy bone, looks like a honeycomb. This is the site of red marrow, where red blood cells are formed.

   d. The center of bone is the medullary canal, filled with yellow bone marrow. This is where white blood cells are formed. This also functions as a storage center for fat.

6. Divisions of the skeletal system (See Figure 4-9.)

   a. Axial skeleton—Skull, spinal column, ribs, sternum, and hyoid bone

   b. Appendicular skeleton—Shoulder and pelvic girdles as well as the upper and lower extremities

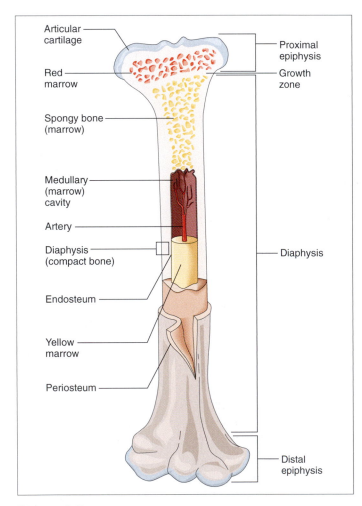

Articular cartilage

Proximal epiphysis

Growth zone

Red marrow

Spongy bone (marrow)

Medullary (marrow) cavity

Artery

Diaphysis (compact bone)

Diaphysis

Endosteum

Yellow marrow

Periosteum

Distal epiphysis

Figure 4-8

Structure of Bone.

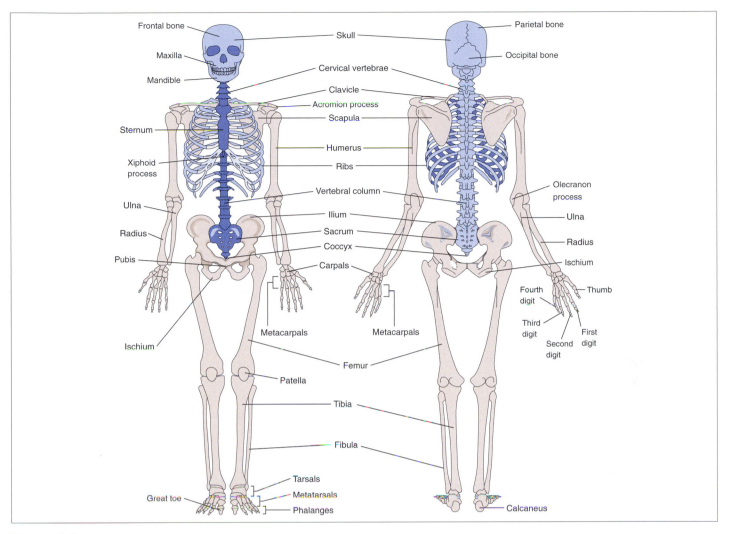

Figure 4-9

Axial and Appendicular Skeleton.

7. Disorders
   a. Arthritis—Inflammatory condition of one or more joints
   b. Bursitis—Inflammation of the fluid-filled sac, the bursa, between muscle attachments and bones
   c. Gout—Increase of uric acid in the bloodstream, caused by faulty protein metabolism affecting most commonly the joints of the feet; a form of arthritis
   d. Osteomyelitis—Inflammation of the bone and the bone marrow, caused by bacterial infection
   e. Osteochondritis—Inflammation of the bone and cartilage
   f. Osteoporosis—Disorder and common condition of aging and loss of nutrients, involving loss of bone density
   g. Rickets—Abnormal bone formation caused by a lack of Vitamin D in the diet; primarily affects children and causes the bones to soften and become malformed
   h. Slipped (herniated) disc—Condition when a disc between the vertebrae of the spine ruptures or protrudes out of place and places pressure on the spinal nerve
   i. Tumor—Abnormal bone growth; may be malignant (cancer) or benign

8. Diagnostic tests
   a. Alkaline phosphatase (ALP)
   b. Calcium
   c. Complete blood count (CBC)
   d. Erythrocyte sedimentation rate (ESR)
   e. Phosphorus (P)
   f. Synovial fluid analysis
   g. Uric acid
   h. Vitamin D

F. The muscular system
1. Nearly half of the body's weight comes from muscle. There are 656 muscles in the human body.
2. Muscles control the voluntary movement of the body as well as the involuntary movement of organs such as the heart and lungs.
3. Adenosine triphosphate (ATP) is manufactured in the mitochondria of cells and produces energy for muscle contraction.
4. Functions
   a. Facilitates body movement.
   b. Gives the body form and shape to maintain posture.
   c. Plays a role in body heating, to maintain body temperature.
5. Types—There are three principle types of muscle tissue: skeletal, cardiac, and smooth (discussed earlier).
6. Muscle characteristics allow the body to perform complex and intricate movements:
   a. Contractility—Ability to shorten or reduce the distance between two parts
   b. Excitability—Ability to respond to stimuli
   c. Extensibility—Ability to lengthen (stretch) and increase the distance between two parts
   d. Elasticity—Ability to return to original form after being stretched or compressed
7. Disorders
   a. Atrophy—Decrease in size or a wasting away
   b. Hernia—Occurs when an organ protrudes through a weak muscle
   c. Muscular dystrophy—A group of diseases in which the muscle cells deteriorate
   d. Myalgia—Tenderness or pain in the muscles. Example, Fibromyalgia, a disease in which chronic muscle pain lasting three months or longer occurs in specific muscle groups. Other symptoms are fatigue, headache, numbness and tingling, and joint pain.
   e. Myasthenia gravis—Progressive muscular weakness and paralysis, sometimes even death; cause is unknown, may be due to a defect in the immune system, which affects myoneural function
   f. Tendonitis—Inflammation of muscle tendons, usually due to overexertion
   g. Tetanus (lockjaw)—Infectious disease characterized by continuous spasms of the voluntary muscles
   h. Torticollis (wryneck)—Inflammation of the trapezius, sternocleidomastoid, or both muscles

8. Diagnostic tests
   a. Creatine phosphokinase (CPK/CK)
   b. CPK/CK isoenzymes
   c. Lactic acid
   d. Lactate dehydrogenase (LDH/LD)
   e. Myoglobin
   f. Electromyography
G. The nervous system
1. Functions
   a. The nervous system controls the communication among and coordination of all body functions. Nerve impulses and chemical substances regulate, control, integrate, and organize body functions.
   b. The brain is the center for intellect and reasoning.
2. The neuron (See Figure 4-10.)

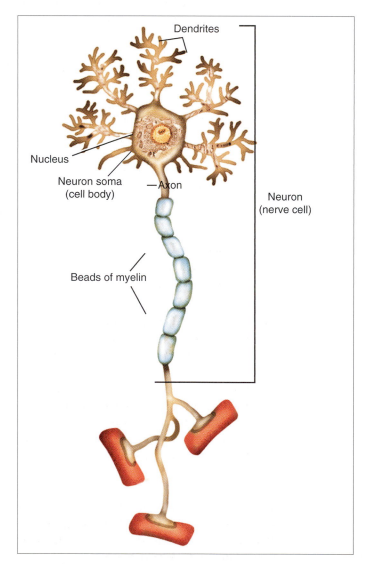

Dendrites

Nucleus

Neuron soma (cell body)

Axon

Neuron (nerve cell)

Beads of myelin

Figure 4-10

Neuron.

a. The nervous system is composed of highly specialized cells called neurons.

b. Neurons are capable of conducting messages in the form of impulses.

c. The body contains over 10 billion neurons, most residing in the brain.

d. The cell body of the neuron contains the nucleus.

e. Neurons have two types of extensions.

   (1) Dendrites are extensions of the neuron. Dendrites differentiate nerve cells from other cells. There may be several dendrites per neuron. The dendrites serve as pathways for impulse conduction.

   (2) Axons are also extensions of the neuron. Each neuron typically has only one axon. They also serve as a passageway for impulse conduction.

      (a) The myelin sheath covers the axon of a neuron and helps to speed up nerve impulse.

      (b) Schwann cells are a fatty substance that the myelin sheath is composed of and that protects the axon.

      (c) The myelin sheath is what makes up the "white matter."

      (d) Nodes of Ranvier are small indentations along the axon that are not covered by the myelin sheath. These structures are important to the conduction of the nerve impulse.

      (e) Nonmyelinated axons are not covered by a myelin sheath, are located in the central nervous system, and make up the "gray matter."

f. Types of neurons

   (1) Sensory, or afferent, neurons—Originate in the skin or sense organs and can carry impulses toward the spinal cord and brain.

   (2) Motor, or efferent, neurons—Carry impulses from the brain and spinal cord to the muscles and glands.

   (3) Associative neurons, or interneurons—Carry impulses from sensory neurons to the motor neurons.

3. Synapse

   a. The synapse is the area between neurons across which impulses literally jump to transmit messages. The "jump" is aided by neurotransmitters (chemicals).

4. The central nervous system (CNS) consists of the brain and spinal cord.

   a. The CNS functions as the command center, interprets all incoming impulses, and dictates responses.

   b. All nerves eventually terminate in the brain via the spinal cord.

   c. The meninges are structures that protect the brain and spinal cord.

      (1) The meninges consist of three layers: dura mater, arachnoid mater, and pia mater.

      (2) Between each layer is a space filled with cerebrospinal fluid.

5. The peripheral nervous system (PNS) is the part of the nervous system that is outside the central nervous system and comprises the cranial nerves, except the optic nerve, the spinal nerves, and the autonomic nervous system.

   a. The PNS can be divided into two smaller systems: the sensory, or afferent, system and the motor, or efferent, system.

      (1) The sensory, or afferent, division serves to convey information from receptors in the periphery of the body to the brain and spinal cord.

      (2) The motor, or efferent, division serves to convey information from the brain and spinal cord to the muscles and glands. This portion of the PNS can be further divided into the somatic nervous system and the autonomic nervous system.

         (a) The somatic nervous system conducts messages from the brain and spinal cord to skeletal muscle.

         (b) The autonomic nervous system conducts messages from the brain and spinal cord to the smooth muscle and cardiac muscle. The organs affected by the autonomic nervous system receive nerve fibers from the sympathetic division, which speeds up activity and energy expenditure, and from the parasympathetic division, which speeds up vegetative activities or slows down other activities.

6. Disorders

   a. Alzheimer's disease—Progressive disease involving confusion, short-term memory loss, anxiety, and poor judgment; progresses into the inability to recognize oneself, weight loss, mood swings, loss of speech, and seizures

   b. Bell's palsy—Condition involving the facial nerve and usually affecting only one side of the face. On the affected side, the eye has difficulty closing, the mouth droops, and there is numbness. Bell's palsy gives the patient the appearance of having had a stroke. The onset may be sudden and the cause is unknown.

   c. Brain tumor—Tumor that may develop in any area of the brain; symptoms vary depending on which area has been damaged and to what extent the tumor has developed

   d. Carpal tunnel syndrome—Disorder of the hand caused by pinching or compression of the median nerve at the wrist. The nerve compression is usually secondary to thickening of the lining or synovium surrounding the tendons that travel through the carpal tunnel alongside the median nerve.

   e. Cerebral palsy—Disturbance in voluntary muscle activity resulting from brain damage

   f. Encephalitis—Inflammation of the brain, most often caused by a virus. The symptoms include fever, lethargy, extreme weakness, and visual disturbances.

   g. Epilepsy—Seizure disorder of the brain, characterized by recurrent and excessive discharge from the neurons

   h. Hydrocephalus—An increased volume of cerebrospinal fluid with the ventricles of the brain; typically apparent at birth, with an enlargement of the infant's head

   i. Meningitis—Inflammation of the meninges lining the brain and spinal cord. Bacteria or a virus may cause it. Symptoms include headache, fever, and stiff neck.

   j. Multiple sclerosis—Chronic inflammatory disease of the central nervous system, in which the patient's own immune cells attack and destroy the myelin sheath of the nerve cell axons

   k. Neuralgia—Severe sharp, stabbing pain with sudden onset along a nerve; usually of short duration

   l. Neuritis—Inflammation of a nerve or nerve trunk. Symptoms may include severe pain, loss of sensation, muscular atrophy, paresthesia, and hypersensitivity.

   m. Parkinson's disease—Disease characterized by tremors, a pill-rolling movement of the thumb and first finger, a shuffling gait, and muscular rigidity

   n. Poliomyelitis—Viral disease affecting the nerve pathways of the spinal cord, which causes paralysis. Due to the Sabin and Salk vaccines this disease has been all but eliminated in the United States.

   o. Sciatica—Type of neuritis, which affects the sciatic nerve. It may be caused by a rupture of a lumbar disc or aggravated by an arthritic condition or trauma.

   p. Shingles—Latent viral infection that is reactivated by the *varicella zoster* virus; characterized by inflammation of a cutaneous nerve

  7. Diagnostic tests

   a. Acetylcholine receptor antibody

   b. Cerebral spinal fluid analysis (cell count, glucose, protein, culture)

   c. Cholinesterase

   d. Drug levels

   e. Serotonin

H. Integumentary system

  1. Skin is called integument, along with its appendages, hair, and nails. It is the largest organ of the body.

  2. Functions

   a. Protects underlying tissues from dehydration, injury, and germ invasion.

   b. Regulates body temperature.

   c. Temporarily stores fats, glucose, water, and salts.

   d. Provides the sense of touch, pain, temperature, and pressure. There are 72 feet of nerves and hundreds of sense receptors per square inch.

   e. Plays a role in the manufacture of Vitamin D.

   f. Screens ultraviolet radiation in sunlight.

   g. Absorbs drugs and chemicals.

  3. Structure

   a. The skin has two basic layers (epidermis and dermis), attached to a third (subcutaneous, or hypodermal). (See Figure 4-11.)

    (1) The epidermis is the outermost layer, made up of stratified, squamous, keratinized, epithelial cells. It is avascular. Melanocytes are cells within the epidermis that create the protein melanin that helps to protect against harmful ultraviolet rays. There are two functionally significant layers in the epidermis.

     (a) Stratum corium is the surface layer consisting of dead cells rich in keratin.

     (b) Stratum germinativum is the deepest layer of the epidermis and is continuously undergoing cell division. The lower edges of the stratum germinativum form the ridges that make up our fingerprints.

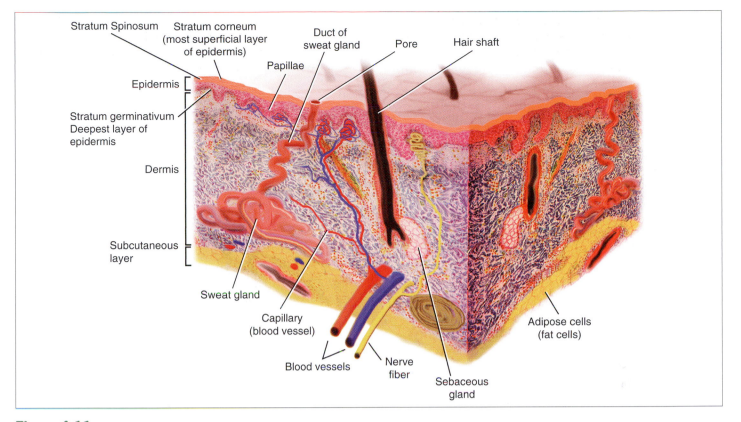

Figure 4-11

Structure of the Skin.

(2) The dermis, also called the "true skin" or corium, is thicker than the epidermis and contains blood and lymph vessels, nerves, sebaceous glands, hair follicles, sudoriferous glands, connective tissue, collagen tissue bands, elastic fibers, and fat cells.

(3) The subcutaneous, or hypodermal, layer lies under the dermis. This layer is not a true part of the integumentary system. It is composed of connective tissue and contains half the body's fat. This layer connects the integumentary system to the underlying muscles.

4. Appendages
   a. Hair is a nonliving tissue that covers most body surfaces except the palms of the hands, the soles of the feet, the glans penis, and the inner surfaces of the vaginal labia. Hair grows from a follicle in the epidermis.
   b. Nails are a nonliving tissue composed of keratin. The nails cover the dorsal surfaces of the ends of the fingers and toes.
   c. Sebaceous glands are connected to hair follicles. These glands secrete an oily substance called sebum.
   d. Sudoriferous glands, or "sweat glands," are located in the dermis. These glands are distributed over the entire skin and are present in larger numbers under the arms, palms of the hands, and soles of the feet. The sudoriferous glands secrete a watery substance called perspiration. Perspiration is 99 percent water, 1 percent waste.

5. Disorders
   a. Acne vulgaris—Common and often chronic inflammatory disorder of the sebaceous glands and hair follicles. Excessive secretion of sebum can cause a skin pore to plug, which prevents further secretions from escaping. Leukocytes (white blood cells) fill the area and cause pus to form.
   b. Athlete's foot—Contagious fungal infection that affects the superficial layers of the skin; characterized by small blisters and by cracking and scaling of the skin, most commonly on the feet
   c. Boils or carbuncles—Very painful bacterial infections of the hair follicles or sebaceous glands, usually caused by a staphylococcal organism
   d. Burns—Of many causes, classified by degrees. Redness, swelling, and pain characterize first-degree burns

e. Cancer—Of several types: basal cell carcinoma, squamous cell carcinoma, and malignant melanomas

f. Dermatitis—Inflammation of the skin, which may be nonspecific; may be caused by emotional stress or by using a different type of laundry soap

g. Eczema—Allergic inflammatory skin disorder, which can be acute or chronic in nature; characterized by itchy, red, scaly, and dry skin

h. Genital herpes—Viral infection that appears as blisters in the genital area; usually spread through sexual contact. Those infected may have periods of remission and exacerbation.

i. Herpes simplex—Viral infection usually seen as a fever blister or cold sore; may be spread orally or through the respiratory tract

j. Hives, or urticaria—Generally a hypersensitive response to an allergen, such as an ingested food or drug; characterized by extreme itching, wheals or welts that typically have a raised white center, surrounded by a pink or red area; can also be triggered by stress

k. Impetigo—A contagious, acute inflammatory skin disease, most commonly affecting infants and small children; caused by staphylococcal or streptococcal organisms; characterized by small vesicles, which rupture and develop a distinct yellow crusty appearance

l. Psoriasis—Chronic inflammatory skin disease that typically affects the skin over the areas of the elbows, knees, shins, scalp, and lower back; characterized dry reddish patches, which are covered with silvery-white scales

m. Ringworm—Highly contagious fungal infection, characterized by itchy, raised, circular patches with crusts

6. Diagnostic tests
   a. Biopsies
   b. KOH prep (potassium hydroxide)
   c. Microbiological cultures
   d. Tissue cultures

I. The digestive system (See Figure 4-12.)
   1. The GI tract (also called the alimentary canal) is continuous, beginning in the mouth and ending at the anus. It is approximately 27 feet long in an adult.
   2. Functions
      a. Physically breaks down food into smaller pieces.
      b. Chemically changes food into fats, carbohydrates, and proteins.

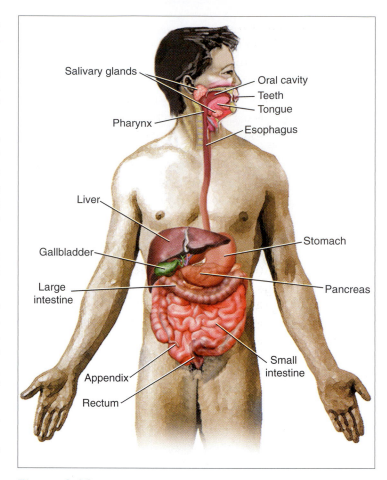

Figure 4-12

Structures of the Digestive System.

c. Absorbs nutrients into the capillaries of the small intestines.
d. Eliminates waste products.

3. Structure
   a. Mouth (oral or buccal cavity)
      (1) Lips
      (2) Uvula
      (3) Tongue, containing the taste buds
      (4) Teeth, which aid in the process of mastication
      (5) Salivary glands
         (a) Parotid
         (b) Submandibular
         (c) Salivary
   b. Pharynx, also known as the throat
   c. Esophagus—Hollow tube, approximately 10 inches long, that begins at the lower end of the pharynx behind the trachea. The upper-third muscles are voluntary while the lower two-thirds consist of involuntary muscle.

d. Stomach
   (1) Fundus
   (2) Cardiac sphincter
   (3) Pyloric sphincter
e. Small intestine—Approximately 20 feet long
   (1) Most nutrients are absorbed into the body from the small intestine. The small intestine is lined with small projections, called villi, which contain lymph and blood capillaries.
   (2) The small intestine is divided into three sections:
      (a) Duodenum—12 inches
      (b) Jejunum—8 feet
      (c) Ileum—10–12 feet
f. Large intestine
   (1) Also known as the colon, this is approximately 5 feet long and 2 inches in diameter. The main function of the large intestine is to absorb water.
   (2) The large intestine has four primary sections:
      (a) Ascending colon
      (b) Transverse colon
      (c) Descending colon
      (d) Sigmoid colon
g. Cecum
h. Vermiform appendix
i. Accessory Organs
   (1) Liver
   (2) Gallbladder
   (3) Pancreas

4. Disorders
   a. Appendicitis—Inflammation of the appendix caused typically by bacterial infections
   b. Cholecystitis—Inflammation of the gallbladder
   c. Cirrhosis—Chronic, progressive, inflammatory disease of the liver. Three-fourths of cirrhosis is caused by excessive alcohol consumption.
   d. Colitis—Also called irritable bowel syndrome (IBS), inflammation of the large intestine (colon)
   e. Colon cancer—Typically from a polyplike lesion. Early detection is critical, and everyone over the age of 50 is encouraged to have a colon cancer screening. Sections of the colon may be removed from patients with colon cancer. A colostomy may be performed.
   f. Diverticulosis—Condition in which small sacs develop in the wall of the colon
   g. Gastritis—Acute or chronic inflammation of the lining of the stomach
   h. Gastroesophageal reflux disease (GERD)—Disorder affecting the lower sphincter muscle connecting the esophagus to the stomach, which relaxes inappropriately, allowing the contents of the stomach to flow up the esophagus
   i. Heartburn—Acid indigestion resulting from a backflow of acid from the stomach
   j. Hepatitis—Inflammation of the liver. There are several types of hepatitis: hepatitis A, hepatitis B, hepatitis C, hepatitis D, and hepatitis E.
      (1) Hepatitis A—Viral infection often referred to as infectious hepatitis and spread through ingestion of contaminated water or food
      (2) Hepatitis B—Serum hepatitis; a virus spread via blood and contact
      (3) Hepatitis C—Mostly associated with a viral infection of the liver; also spread via blood and contact with body fluids; also commonly a result of needles shared by IV drug users
      (4) Hepatitis D—Requires a coinfection with hepatitis B
      (5) Hepatitis E—Transmitted through intestinal excrements; not common in the United States
   k. Hiatal hernia—Protrusion of stomach through a weak area in the diaphragm
   l. Pancreatitis—Inflammation of the pancreas
   m. Peptic ulcer—Erosion in the lining of the stomach or duodenum; most frequently caused by a bacterial infection. Peptic ulcer may also form due to a patient's lifestyle and stress levels.
   n. Peritonitis—Inflammation of the lining of the abdominal cavity
   o. Stomach cancer—Cancer cells in the stomach, which rapidly grow into tumors Malignant stomach cancer can spread to other parts of the body, even if the original mass is surgically removed.

5. Diagnostic tests
   a. Amylase
   b. Bilirubin
   c. Carcinoembryonic antigen (CEA)
   d. Carotene
   e. Cholesterol
   f. Complete blood count (CBC)
   g. Glucose

h. Glucose tolerance test (GTT)

i. Lipase

j. Occult blood

k. Ova and parasite (O&P)

l. Triglycerides

J. The endocrine system

1. Function

a. Secretes hormones directly into the bloodstream to be carried to the appropriate target organs and tissues.

2. Types

a. There are two types of glands in the endocrine system: endocrine and exocrine.

(1) Endocrine glands are ductless; they secrete hormones directly into the bloodstream to be carried to all areas of the body. Each endocrine gland secretes one or more specific hormones that regulate a specific body function, such as metabolism, growth, reproduction, or acid-base balance. (See Figure 4-13.)

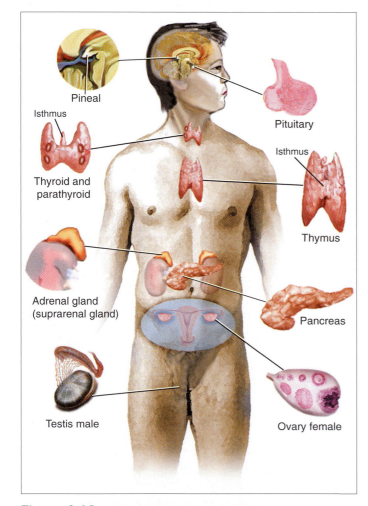

Figure 4-13

Structures of the Endocrine System.

(a) Pituitary—Known as the master gland, influences body activities such as growth of tissues, production of estrogen and progesterone in women and testosterone in men, and increases skin pigmentation.

(b) Thyroid—Regulates body metabolism.

(c) Parathyroid—Maintains the body's calcium-phosphorus balance.

(d) Thymus—Produces hormones, specifically those that produce T-cells and aid in fighting certain diseases.

(e) Adrenals—Increases heart rate, blood pressure, and blood flow; decreases intestinal activity; affects metabolism of fat, protein, and glucose; controls electrolyte balances; governs sex characteristics.

(f) Pineal—Regulates the sleep cycle.

(g) Pancreas—Metabolizes carbohydrates; controls blood sugar levels.

(h) Gonads—Develop primary and secondary sex characteristics.

(2) Exocrine glands have ducts that carry secretions to a body surface or an organ. Exocrine secretions include sweat, saliva, mucus, and digestive juices. There are four types of exocrine glands:

(a) Sweat glands

(b) Sebaceous glands

(c) Mammary glands

(d) Salivary glands

3. Disorders

a. Acromegaly—Overdevelopment of the bones of the face, hands, and feet; caused by an oversecretion of the growth hormone that occurs during adulthood

b. Addison's disease—Caused by hypofunctioning of the adrenal cortex. Symptoms include excessive pigmentation (bronzing of the skin), decreased levels of blood glucose, hypoglycemia, low blood pressure, muscular weakness, fatigue, diarrhea, weight loss, vomiting, and decrease in sodium levels causing an imbalance of electrolytes.

c. Cretinism—Congenital hypothyroidism, characterized by lack of mental and physical growth, resulting in mental retardation and malformation. Sexual development and physical growth do not progress beyond that of a 7- or 8-year-old child.

d. Cushing's syndrome—Caused by the hypersecretion of the glucocorticoid hormones from the adrenal cortex, which may be caused by an adrenal cortical tumor or the prolonged use of prednisone

e. Dwarfism—Hypofunctioning of the pituitary gland (growth hormone) during childhood. Growth of the long bones is abnormally decreased.

f. Diabetes insipidus—Condition characterized by increased thirst and increased urine production because of an inadequate production of antidiuretic hormone (ADH)

g. Diabetes mellitus—A condition caused by decreased secretion of insulin from the islet of Langerhans cells of the pancreas or by ineffective use of insulin

h. Gigantism—Hyperfunctioning of the pituitary gland; hypersecretion of the growth hormone, causing an overgrowth of the long bones during preadolescence and leading to excessive tallness

i. Hypothyroidism—Condition in which the thyroid gland does not secrete sufficient thyroxine. Adult hypothyroidism may be caused by an insufficient dietary intake of iodine. This condition may also be the result of an autoimmune disorder.

j. Hyperthyroidism—Condition due to over activity of the thyroid gland. Too much thyroxine is secreted.

4. Diagnostic tests
   a. Adrenocorticotropic hormone levels (ACTH)
   b. Aldosterone levels
   c. Antidiuretic hormone levels (ADH)
   d. Cortisol levels
   e. Erythropoietin
   f. Fasting blood sugar (FBS)
   g. Glucagon
   h. Glucose tolerance tests (GTTs)
   i. Growth hormone (GH)
   j. Glycosylated hemoglobin
   k. Insulin
   l. Renin
   m. Serotonin
   n. Thyroid function—Triiodothyronine (T3), thyroxine (T4), thyroid stimulating hormone (TSH)

K. The urinary system
   1. Functions
      a. Filters metabolic waste products from the body.
      b. Secretes waste products in the urine.

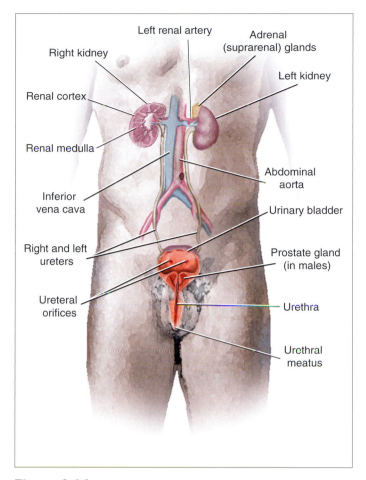

Figure 4-14

Structures of the Urinary System.

   c. Eliminates urine from the bladder.
   d. Helps to maintain acid-base balance.

2. Structures (See Figure 4-14.)
   a. Kidneys—Bean-shaped organs; two in the body. The kidneys function to maintain water and electrolyte balance and eliminate urea.
      (1) The nephron is the functional unit of the kidneys and is predominantly located in the cortex. A double-walled hollow capsule, called Bowman's capsule, and a knotty ball of capillaries, called the glomerulus, make up the nephron.
      (2) Renal tubules branch from the nephron and form a loop, called the loop of Henle. The loop descends from the nephron into the medulla and then back up into the cortex before continuing down again into the collecting tubule.
      (3) Renal pelvis is the structure that the collecting tubule empties into.
   b. Ureters—Approximately 10–12 inches long. There are two ureters that pass out of each kidney and carry urine into the bladder.

c. Bladder—Hollow organ that collects urine until a sufficient amount (approximately 500 milliliters) triggers the elimination response.

d. Urethra—Narrow tube that extends from the bladder to the urinary meatus. In women it is approximately 1½–2 inches long, while in men it is approximately 5–6 inches long.

3. Disorders

a. Cystitis—Inflammation of the mucous membrane lining of the urinary bladder

b. Glomerulonephritis—Inflammation of the glomerulus of the nephron; affects the filtration process, allowing protein and red blood cells to pass through to the urine

c. Kidney failure—May be of acute or sudden onset; may be caused by nephritis (inflammation of the nephron), shock, sudden heart failure, poisoning, or bleeding

d. Kidney stones—Also called renal calculi, stones that are formed in the kidneys

e. Pyelonephritis—Inflammation of the kidney tissue and the renal pelvis; generally resulting from an ascending cystitis

f. Urinary tract infection (UTI)—A term that describes an infection involving the organs or ducts of the urinary system is present

4. Diagnostic tests

a. Albumin

b. Ammonia

c. Blood urea nitrogen (BUN)

d. Creatinine clearance

e. Electrolytes

f. Osmolality

g. Urinalysis (UA)

h. Urine culture and sensitivity (C&S)

L. The lymphatic system

1. Functions

a. Maintains fluid balance in the tissue by filtering blood and lymph fluid.

b. Protects by filtering out harmful microorganisms; produces lymphocytes to help provide immunity and fight off disease.

c. Absorbs fats from the small intestine and transports them to the bloodstream.

2. Structures (See Figure 4-15.)

a. Lymph is a straw-colored fluid composed of water, lymphocytes, oxygen, digested nutrients, hormones, salts, carbon dioxide, and urea.

b. Lymphatic vessels run parallel to the veins of the circulatory system. There are two main lymphatic vessels, or lymphatics:

(1) The thoracic duct receives lymph from the left side of the chest, head, neck, abdominal area, and lower limbs.

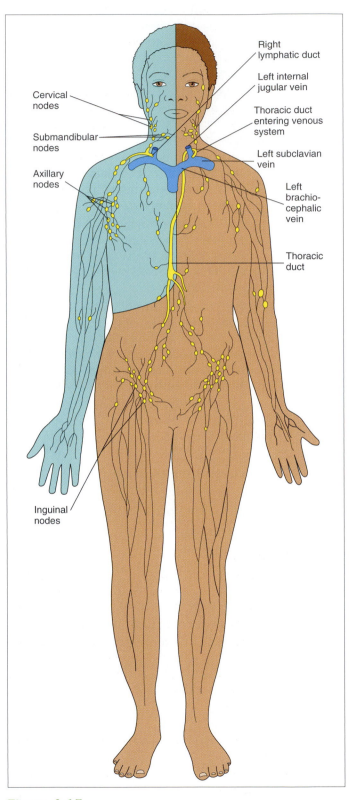

Figure 4-15

Structures of the Lymphatic System.

(2) The right lymphatic duct receives lymph from the right arm, right side of the head, and upper trunk.

c. Lymph nodes are tiny oval-shaped structures comprised of special tissue called lymphoid tissue. The lymph nodes provide a site for lymphocyte production and filter out harmful substances.

d. Other components of the lymphatic system:

(1) The thymus gland is located in the upper anterior part of the thorax above the heart. It functions as a source of lymphocytes prior to birth and then in the maturation and differentiation of lymphocytes as they leave the thymus and circulate to the spleen, tonsils, and other lymph nodes. These lymphocytes are called T-cells and are critical to the role of immunity. It is an endocrine gland that secretes the hormone thymosin, which stimulates the production of lymphoid cells.

(2) The spleen is located in the upper left quadrant of the abdominal cavity, below the diaphragm. The spleen is capable of storing large numbers of red blood cells, lymphocytes, and monocytes. The spleen functions to rid the body of old or damaged red blood cells. It also forms embryonic erythrocytes.

(3) The tonsils produce lymphocytes and filter bacteria. There are three pairs of tonsils:

(a) Palatine tonsils—Located on both sides of the soft palate of the mouth

(b) Adenoids—Upper part of the throat

(c) Lingual tonsils—Back of the tongue

3. Disorders

a. Acquired immunodeficiency syndrome (AIDS)—Disease that suppresses the body's natural immune system; caused by the human immunodeficiency virus (HIV)

b. Autoimmune disorders—Occur when the body's immune system goes haywire and the body forms antibodies to its own tissues, which destroy the tissues

c. Hodgkin's disease—Cancer of the lymph nodes. The most common early symptom of Hodgkin's disease is a painless swelling of the lymph nodes.

d. Human immunodeficiency virus (HIV)—Causative agent of AIDS

e. Hypersensitivity or allergic response—Occurs when the body's defense system fails to protect itself against invasion of foreign substances, causing an allergic response

f. Infectious mononucleosis—Caused by the Epstein-Barr virus; typically occurs in children and young adults

g. Lymphadenitis—Enlargement of the lymph nodes; may occur whenever the body is fighting an infection

h. Lymphadenopathy—Disease of the lymph nodes, often associated with enlargement of the lymph nodes, such as in mononucleosis

i. Lymphangitis—Inflammation of the lymph vessel

j. Lymphoma—Term used for any lymphoid tumor, either benign or malignant

k. Lymphosarcoma—Malignant lymphoid tumor

l. Spleenomegaly—Enlargement of the spleen

4. Diagnostic tests

a. Biopsy

b. Complete blood count (CBC)

c. Mononucleosis test (Monospot)

d. Culture and sensitivity (C&S)

e. Bone marrow biopsy

M. The reproductive system

1. Functions

a. Provides the organs necessary for reproduction.

b. Manufactures the hormones necessary for development of reproductive organs and secondary sex characteristics.

2. Structures

a. Female (See Figure 4-16.)

(1) Ovaries are the size and shape of an almond (3 centimeters long, 1.5–3 centimeters wide) and are located on both sides of the uterus. The ovaries function to produce female germ cells (ova), estrogen, and progesterone.

(2) Fallopian tubes are approximately 10 centimeters in length. They are not directly attached to the ovaries.

(3) The uterus is a hollow, thick-walled, pear-shaped, muscular organ. It lies behind the urinary bladder in front of the rectum. The uterus is divided into three parts: fundus, body, and cervix.

(4) The vagina consists of smooth muscle and is a canal that extends from the cervix to the vulva.

(5) The vulva is the external genitalia and consists of the mons pubis, clitoris, labia minora, and labia majora.

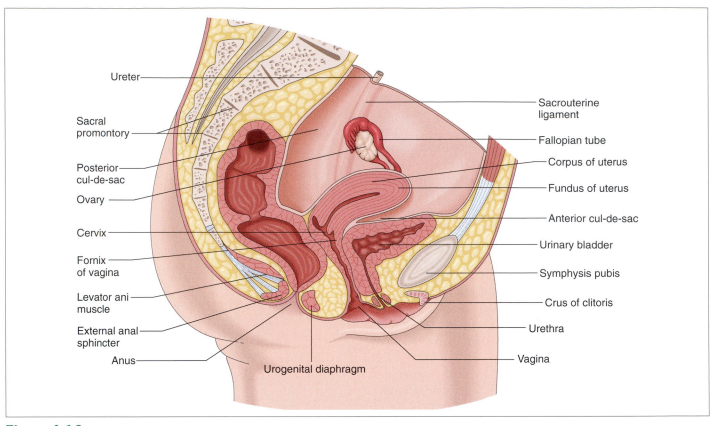

Figure 4-16

Female Reproductive System.

(6) Perineum is the area between the anus and the posterior part of the external genitalia, especially in the female.

(7) Breasts are accessory organs of female reproduction. The mammary glands in the breast secrete milk after childbirth.

b. Male (See Figure 4-17.)

(1) The testes produce the male gametes, spermatozoa. They are enclosed in the scrotum and are approximately 4 centimeters long, 2.5 centimeters wide, and 2 centimeters thick.

(2) The epididymis is attached to the testes and consists of a convoluted tube 13–20 feet long. It functions as the secretory duct of each testis.

(3) The right and left vas deferens are continuous with the epididymis and serve as storage sites for sperm and as excretory ducts.

(4) The seminal vesicles are two highly convoluted membranous tubes, which produce secretions that help to nourish and protect the sperm. A duct leads from the seminal vesicles to the ductus deferens to form the ejaculatory ducts.

(5) The ejaculatory ducts are very short and narrow. They descend into the prostate gland and join the urethra, where they discharge semen.

(6) The prostate gland is located in front of the rectum under the bladder. It is about the size and shape of a chestnut. It secretes a thin, milky alkaline fluid that enhances sperm motility.

(7) The external male genitalia consists of the scrotum and the penis.

(a) The penis contains erectile tissue. The foreskin, or prepuce, covers the end of the penis; it is sometimes surgically removed by circumcision.

(b) The scrotum is divided into two sacs, each containing a testicle.

(8) The urethra serves two functions: to empty the bladder of urine and to expel semen during sexual intercourse. The ureter runs the length of the penis.

(9) Bulbourethral glands, or Cowper's glands, lie on either side of the urethra, below the prostate. These glands function to add an alkaline secretion to the semen.

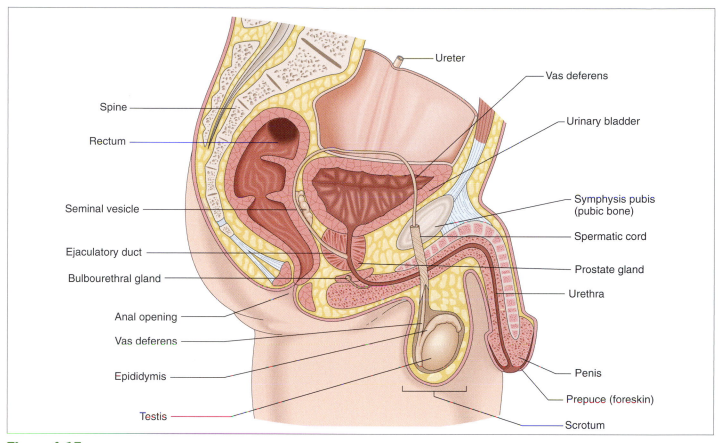

Figure 4-17

Male Reproductive System.

3. Disorders
   a. Cancer of the reproductive organs— Cervical, ovarian, uterine, testicular, prostate
   b. Infertility—The inability to conceive
   c. Impotence—The inability to have or sustain an erection during intercourse
   d. Ovarian cyst—A fluid-filled sac that develops on the ovary
   e. Sexually transmitted diseases (STDs)— Transmitted through the exchange of body fluids such as semen, vaginal fluid, or blood. There is a wide variety of STDs; some of the more common are:
      (1) Chlamydia
      (2) Genital warts
      (3) Gonorrhea
      (4) Genital herpes
      (5) Syphilis
      (6) Trichomoniasis vaginalis
4. Diagnostic tests
   a. Acid phosphatase
   b. Estrogen
   c. Follicle-stimulating hormone (FSH)
   d. Human chorionic gonadotropin (hCG)
   e. Luteinizing hormone (LH)
   f. Microbiological cultures
   g. Pap smear
   h. Prostate-specific antigen (PSA)
   i. Rapid plasmin reagin (RPR)
   j. Testosterone
   k. Tissue analysis

N. The respiratory system
   1. Functions
      a. Provides the structures for the exchange of oxygen and carbon dioxide in the process of respiration.
         (1) External respiration occurs between the lungs and the outside environment.
         (2) Internal respiration takes place at a cellular level.
         (3) Cellular respiration occurs inside the cell.
      b. Provides the structures allowing the body to produce sound.
   2. Structures (See Figure 4-18.)
      a. The nasal cavity is the main route of respiration.

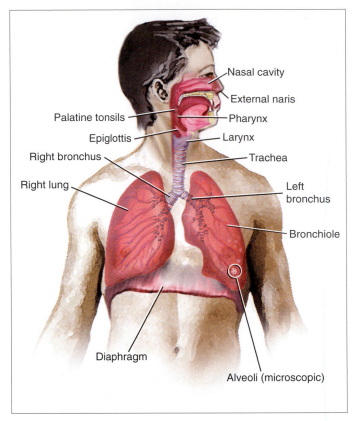

Figure 4-18

Structures of the Respiratory System.

    (1) The nose is divided into two cavities by the nasal septum.

    (2) It is lined with mucous membranes that help to warm inhaled air.

    (3) Small hairs within the nose, called cilia, trap larger dirt particles.

    (4) The nose contains the sensory receptors for the sense of smell. It also provides the voice with resonance.

  b. The pharynx, or throat, is a funnel-shaped passage approximately 5 inches long, used as a passageway for both food and air.

    (1) The epiglottis covers the opening to the larynx so that food goes down the esophagus instead of the trachea.

  c. The larynx, or voice box, contains small rings of cartilage.

    (1) The largest of these rings is called the Adam's apple.

    (2) The larynx divides the upper respiratory tract and the lower respiratory tract.

  d. The trachea, or windpipe, is approximately 4.5 inches long. This is a tubelike passageway that branches into the bronchi.

  e. Bronchi and bronchioles are composed of mucous membrane, cartilage, and cilia. The right and left divisions form a Y-shaped structure. They continue to branch and become smaller and smaller. The smallest divisions are called bronchioles.

  f. The alveoli extend from the bronchioles and form a saclike structure called the alveolar sac.

    (1) The lungs contain thousands of alveoli.

    (2) Gas exchange takes place within the alveoli and the capillaries that surround each alveolus.

  g. There are two lungs.

    (1) The right lung has three lobes.

    (2) The left lung has two lobes to allow space for the heart.

    (3) The lungs are separated by the mediastinum.

    (4) The lungs are covered with a thin, moist, slippery membrane, called the pleural membrane. The pleural membrane is composed of two layers:

      (a) Visceral

      (b) Parietal

    (5) Fluid prevents the two linings from rubbing against each other.

3. Gas exchange occurs when red blood cells transport oxygen and carbon dioxide throughout the body using the protein molecule called hemoglobin.

4. Disorders

  a. Adult respiratory distress syndrome—Respiratory failure in adults or children that results from diffuse injury to the endothelium of the lung; characterized by pulmonary edema with an abnormally high amount of protein in the edematous fluid and by difficult rapid breathing and hypoxemia

  b. Apnea—The temporary stoppage of breathing

  c. Asthma—Obstruction of the airway due to an inflammatory response to a stimulus

  d. Bronchitis—Inflammation of the mucous membrane of the trachea and the bronchial tubules, producing excess mucus

  e. Cancer—Abnormal cell growth that can spread rapidly to other organs

  f. Diphtheria—An infectious disease caused by the *Corynebacterium diphtheriae* bacterium

  g. Dyspnea—Difficult, labored, or painful breathing

  h. Emphysema—Overdilation of the alveoli of the lungs, causing them to lose their elasticity

i. Hyperpnea—An increase in the rate and depth of breathing, accompanied by abnormal exaggeration of respiratory movements

j. Hyperventilation—Rapid breathing that causes the body to lose carbon dioxide too quickly

k. Hypoxia—An oxygen deficiency

l. Infant respiratory distress syndrome (IRDS)—A breathing disorder present at birth

m. Influenza—A viral infection characterized by inflammation of the mucous membrane of the respiratory system

n. Laryngitis—Inflammation of the larynx

o. Pertussis—Also known as whooping cough, severe coughing attacks and dyspnea

p. Pleurisy—Inflammation of the pleura

q. Pneumonia—Infection of the lung

r. Pulmonary edema—Swelling of the pulmonary blood vessels; a life-threatening condition

s. Tuberculosis (TB)—Infectious disease of the lungs

t. Rhinitis—Inflammation of the nasal mucous membrane, causing swelling and increased secretions

u. Tachypnea—Abnormally rapid and shallow rate of breathing

v. Tonsillitis—Infection and swelling of the tonsils

w. Upper respiratory infection (URI)—Any infectious disease process infecting the nasal passages, pharynx, and bronchi

5. Diagnostic tests
   a. Alkaline phosphatase (ALP)
   b. Arterial blood gases (ABGs)
   c. Bronchial washings
   d. Capillary blood gases (CBGs)
   e. Complete blood count (CBC)
   f. Drug levels
   g. Electrolytes ('lytes)
   h. Microbiology cultures
   i. Pleuracentesis
   j. Skin tests (PPD)
   k. Sputum cultures

O. Cardiovascular system
   1. All systems of the body are connected by the cardiovascular system. *This is the most important system to the phlebotomist.* There are three elements of the cardiovascular system: the heart, the blood, and the vessels.

P. The heart
   1. Function
      a. Pumps circulating blood to all parts of the body. Approximately 2 ounces of blood are pumped with each heartbeat, or 5 quarts per minute.
   2. Structures (See Figure 4-19.)
      a. The heart is a hollow muscular organ, slightly larger than a closed fist and weighing less than 1 pound. It is located slightly left of the midline thoracic cavity.

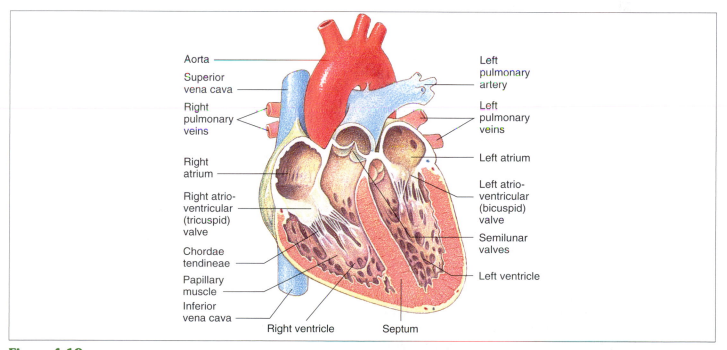

Figure 4-19

Structures of the Heart.

b. The heart has four chambers divided by a wall of cartilage, called the septum.
  (1) The receiving chambers are the atria. The right atrium receives deoxygenated blood from the body, and the left receives oxygenated blood from the lungs.
  (2) The pumping chambers are the ventricles. The right pumps deoxygenated blood to the lungs, and the left pumps oxygenated blood to the body.
c. The heart has four valves that open and close with the contraction of the heart:
  (1) The tricuspid valve
  (2) The bicuspid valve
  (3) The pulmonary semilunar valve
  (4) The aortic semilunar valve.
d. Layers of the heart
  (1) Pericardium surrounds the heart and is a double layer of fibrous tissue.
    (a) The thin layer covering the heart is the visceral pericardium.
    (b) The outer layer is the parietal pericardium.
    (c) Between these two layers lies pericardial fluid, which keeps the layers from rubbing against one another.
  (2) Myocardium is the cardiac muscle tissue and makes up the major portion of the heart.
  (3) Endocardium covers the inner layer of the heart, providing smooth transit for blood through valves and vessels.
3. Electrical conduction system
  a. The heart has the ability to generate the heartbeat and conduct an impulse.
    (1) The time it takes for the impulse to be generated and for the process to begin again is one heartbeat.
    (2) The impulse originates in the sinoatrial (SA) node and stimulates the contraction of the atria.
    (3) Blood flows from the atria into the ventricles.
    (4) The relaxed ventricles fill with blood.
  b. The impulse travels to the atrioventricular (AV) node, which stimulates the ventricles to contract.
    (1) Blood from the ventricles is pumped into the pulmonary artery and the aorta.
    (2) The heart rests briefly before the cycle begins again.

4. Disorders
  a. Angina pectoris—Severe chest pain that occurs when the heart does not receive enough oxygen
  b. Arrhythmia—Any change or deviation from the normal heart rate or rhythm
  c. Bacterial endocarditis—Inflammation of the membrane that lines the heart and covers the valves
  d. Bradycardia—Slow heart rate
  e. Congestive heart failure (CHF)—Similar to heart failure with the addition of edema in the lower extremities
  f. Heart failure—Pooling of blood in the heart, resulting from the inability of the ventricles to adequately contract
  g. Murmers—Defects in the valves of the heart
  h. Myocardial infarction—Lack of blood supply to the heart muscle
  i. Arteriosclerosis—Narrowing of the artery
  j. Atherosclerosis—Plaque buildup in the arterial walls
  k. Pericarditis—Inflammation of the outer membrane covering the heart
  l. Tachycardia—Rapid heart rate
5. Diagnostic tests
  a. Arterial blood gases (ABGs)
  b. Aspartate aminotransferase (AST), serum glutamic oxaloacetic transaminase (SGOT)
  c. Cholesterol
  d. creatine kinase (CK), creatine phosphokinase (CPK)
  e. electrocardiogram (ECG)
  f. Potassium
  g. Triglycerides
Q. Blood
  1. The average adult human contains approximately 8–10 pints, or 4–5 quarts, of blood.
  2. Functions
    a. Provides the body with oxygen, nutrients, hormones, and removal of waste products by means of a viscous transporting fluid.
    b. Aids in the maintenance of body temperature.
    c. Is important in regulating the acid-base balance.
    d. Fights infection.
  3. Structure—Blood is composed of plasma and cellular elements.
  4. Plasma
    a. Plasma makes up 55 percent of total blood volume.

b. It is the straw-colored liquid portion of blood minus the cellular elements.

c. Approximately 92 percent of plasma is water; the remaining substances are called solutes.

d. The most abundant plasma proteins found in plasma are fibrinogen (necessary for blood clotting), albumin (maintains osmotic pressure and volume), and globulin (helps in the synthesis of antibodies).

e. Plasma also contains:

   (1) Nutrients (glucose, fatty acids, cholesterol, and amino acids) are absorbed in the plasma from the digestive tract.

   (2) Electrolytes also come from food and are found in the plasma (sodium, calcium, magnesium, and potassium).

   (3) Hormones, vitamins, and enzymes are found in very small portions in the plasma.

   (4) Gases such as oxygen, carbon dioxide, and nitrogen are found in the plasma.

5. Cellular elements—The formed elements found in the blood

   a. When blood has been allowed to clot for 30–60 minutes after being removed from the body in preparation for separating the formed elements from the liquid portion, the liquid portion is called serum.

   b. The formed elements consist of erythrocytes, leukocytes, and thrombocytes.

      (1) Erythrocytes—RBC biconcave, disc-shaped cells.

         (a) The main function of erythrocytes is to carry oxygen from the lungs to the cells as well as to carry carbon dioxide from the cells back to the lungs.

         (b) They are 7–8 microns in diameter and anuclear.

         (c) The average adult has 4.5–5 million RBC per cubic millimeter of blood.

         (d) Erythrocytes are produced in the bone marrow.

         (e) They have a life span approximately 120 days.

         (f) Hemoglobin gives RBCs their typical red color. RBCs are composed of globins and iron compounds.

         (g) Hemolysis occurs when cells rupture.

      (2) Leukocytes—White blood cells (WBCs) that are larger than RBCs and vary in size.

         (a) The main function of leukocytes is to destroy pathogens.

         (b) The average adult has approximately 5,000–10,000 per cubic millimeter of blood.

         (c) Leukocytes are formed in the bone marrow and lymphatic tissue. They can travel into surrounding tissues.

         (d) Their life span varies from 6 to 8 hours in the bloodstream and weeks, months, even years in the tissues.

         (e) There are two classifications of leukocytes: granulocytes and agranulocytes.

            (i) Granulocytes—There are three types of granulocytes: neutrophils, eosinophils, and basophils.

            Neutrophils make up 65 percent of all WBCs. They are fine granules in the cytoplasm and they stain lavender. They are polymorphonuclear, meaning the nucleus has many lobes. Neutrophils phagocytize (engulf) bacteria and increase in number in the presence of bacterial infections. The life span of a neutrophil is 6 hours to a few days.

            Eosinophils make up 3 percent of total WBCs. They contain beadlike granules and stain bright orange-red. The nucleus has two lobes. The number of eosinophils increases in allergic reactions and parasitic infestations and their primary function is in defense of invading organisms. Their life span is 8–12 days.

            Basophils make up 1 percent of total WBCs. They form large granules and stain dark blue purple to black, often obscuring the nucleus. The nucleus is often S-shaped. Basophils release histamine and heparin to help in inflammatory processes. Their life span is a few days.

            (ii) Agranulocytes are divided into monocytes and lymphocytes.

            Monocytes form 1–7 percent of the total WBC. They are formed in the bone marrow and the spleen. They are the largest

WBC and stain blue-gray, with a large dark nucleus. The cytoplasm contains vacuoles. They aid in phagocytosis and have a life span of several days.

Lymphocytes are 15–30 percent of the total WBC. They are the most numerous. Lymphocytes are large, round, and have a dark purple nucleus that occupies the bulk of the cell. There is a thin rim of robin's egg blue cytoplasm. Two types of T-cells attack infected cells and B-cells, which produce antibodies. Leukocytes play a major role in immunity. They have a life span from a few hours to several years.

(3) Thrombocytes—The smallest of the solid components of blood.

    (a) They start as part of a larger cell, the megakaryocyte, which is formed in the red bone marrow.

    (b) The average adult has approximately 250,000– 450,000 per cubic millimeter.

    (c) The life span is approximately 10 days. Thrombocytes play a role in coagulation.

c. Thrombocytes play a role in coagulation.

    (1) Coagulation, or hemostasis—The process whereby blood coagulates (clots) and bleeding stops. There are four stages:

    (a) Vasoconstriction—The flow of blood to the injured area decreases as the vessel constricts.

    (b) Platelet aggregation—Thromboplastin is released, causing the platelets to clump and stick to one another and forming a platelet plug.

    (c) Fibrin clot—Thromboplastin and calcium act together as an enzyme, causing a reaction that converts the prothrombin into thrombin; gel-like fibrin threads layer themselves over the cut, creating a fine mesh-like network.

    (d) Scab formation—The fibrin network traps red blood cells, platelets, and plasma, and forms a blood clot; serum oozes out of the injury and, as it dries, a crust (scab) forms over the fibrin threads, completing the clotting process.

6. Blood types

  a. Antigens and antibodies

    (1) Blood type is inherited and determined by the presence or absence of two blood proteins (antigen A and antigen B), located on the surface of red blood cells.

    (2) There is also a protein present in the plasma of a person's blood, referred to as agglutinin or antibody. A person with type A blood has B antibodies. Type B blood has A antibodies; type AB has no antibodies, and type O contains both A and B antibodies.

    (3) The antigens in the blood react with antibodies of the same type. These reactions cause red blood cells to clump together in a process called agglutination.

      (a) Example: If a person with type B blood were transfused with type A blood, the A antibodies of the recipient would clump with the A antigens of the donor.

      (b) In an emergency, a person with type A blood could receive type A and type O blood, because type O blood carries no A or B antigens; therefore there would be no reaction because of the lack of antigens.

  b. Matching blood types

    (1) Universal donor—Because type O blood lacks antigens, it can be donated to all four blood types. Therefore, type O blood is the universal donor. By the same token, type AB blood lacks antibodies in its plasma, so it cannot agglutinate the red blood cells of any donor.

    (2) Universal recipient—Type AB blood is the universal recipient. It can receive all four blood types.

      (a) This is done only in emergency situations, because the same blood type should be given to avoid serious complications.

    (3) Type and cross-match—This is why it is vitally important to know a patient's blood type before surgeries or blood transfusions. A test called type and cross-match is performed prior to a blood transfusion or surgery. This test identifies the blood type of both the recipient and the donor so that they are properly matched and mismatch emergencies do not occur.

c. Percentages of blood types by population in the United States:
   (1) Type A—41%
   (2) Type B—12%
   (3) Type AB—3%
   (4) Type O—44%

7. Rh factor
   a. The outer membrane of human blood cells may also contain a D antigen, known as the Rh factor. This was first discovered in Rhesus monkeys.
   b. An individual is Rh+ if the Rh factor is present and Rh− if the Rh factor is absent.
   c. It is critical that the same Rh type be given from donor to recipient.
      (1) If Rh+ blood is transfused to an Rh− patient, he or she may develop antibodies to it. The antibodies take approximately two weeks to develop. There is usually no problem with the first transfusion, but if subsequent transfusions occur, the accumulated Rh antibodies in the patient's blood could react with the Rh antigen of the donor's blood. Clumping and its potentially lethal consequences could occur.
      (2) The same problem may arise when an Rh− mother is pregnant with an Rh+ fetus. The mother's blood can develop anti-Rh antibodies to fetal Rh antigens. This typically does not affect the first-born child. However, subsequent pregnancies may be affected because the mother's accumulated anti-Rh antibodies clump with the fetus's red blood cells.
      (3) If the condition is left untreated, the baby could be born with a condition called erythroblastosis fetalis (hemolytic disease of the newborn).
      (4) This condition is preventable because a special injection of immune globulin, RhoGAM can be given to Rh− mother within 72 hours after delivery of a viable or nonviable fetus or a miscarriage. The RhoGAM antibodies destroy any Rh+ fetal cells that may have entered the mother's bloodstream; therefore the mother's immune system is not stimulated to produce antibodies.

8. Disorders
   a. Anemia—A deficiency in the number and/or percentage of red blood cells and the amount of hemoglobin in the blood
   b. Hemophilia—A hereditary disease in which the blood clots slowly or abnormally; can cause prolonged bleeding
   c. Leukemia—A cancerous or malignant condition in which there is a great increase in the number of white blood cells
   d. Leukocytosis—An increase in the white blood cell count
   e. Leukopenia—A decrease in the normal number of white blood cells
   f. Polycythemia—Too many red blood cells
   g. Septicemia—The presence of pathogenic organisms or toxins in the blood
   h. Thrombocytosis—An increase in the number of blood platelets
   i. Thrombocytopenia—A decrease in the number of platelets (thrombocytes)

9. Diagnostic tests
   a. ABO and Rh Type
   b. Bone marrow
   c. Complete blood count (CBC)
   d. Type and cross-match
   e. Differential
   f. Eosinophil (Eos) count
   g. Erythrocyte sedimentation rate (ESR)
   h. Ferritin
   i. Hematocrit (Hct)
   j. Hemoglobin (hgb)
   k. Hemogram
   l. Indices (MCH, MCV, MCHC)
   m. Iron (Fe)
   n. Reticulocyte (retic) count
   o. Total iron binding (TIBC)

10. Circulation (See Figure 4-20.)
   a. Cardiopulmonary circulation is the process whereby blood circulates through the heart. Deoxygenated blood from the heart travels through the lungs, where carbon dioxide is exchanged for oxygen and oxygenated blood is then pumped out to the body.
   b. Types of circulation
      (1) Systemic circulation is the process that circulates oxygen, water, nutrients, and secretions to the body's tissues and back to the heart.
      (2) Coronary circulation is the process that takes oxygenated blood directly to the cells of the heart muscle. Coronary arteries branch off the aorta and encircle the heart muscle.
      (3) Portal circulation is a division of systemic venous circulation. Veins from the

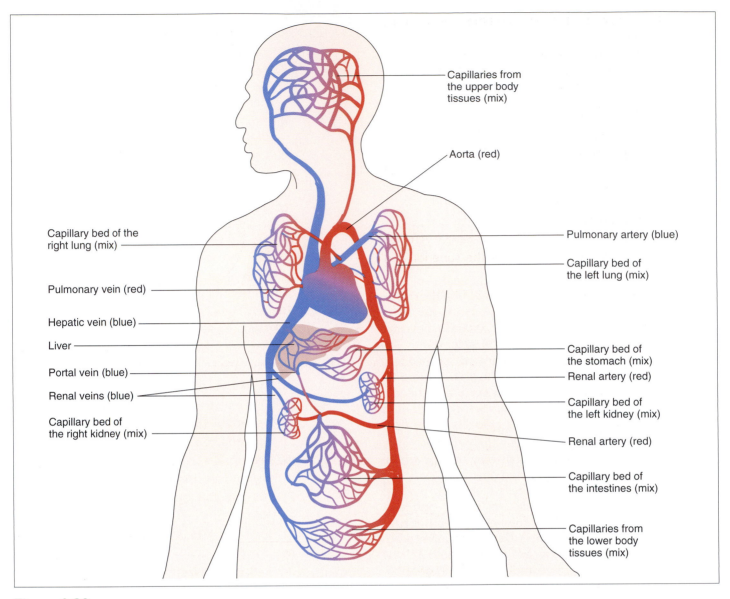

Capillaries from the upper body tissues (mix)

Aorta (red)

Capillary bed of the right lung (mix)

Pulmonary vein (red)

Hepatic vein (blue)

Liver

Portal vein (blue)

Renal veins (blue)

Capillary bed of the right kidney (mix)

Pulmonary artery (blue)

Capillary bed of the left lung (mix)

Capillary bed of the stomach (mix)

Renal artery (red)

Capillary bed of the left kidney (mix)

Renal artery (red)

Capillary bed of the intestines (mix)

Capillaries from the lower body tissues (mix)

Figure 4-20

Circulatory System.

pancreas, stomach, small intestines, colon, and spleen empty blood into the portal vein, which travel to the liver.

(a) Blood needs to take this detour through the liver before it returns to the heart because the liver removes excess glucose from digested food, converting it to glycogen for later use.

(4) Fetal circulation takes place in a fetus. The fetus obtains blood, oxygen, and nutrients from its mother's blood. The blood of the fetus and the blood of the mother never mix.

R. Blood vessels

1. Types

a. Arteries carry oxygenated blood away from the heart to the body's tissues, except the pulmonary arteries, which carry deoxygenated blood from the right ventricle to the lungs.

(1) The arteries have thick, elastic, muscular walls. They are the strongest blood vessels in the body.

(2) Blood of the arteries is bright red in color.

(3) Smaller branches of arteries are called arterioles.

(4) The largest artery is the aorta.

b. Veins carry deoxygenated blood toward the heart.
   (1) The exception is the pulmonary vein, which carries oxygenated blood from the lungs back to the heart.
   (2) Veins have thinner walls than arteries, and they do not have the pressure behind them of ventricular contractions.
   (3) Movement of blood through veins occurs mainly due to the movement of skeletal muscles. Veins contain valves to help prevent backflow of blood.
   (4) Venous blood is dark red in color.
   (5) The smallest veins are called venules.
   (6) The largest veins are the superior and inferior vena cava.
   (7) The longest vein is the great saphenous vein, located in the leg.
c. Capillaries are microscopic vessels, one cell thick.
   (1) They connect with arterioles and venules.
   (2) Blood in capillaries is both venous and arterial.
   (3) Walls are thin enough to allow for the exchange of oxygen and nutrients and carbon dioxide and waste products.
2. Structure of blood vessels (See Figure 4-21.)
   a. Blood vessels are composed of three layers with an internal opening called a lumen.
      (1) Tunica adventitia is the outer layer. It is composed of fibrous connective tissue.
      (2) Tunica media is the middle layer. It is made up of smooth muscle tissue.
      (3) Tunica intima is the inner layer. It is composed of three smaller layers.
3. Disorders
   a. Aneurysm—The ballooning out of an artery accompanied by a thinning arterial wall
   b. Arteriosclerosis—Thickening of the arterial wall due to loss of elasticity
   c. Atherosclerosis—Fatty deposits on the walls of the artery that cause narrowing of the lumen
   d. Cerebrovascular accident (CVA, or stroke)—The sudden interruption of blood flow to the brain
   e. Embolism—A traveling blood clot
   f. Hemorrhoids—Varicose veins in the walls of the lower rectum and tissues around the anus
   g. Phlebitis—Inflammation of a vein with or without infection and thrombus formation

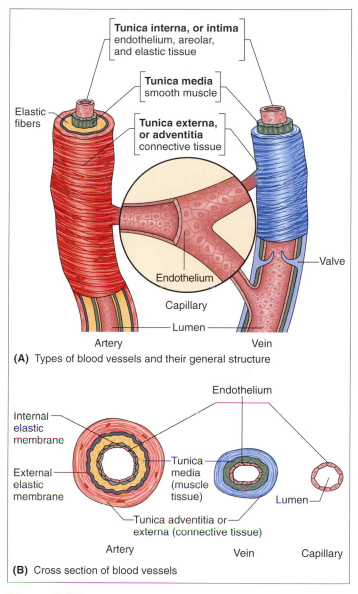

(A) Types of blood vessels and their general structure

(B) Cross section of blood vessels

Figure 4-21

Structures of Blood Vessels.

h. Thrombophlebitis—Inflammation of a vein in conjunction with the formation of a thrombus
i. Thrombus—Blood clot formed in a blood vessel
j. Transient ischemic attack (TIA)—Temporary interruption of blood flow of short duration to the brain
k. Varicose veins—Swollen veins that result from a slowing of blood flow back to the heart
4. Diagnostic tests
   a. Disseminated intravascular coagulation (DIC) screen
   b. Lipoproteins
   c. Prothrombin time (PT)

d. Partial thromboplastin time (PTT/APTT)

e. Triglycerides

5. Vessels related to venous and arterial puncture (See Figure 4-22.)

   a. Venous punctureThe veins most frequently used for venipuncture are located in the antecubital fossa.

      (1) The antecubital veins are the medial cubital, cephalic, and basilic.

      (2) The median cubital vein is usually large and well anchored. This makes it the first choice for venipuncture.

      (3) It is acceptable to use the other veins of the arms and hands for venipuncture.

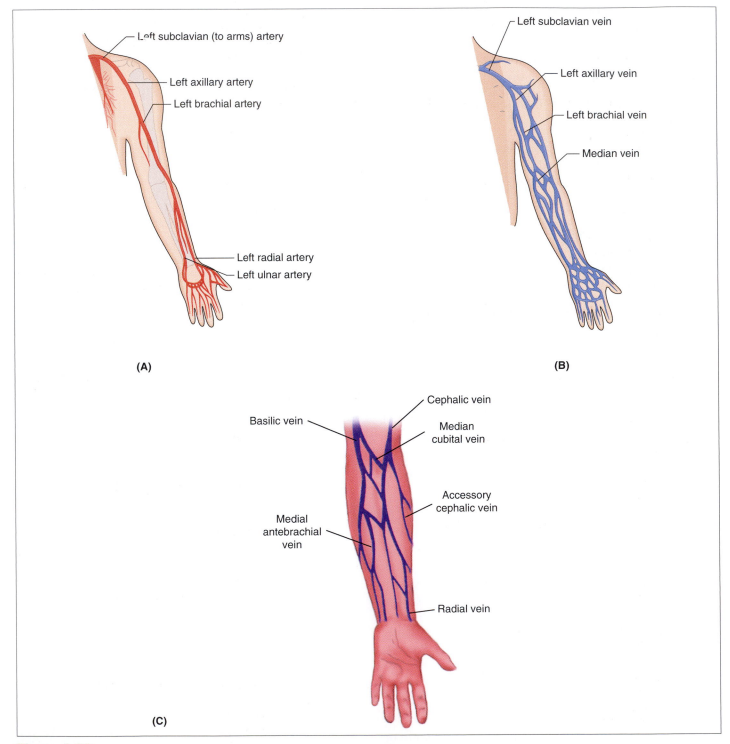

(A)

- Left subclavian (to arms) artery
- Left axillary artery
- Left brachial artery
- Left radial artery
- Left ulnar artery

(B)

- Left subclavian vein
- Left axillary vein
- Left brachial vein
- Median vein

(C)

- Basilic vein
- Cephalic vein
- Median cubital vein
- Accessory cephalic vein
- Medial antebrachial vein
- Radial vein

Figure 4-22

Arteries and Veins of Common Venipuncture Sites.

(4) The veins of the leg, ankle, and foot are used only with permission of the practitioner ordering the test.

b. Arterial puncture—This site is used for ABGs. Radial and brachial arteries can be used as well as the femoral artery of the leg in an emergency or when no other arterial sites are available.

PRACTICE

Identify the letter of the choice that best completes the statement or answers the question.

1. A _____ establishes the basic meaning of a medical term.
   a. prefix
   b. suffix
   c. combining form
   d. word root

2. The letter "o" or "i" used with a word root is called a _____.
   a. combining word
   b. combining vowel
   c. word part
   d. word form

3. The medical abbreviation for arterial blood gases is _____.
   a. aBgs
   b. Abgs
   c. AbGs
   d. ABGs

4. The word root with the combining vowel "thromb/o" refers to a(n) _____.
   a. vein
   b. clot
   c. little body
   d. artery

5. The medical abbreviation for hemoglobin is _____.
   a. hgb
   b. Hg
   c. hGb
   d. HBG

6. The longitudinal imaginary line dividing the body into equal right and left parts is called the _____.
   a. sagittal plane
   b. midsagittal plane
   c. frontal plane
   d. transverse plane

7. The _____ is a small cavity or chamber of the heart or brain.
   a. ventricle
   b. atria
   c. Purkinje fiber
   d. bundle of His

8. The _____ is also called the mitral valve and is an atrioventricular valve of the left side of the heart.
   a. tricuspid valve
   b. bicuspid valve
   c. pulmonary semilunar valve
   d. aortic semilunar valve

9. The _____ is the muscle layer of the heart.
   a. pericardium
   b. myocardium
   c. endocardium
   d. epicardium

10. The outermost layer of a vein is called the _____.
    a. tunica adventitia
    b. tunica media
    c. tunica intima
    d. lumen

11. A(n) _____ is the inflammation of the lining of a vein, accompanied by clotting of blood in the vein.
    a. aneurysm
    b. CVA
    c. hemorrhoid
    d. phlebitis

12. The average adult has _____ million RBCs per cubic millimeter of blood.
    a. 2.0 to 3.5
    b. 3.0 to 4.0
    c. 4.5 to 5.0
    d. 5.5 to 6.0

13. _____ is an arrest of bleeding or of circulation.
    a. Hemostasis
    b. Homeostasis
    c. Hemopoiesis
    d. Hemolysis

14. An individual belonging to the _____ blood group can accept blood from all blood types.
    a. A
    b. B
    c. AB
    d. O

15. _____ is an abnormal decrease in WBCs.
    a. Anemia
    b. Leukocytosis
    c. Leukopenia
    d. Polycythemia

16. _____ is a cancer or malignant condition in which there is a great increase in the number of white blood cells.
    a. Anemia
    b. Hemophilia
    c. Leukemia
    d. Polycythemia

17. The outer membrane of human red blood cells may also contain a(n) _____ antigen, better known as the Rh factor.
    a. D
    b. R
    c. Q
    d. X

18. _____ carry deoxygenated blood toward the heart.
    a. Arterioles
    b. Arteries
    c. Capillaries
    d. Veins

19. _____ is/are blood that has been removed from the body and allowed to clot 30–60 minutes before centrifuging.
    a. Electrolytes
    b. Plasma
    c. Serum
    d. Whole blood

20. _____ circulation is a division of systemic venous circulation.
    a. Coronary
    b. Fetal
    c. Caudal
    d. Portal

21. The _____ vein is usually large and well anchored and therefore the first choice for venipuncture.
    a. basilic
    b. cephalic
    c. median cubital
    d. radial

22. _____ are the upper two chambers of the heart.
    a. Atria
    b. Atrium
    c. Ventricles
    d. Pericardium

23. The medical prefix "infra-" means _____.
    a. inferior to
    b. without
    c. within
    d. in front of

24. _____ occurs when red blood cells rupture.
    a. Hemopoiesis
    b. Hemolysis
    c. Hemocytosis
    d. Hemostasis

25. The medical suffix that means dilation is _____.
    a. -iasis
    b. -ectasis
    c. -exis
    d. -esis

26. _____ numbers increase in allergic reactions and parasitic infestations, and their primary function is in the defense of invading organisms.
    a. Neutrophil
    b. Basophil
    c. Monophil
    d. Eosinophil

27. Which blood type is considered the universal donor?
    a. AB
    b. O
    c. A
    d. B

28. Type _____ blood accounts for 12 percent of the U.S. population.
    a. AB
    b. O
    c. A
    d. B

29. In the prevention of erythroblastosis fetalis, a special injection of immune globulin, RHO-gam, can be given to an RH− mother within _____ hours after delivery.
    a. 24
    b. 48
    c. 72
    d. 12

30. Plasma makes up about 55 percent of the total blood volume and is approximately _____ percent water.
    a. 80
    b. 50
    c. 92
    d. 98

CRITICAL THINKING

1. Dr. Jones left you the following order for Sandra Henderson.

   Pt c/o **LLQ** pain **pc**, her **LOC** is 80%. **Pt** has a **Hx** of **HBV**. I will need a **CBC**, **Ca**, et **H&H**. Will perform an **ALT** in **am**. **Pt** is to be **NPO pre-op and 4 h. post-op.** Identify and define all terms or abbreviations in bold.

2. Mike and Vicki are expecting their first child. They have anxiously been looking forward to the birth of Baby Lori. Once they arrived at the hospital and were taken to **L&D**, everything seemed to be

progressing smoothly. Vicki was in labor for 12 hours and the baby was delivered **w/o** complications. However, baby Lori was born with a very blue tinge to her skin. Baby Lori was rushed to the **NICU STAT,** and neither Mike nor Vicki were able to hold the baby. You are called to the NICU to draw an **AST,** Potassium, and **CK.** The nurses have an **ECG** monitor attached, and an ECG is being performed. Mike and Vicki are told that Lori has a heart murmur and will need to be monitored closely in an oxygen tent for a few days. They are also informed that some heart murmurs repair on their own a few days after birth. If hers doesn't, she may require surgery.

- Identify and define all terms or abbreviations in bold.
- Explain to Mike and Lori what a heart murmur is and what caused baby Lori's skin to look blue when she was born?

3. Jamie has been asked to draw the patient in room 312's blood. Jaimie gathers her supplies and reports to the room. The patient is overweight and has recently been on a crash diet and not eating properly. She has been lethargic and nauseated, and she has had stomach cramps for the past two days. She appears dehydrated, and Jamie thinks this might be a tough stick. Jamie palpates and inspects her arms for a good vein. With her choice made, she prepares the patient for the collection. Jaimie performs the stick and inserts the evacuated tube onto the needle. Bright red blood spurts into the tube. Jamie realizes it looks a little different than blood she has drawn from other patients, assumes it is because of the patient's extreme dieting and the dehydration, and continues with the collection. Just as Jaimie begins changing tubes, Dr. Smart walks into the room. Dr. Smart yells at Jamie to stop the draw and remove the needle immediately. Jamie is startled by the outburst from the physician and pulls the needle out of the patient's arm but has forgotten to remove the tourniquet. Bright red blood is spurting everywhere. Dr. Smart pulls Jamie out of the way, telling her to get a nurse immediately. Jamie is confused; she was getting blood in the right color tubes and in the right order.

- Why is Dr. Smart alarmed?
- What steps will Dr. Smart take to complete the procedure?
- What should Jamie do?

MODULE 5

The Health Care System

I. HOSPITAL DEPARTMENTS

A. Anesthesiology—Department responsible for the administration of anesthesia to provide partial or complete loss of sensation

B. Cardiology—Subspecialty of internal medicine dealing with the blood vessels and the heart

C. Emergency room (ER)—Specializes in the emergency care of the acutely ill and injured

D. Intensive care unit (ICU)—Department for patients who require continuous monitoring by specially trained personnel

E. Internal medicine—Department that treats diseases of the internal organs

F. Obstetrics/gynecology (Ob/Gyn)—Department concerned with the management of women's health

G. Oncology—Department specializing in the diagnosis and treatment of malignant tumors and blood disorders

H. Orthopedics—Department that works with disorders of the musculoskeletal system

I. Pathology/laboratory—Department specializing in the study of the nature and cause of disease through clinical laboratory test results

J. Pediatrics—Department specializing in the treatment and care of children from birth to adolescence

K. Physical medicine—Department concerned with the diagnosis and treatment of diseases and disorders of the neuromuscular system

L. Psychiatry/neurology—Department concerned with the diagnosis, treatment, and prevention of mental illness and disorders of the brain

M. Radiology/medical imaging—Department concerned with the diagnosis, treatment, and prevention of disease through the use of X-rays, radioactive isotopes, ionizing radiations, ultrasonography, and magnetic resonance imaging

N. Surgery—Department concerned with the manual and operative procedures for the correction of deformities and defects, repair of injuries, and diagnosis and cure of certain diseases

II. HEALTH CARE PERSONNEL

A. Physician—Doctor; an individual who has been educated, trained, and state-licensed to practice the art and science of medicine

B. Physician's assistant (PA)—Works under the supervision of a physician and provides patient services ranging from physical examinations to surgical procedures. A PA receives two years of postcollege training and is licensed by the state where he or she works.

C. Registered nurse (RN)—Nurse who graduated from an accredited nursing program, passed the state examination for licensure, and is registered and licensed to practice by state authority

D. Nurse practitioner (NP) or advanced practice registered nurse (APRN)—Registered nurse with a minimum of a master's degree in nursing and advanced education in a particular health care specialty from family practice to midwifery in collaboration with a physician

E. Licensed practical nurse (LPN)—Nurse who graduated from an accredited school of practical nursing, passed the state examination for licensure, and is licensed to practice by a state authority

F. Certified nursing assistant (CNA)—Unlicensed nursing staff member who assists with basic patient care and who usually must complete a training course

G. Anesthesiologist—Physician specializing solely in anesthesiology and related areas; has a medical degree and is board-certified and state-licensed to administer anesthetics and apply related techniques

H. Pharmacist—Specialist in formulating and dispensing medications, with two years of postgraduate study in pharmacology and licensed by individual states to practice.

I. Respiratory therapist (RT)—Licensed allied health professional trained to provide respiratory care; works under the direction of a physician, educating patients, treating and assessing patient response to therapy, and managing and monitoring patients with deficiencies and abnormalities of cardiopulmonary function

J. Physical therapist (PT)—Medical practitioner with either a bachelor's or master's degree in physical therapy; treats patients for the restoration of physical strength and endurance, coordination, and range of motion through exercises, heat or cold therapy, and massage

K. Occupational therapist (OT)—Medical practitioner with either a bachelor's or master's degree in occupational therapy; helps people with physical or mental disabilities to use the activities of everyday living to achieve maximum functioning and independence at home and in the workplace

L. Radiologist—Physician trained in the diagnostic and/or therapeutic use of X-rays and radionuclides, radiation physics, and biology and in diagnostic ultrasound and magnetic resonance imaging and applicable physics

III. LABORATORY PERSONNEL

A. Laboratory director/pathologist
   1. Ph.D. or physician
   2. Practicing, evaluating, or supervising diagnostic tests, using materials removed from living or dead patients

B. Laboratory manager
   1. Bachelor's degree in health science, plus additional years of clinical laboratory experience or the equivalent combination of education and experience
      a. Some states require the laboratory manager to be a bioanalyst, which is a licensed position requiring extensive postgraduate work.
   2. Overseeing all business operations of the laboratory

C. Medical technologist (MT) or clinical laboratory scientist (CLS)
   1. Four-year bachelor's degree in medical technology
   2. MTs or CLSs are authorized to perform any and all clinical laboratory tests.

D. Medical laboratory technicians (MLT) or clinical laboratory technician (CLT)
   1. Two-year associate degree program and completion of the required credit hours of hands-on clinical training as part of the degree. Under the supervision of the medical technologist, performs general laboratory tests.

E. Phlebotomist
   1. Technician and clinical laboratory employee who has graduated from an accredited phlebotomy technician program or has been cross-trained from another medical profession.
   2. Collects blood samples and other specimens to be used in many laboratory tests to detect and monitor treatment.

F. Clinical laboratory clerical staff
   1. Generally required to have a high school diploma and some prior clinical training.
   2. The clinical laboratory clerical staff may answer telephones, take messages, perform data entry of test results and retrieve test results, file laboratory reports, and distribute reports to physicians or the medical records department

IV. DEPARTMENTS IN THE LABORATORY

A. Administrative
   1. Processing telecommunications
   2. Handling specimen requests
   3. Overall clerical functions of the department

B. Biochemistry
   1. Branch of biology dealing with the chemical compounds and processes occurring in organisms
   2. Usually receipt of serum and testing it for different chemical characteristics

C. Cytogenetics
   1. Branch of biology that deals with the study of heredity and variation by the methods of both cytology and genetics
   2. Using blood and other cells to get a karyotype, which can be helpful in prenatal diagnosis (e.g., Down's syndrome) and in cancer diagnosis

D. Cytology
   1. Branch of biology dealing with the structure and function, multiplication, pathology, and life history of cells
   2. Examination of smears of cells (such as from the cervix) for evidence of cancer and other conditions

E. Hematology
   1. Department dealing with the blood and blood-forming organs
   2. Receipt of whole blood and citrated plasma for full blood counts, blood films, and coagulation investigations

F. Histology
   1. Department that prepares body samples for microscopic examination by the pathologist using sophisticated techniques such as immunohistochemistry
   2. Processing of solid tissue removed from the body to make slides and examine cellular detail

G. Immunology
   1. Department dealing with the immune system and the cell-mediated and humoral aspects of immunity and immune responses
   2. Testing for antibodies and antigens and immune responses of the human body

H. Microbiology
   1. Branch of biology dealing especially with microscopic forms of life (bacteria, protozoa, viruses, and fungi)
   2. Receipt of swabs, feces, urine, blood, sputum, medical equipment, as well as possible infected tissue, and checking for pathogenic microbes

I. Phlebotomy
   1. Handles specimen collections, transportation of specimens, and processing specimens within the scope of practice.

J. Serology
   1. Branch of biology dealing with blood sera and especially their immunological reactions and properties
   2. Receipt of serum samples to look for evidence of diseases, such as hepatitis or HIV

K. Virology
   1. Branch of biology dealing with viruses
   2. DNA analysis is also done in the large medical laboratories.

PRACTICE

1. A(n) _____ administers anesthesia to provide partial or complete loss of sensation prior to surgical procedures.
   a. anesthesiologist
   b. oncologist
   c. neurologist
   d. surgeon

2. _____ is the branch of medicine dealing with manual and operative procedures for the correction of deformities and defects, repair of injuries, and diagnosis and cure of certain diseases.
   a. Internal medicine
   b. Intensive care unit
   c. Surgery
   d. Emergency room

3. A(n) _____ is a nurse who graduated from an accredited nursing program (typically with a bachelor-level degree), passed a state examination for licensure, and is registered and licensed to practice by state authority.
   a. registered nurse
   b. licensed practical nurse
   c. nurse practitioner—Advanced practice registered nurse
   d. certified nursing assistant

4. _____ provides diagnosis and treatment of malignant tumors and blood disorders.
   a. Internal medicine
   b. Oncology
   c. Radiology
   d. Neurology

5. The _____ is a clinical employee whose primary responsibility is the collection of blood samples from patients.
   a. medical laboratory technician/clinical laboratory technician
   b. medical technologist/clinical laboratory scientist
   c. phlebotomist
   d. pharmacist

6. The _____ is a physician who practices, evaluates, or supervises diagnostic tests, using materials removed from living or deceased patients.
   a. medical technologist or clinical laboratory scientist
   b. pathologist
   c. medical laboratory technician or clinical laboratory technician
   d. phlebotomist

7. A _____ has a four-year degree in medical technology.
   a. clinical laboratory clerical staff person
   b. medical laboratory technician or clinical laboratory technician
   c. medical technologist or clinical laboratory scientist
   d. phlebotomist

8. A _____ is a health care professional who provides patient services ranging from physical examination to surgical procedures and works under the supervision of a physician.
   a. medical assistant
   b. licensed practical nurse
   c. physician's assistant
   d. registered nurse

9. _____ is a subspecialty of internal medicine dealing with the blood vessels and the heart.
   a. Cardiology
   b. Neurology
   c. Physiology
   d. Oncology

10. The responsibilities of the _____ include the overseeing of all the business operations of the laboratory.
   a. laboratory director
   b. laboratory manager
   c. laboratory technicians
   d. phlebotomist

11. A(n) _____ is a registered nurse with a minimum of a master's degree in nursing who provides patient services ranging from family practice to midwifery in collaboration with a physician.
   a. APRN
   b. LPN
   c. PT
   d. RT

12. _____ is the department concerned with women's health issues.
   a. Internal medicine
   b. Gynecology
   c. Oncology
   d. Neurology

13. A _____ is a person who has been educated, trained, and state-licensed to practice the art and science of medicine.
   a. registered nurse
   b. phlebotomist
   c. physician
   d. medical laboratory technician/clinical laboratory technician

14. A _____ is generally required to have a high school diploma and some prior clinical training.
   a. clinical laboratory clerical staff person
   b. medical laboratory technicians/clinical laboratory technician
   c. medical technologist
   d. laboratory manager

15. _____ help people with physical or mental disabilities using the activities of everyday living to achieve maximum functioning and independence at home and in the workplace.
   a. Occupational therapists
   b. Physical therapists
   c. Respiratory therapists
   d. Physician's assistants

16. _____ graduated from a two-year associate degree program and completed several semesters of hands-on clinical training as part of their degree.
   a. Laboratory managers
   b. Medical technologists or clinical laboratory scientists
   c. Medical laboratory technicians or clinical laboratory technicians
   d. Pharmacists

17. All of the following skills are required of entry-level phlebotomists *except* _____.
   a. CPR and AED certifications
   b. ability to obtain blood samples
   c. electrocardiography
   d. administering medications by injection

18. The certified nursing assistant is an unlicensed nursing staff member who assists with all of the following except _____.
   a. the patient's personal hygiene
   b. vital signs
   c. specimen collection and processing
   d. patient positioning and bed making

19. A(n) _____ educates patients, treats and assesses patient responses to therapy, and manages and monitors patients with deficiencies and abnormalities of cardiopulmonary function.
   a. physical therapist
   b. cardiologist
   c. respiratory therapist
   d. oncologist

20. _____ is the study of the nature and cause of disease through clinical laboratory test results.
   a. Radiology
   b. Oncology
   c. Gynecology
   d. Pathology

CRITICAL THINKING

Fill in the blanks by identifying the correct hospital departments and/or hospital personnel.

1. Stan woke at 2:00 a.m. He was having a very difficult time breathing, his chest hurt every time he took a breath, and he was drenched with sweat. He slowly got out of bed, pulled on some clothes, and decided he probably should go to the _____ at the hospital. Stan found his car keys and, after an attack of coughing, got into his car and drove himself to the hospital. The _____ on call at the hospital wanted Stan to have a chest X-ray, ECG, and blood tests. Stan was taken to the _____ department and the chest X-ray was taken. This

X-ray will be read by a _____. The ECG technician hooked Stan up to the machine and ran the ECG. Stan was diagnosed with pneumonia and admitted to the hospital. A hospital volunteer took Stan to his room in a wheelchair. Blood tests were ordered, and the _____ came to collect the specimens while the _____ was providing Stan with basic care items (water, ice, toothbrush, toothpaste etc.) and demonstrating to Stan how to adjust the bed for his comfort. Once Stan was settled in and the blood tests completed, a _____ arrived in Stan's room with orders to assist Stan with his breathing. After a few days, Stan's health began to improve and he started to feel much better. His physician decided that he could go home as long as he continued to take it easy for a few more days and take the prescribed medication. The hospital _____ filled the prescription and had it delivered to Stan's room. On his way out of the hospital, Stan stopped by the _____ station to thank everyone for all the help, support, and kindness. Stan told the nurse to be sure and thank the lady who drew his blood; it was the best and least painful blood draw he could remember.

2. Quinn has an appointment today with his _____. Quinn has a history of lymphoma, and his doctor decides it is in Quinn's best interest to remove a small mass from the corner of Quinn's right eye. After removing the mass, the physician's staff prepares the specimen to be sent to the _____ department of the hospital laboratory. The physician informs Quinn that it will be a few days before the lab has the biopsy results and that she will call Quinn as soon as she has them.

3. Mary is your 90-year-old grandmother and a long-time patient of Dr. Jorgensen's. She has a very bad cold; so she calls Dr. Jorgensen's office for an appointment. She is informed that Dr. Jorgensen won't be in the office for two weeks. She tells the receptionist thank you and calls you to help her. You have been a phlebotomist at the hospital laboratory for the past five years and you are familiar with Dr. Jorgensen's staff. You call Dr. Jorgensen's office and speak with Shelly, Dr. Jorgensen's receptionist. Shelly explains to you that Dr. Jorgensen is out of the office for two weeks but that she can get your grandmother in to see Thai, the PA who works for the practice. You make an appointment and call your grandmother back. Your grandmother only wants to see Dr. Jorgensen, the "real" doctor. You explain to your grandmother what a PA is and her qualifications.

What would you tell your grandmother to help her understand and keep the appointment?

Specimen Collection, Processing, and Handling

I. PERSONAL PROTECTIVE EQUIPMENT (PPE)

A. Includes gloves, gowns, lab coats or aprons, and protective face gear (such as masks, face shields, and goggles).

B. PPE is required by OSHA to be worn when handling body fluids and when there is a sufficient potential for exposure to body fluids to warrant its use.

C. Employers must provide this equipment, maintain it, and keep it clean at no charge to the phlebotomist.

D. Gloves
1. Act as a barrier precaution.
2. OSHA has mandated that gloves be worn by health care providers during every invasive procedure.
3. If the phlebotomist or the patient is allergic to latex, vinyl or nitrile gloves may be used. Some phlebotomists prefer nitrile gloves because they are more durable, harder to tear, and more comfortable to wear.

E. Lab coats/gowns/aprons
1. Prevent contamination of the phlebotomist's clothing/uniform.
2. Protect the skin of personnel from blood or body fluid exposure.
3. Gowns are specially treated to make them impermeable to liquids and provide a greater protection of the skin when splashes of large quantities of contaminated material are present or anticipated.
4. Lab coats and aprons are never worn outside the clinical setting, at lunch, or on breaks.

F. Protective eyewear
1. Masks, face shields, and safety goggles protect the phlebotomist from possible aerosol exposure or splashing of blood or other body fluids into the eyes.

II. GENERAL BLOOD COLLECTION EQUIPMENT AND SUPPLIES

A. The primary responsibility of the phlebotomist is to collect blood specimens safely, accurately, and in the most cost-effective manner. To perform these tasks efficiently, the phlebotomist must have the correct "tools of the trade."

B. General blood collection equipment and supplies are used for both capillary and venipuncture.
1. Specific equipment and supplies for capillary punctures and venipunctures are outlined separately.

C. Antiseptics
1. Alcohol pads or alcohol wipes, containing a 70 percent isopropyl alcohol solution, are used prior to most routine blood collections to disinfect the patient's skin at the site of needle insertion.
2. Povidone-iodine (Betadine), hexachlorophene, or chlorhexidine can also be used as an antiseptic prior to a puncture.
   a. Povidone-iodine is specifically used prior to a collection for blood cultures or blood alcohol levels.

D. Gauze pad
1. Gauze pads are made of loosely woven cotton fabric.
2. They come in a variety of sizes.
   a. 2 × 2-inch squares are the most common.

E. Bandages
1. After the collection of a blood specimen, a slight pressure bandage dressing is applied until it has been determined that bleeding at the site has ceased.
2. Instruct patients to remove the bandage 5 to 10 minutes after the draw.
3. Bandages should not be used on children under the age of 2, because the child may put the

bandage into the mouth, which may result in aspiration and suffocation.

   4. The most common dressing is a sterile 2 × 2-inch gauze square, folded into quarters, placed directly over the site, and secured in place with a prepackaged adhesive bandage or a piece of tape.

   5. If the patient is allergic to tape, nonallergenic tape is used.

F. Needle disposal equipment
   1. To aid in the prevention of contaminated needle sticks, the phlebotomist always disposes of needles in specially designed puncture-proof containers, commonly referred to as *sharps containers*.
   2. OSHA requires that the needles are never recapped after their use and, prior to disposal, that they are never bent, cut, or unscrewed from the tube adapter or syringe.

III. CAPILLARY PUNCTURE

A. Capillary puncture, also referred to as a skin puncture, microcapillary stick, finger stick, or heel stick, is the procedure by which the skin is punctured with a lancet.

B. Capillary blood is blood that moves into the capillaries from the arterioles and moves to the venules.
   1. In the capillaries the exchange of oxygen and carbon dioxide occurs, along with the transfer of ions, nutrients, and waste material.
   2. Glucose levels are higher in capillary blood specimens; potassium, calcium, and total proteins are lower.
   3. Interstitial fluid is released into the blood during the process of a capillary puncture and contaminates the blood sample.
   4. Blood specimens that have been contaminated by interstitial fluid do not produce accurate test results, because the specimen is diluted.

C. Equipment and supplies
   1. Lancets
      a. Lancets are small, sterile, single-use instruments used to puncture the capillaries of the skin.
      b. The simple one-handed activation releases a surgical blade, providing a precise and consistent incision, after which the blade retracts into its casing, helping to protect the phelbotomist and the patient.
      c. They are primarily used on infants, children, and the elderly or when microcollection techniques are required.

   d. Lancets are available in a variety of point lengths, which are especially important when performing capillary punctures on infants.
      (1) The point length for capillary punctures on infants, particularly newborn infants, should not exceed 2.4 millimeters. A puncture deeper than this can penetrate the calcaneous bone, which can cause complications such as sepsis and osteomyelitis.
      (2) For premature infants, lancet length is even shorter. The phlebotomist must use a special preemie-length lancet on these babies.

   2. Spring-loaded puncture devices
      a. The advantage of using a spring-loaded puncture device is the consistency of the puncture depth.
      b. These devices are very useful to patients who need to perform routine blood glucose tests at home.

   3. Microhematocrit tubes
      a. Microhematocrit tubes are commonly referred to as capillary tubes, because they fill with blood by capillary action.
      b. Microhematocrit tubes are available with and without anticoagulants and are color coded for easy identification.
         (1) Ammonium-heparin–coated tubes have a red band at one end.
         (2) Plain tubes have a blue band.

   4. Clay sealer trays
      a. A clay sealer tray is a small plastic tray filled with clay, used to:
         (1) Plug the open ends of microhematocrit tubes.
         (2) Hold filled tubes until the specimens are ready to be centrifuged.

   5. Microcollection systems
      a. Microcollection containers provide for the easy measuring, storing, color coding, and centrifugation of the capillary specimen.
      b. These containers are typically plastic disposable tubes with an integrated collection scoop.
      c. The containers are color coded to match the additives of evacuated tube systems.
      d. The microcollection container order of draw is:
         (1) Blood gases.
         (2) Slides and smears, including PKUs.
         (3) EDTA tubes.
         (4) Other additive tubes.
         (5) Serum tubes.

D. Specimen collection process
1. Capillary punctures are more appropriate than venipuncture when:
   a. Only a small volume of blood is required, based on the tests ordered.
   b. Collecting specimens on children and infants.
   c. A substantial vein cannot be located.
   d. A patient is not cooperative or is overly apprehensive about having a venipuncture.
   e. The patient has severe burns or scar tissue over venipuncture sites.
   f. The patient has very fragile or superficial veins.
2. Patient identification and preparation
   a. Assemble the equipment and supplies.
   b. Identify the patient.
      (1) Ask the patient to state his or her full name. A patient on medication may not be able to respond appropriately.
      (2) Inpatient
         (a) Verify the information on the patient's identification bracelet against the laboratory orders and the information supplied by the patient.
         (b) If an identification bracelet is not present, the patient's nurse or physician must be asked to confirm the patient's identification. The nurse's or physician's name is then documented on the requisition form.
      (3) Outpatient—for verification of identification, the Clinical and Laboratory Standards Institute (CLSI) guidelines require the patient to state his or her:
         (a) Name.
         (b) Date of birth (DOB).
         (c) Address.
      (4) Patients who are unable to verbally communicate (i.e., unconscious, in shock, mentally or physically disabled) often come into the emergency room.
         (a) A temporary identification number is assigned by the hospital, and a temporary identification bracelet is issued.
         (b) The temporary identification number is later cross-referenced with a permanent identification number when the patient's identity is confirmed.
   c. Introduce yourself.
   d. Wash your hands and put on gloves.
   e. Select the appropriate capillary site.
3. Site identification (See Figure 6-1.)
   a. Conditions to avoid—Areas that are swollen, scarred, cyanotic, or cold. Blood obtained from these sites may cause inaccurate test results, such as elevated hemoglobins or cell count values.
   b. Capillary punctures may be performed on fingertips, heels, toes, or earlobes.
      (1) Fingertips
         (a) The recommended sites for adults and older children.
         (b) All fingertips may be used, except the 5th digit.
         (c) The tissue on the 5th digit is much thinner and generally more painful when punctured.
         (d) The 3rd and 4th digits are commonly used.
         (e) The puncture should be made perpendicular to the fingerprint, causing a drop to form. Punctures made horizontal to the fingerprint cause blood to run down the finger instead of forming a drop.

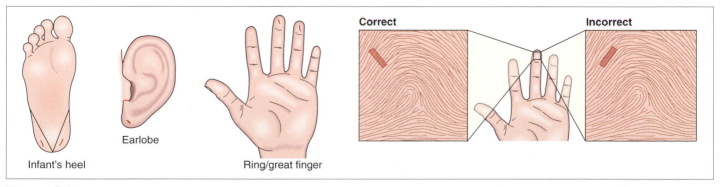

Correct   Incorrect

Earlobe

Infant's heel   Ring/great finger

Figure 6-1
Capillary Blood Collection Sites.

(2) Heels—Infants less than 1 year old

    (a) The lateral edge of the heel is the recommended site for capillary punctures.

    (b) Care should be taken when performing the puncture, so that an area is not used that is directly over bone. The calcaneous bone of an infant's heel can be as little as 2.4 millimeters below the skin surface. The puncture should not exceed 2.4 millimeters in depth, per CLSI guidelines.

    (c) Puncturing the bone is not only painful but can cause osteomyelitis and/or osteochondritis.

    (d) Additional punctures at the same site can spread the infection.

(3) Toes—May be used instead of fingers when fingers are either not available or not usable

(4) Earlobes are *not* recommended as a site of choice but may be used in extreme cases, such as severe burn victims.

4. Performing the puncture

  a. Finger stick

    (1) Assemble the supplies.

    (2) Wash your hands. Put on PPE.

    (3) Identify the patient.

    (4) Explain the procedure to the patient.

    (5) Position the patient seated or lying down, with the palmar side of the hand facing up. Support the arm.

    (6) Select the puncture site.

    (7) Warm the site as needed. Blood flow can be greatly increased when the site is warm. Warming can be accomplished by:

      (a) Massaging the finger.

      (b) Wrapping the finger in a warm moist towel no hotter than 42 degrees Celsius (108 degrees Fahrenheit).

      (c) Running the hand under warm water.

      (d) Use care with infants; their skin burns easily.

      (e) Commercially prepared heel warmers may also be used, especially for infants.

    (8) Clean the site. Use a 70 percent isopropyl alcohol prep pad.

    (9) Allow the site to air-dry.

(10) Perform the puncture.

    (a) Grasp the patient's finger firmly but gently between your thumb and index finger.

    (b) Perform the puncture by resting the safety lancet on the skin over the puncture site, engaging the blade by activating the spring-loaded lancet.

    (c) To assure a proper puncture depth, pressure should not be applied to the lancet against the skin.

(11) Dispose of the lancet.

(12) While applying gentle pressure to the patient's finger, wipe away the first drop of blood with a sterile 2 × 2-inch gauze pad. Remember that the first drop of blood contains interstitial fluid that can dilute the sample.

(13) To ensure a steady blood flow, continue to apply a firm, even pressure proximally to the puncture site.

(14) Collect the blood samples in the appropriate microcollection containers.

(15) Once the specimens have been collected, place a clean, dry 2 × 2-inch gauze pad over the puncture site.

(16) Place a bandage over the puncture site of an adult or older child.

(17) Mix any collection containers that contain an additive.

(18) Dispose of contaminated material in the appropriate biohazardous waste container and remove all equipment from the area.

(19) Label the specimens with the appropriate information.

(20) Remove your gloves and dispose of them in the appropriate biohazardous waste container.

(21) Wash your hands.

(22) Transport the specimens to the lab for testing, or put on a new pair of gloves and perform point-of-care testing.

  b. Heel stick (See Figure 6-2.)

    (1) In the hospital nursery

      (a) Isolation techniques are not required.

      (b) Never take the blood drawing tray into the nursery with you. The nursery has its own equipment and supplies.

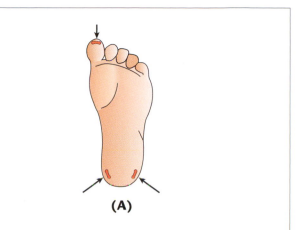

(A)

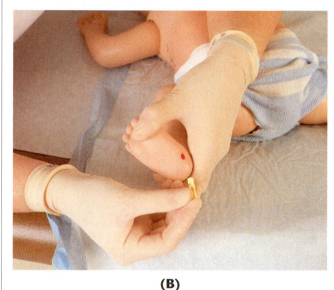

(B)

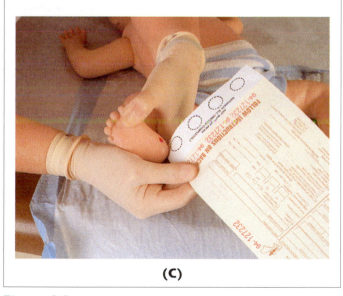

(C)

Figure 6-2

(A) Capillary blood collection sites on the infant's foot. (B) Hold the infant's leg securely with the nondominant hand while the dominant hand uses a pediatric lancet to perform the puncture. (C) Transfer the drops of blood to the filter paper test card.

    (c) Hand washing must be performed thoroughly for a minimum of three minutes.

    (d) Don a gown and mask as required.

    (e) Follow all hospital protocols for working with infants.

  (2) Capillary blood collection sites on an infant's foot

    (a) The most common site is the side of the infant's heel pad.

    (b) Never puncture areas that are bruised or that have been previously punctured.

    (c) Ensure that the infant's heel is warmed adequately prior to the puncture. If not, use a commercially prepared heel warmer.

  (3) Performing the puncture

    (a) The infant's leg should be held securely with the nondominant hand and arm, while the dominant hand uses a pediatric lancet to perform a capillary heel stick.

    (b) Drops of blood are transferred from the capillary puncture to all circles on the filter paper test card, or the specimen is collected into a microcollection container appropriate for the test ordered.

5. Processing the microcollection specimen

  a. Order of draw

    (1) It is important to collect specimens in the correct order.

    (2) The microcollection container order of draw is:

      (a) Blood gases.

      (b) Slides and smears, including PKUs.

      (c) EDTA tubes.

      (d) Other additive tubes.

      (e) Serum tubes.

  b. Microcollection containers

    (1) The proper collection container must be selected according to the type of test requested.

    (2) Refer to the previous section on equipment and supplies.

  c. Blood smears

    (1) A blood smear is a drop of blood that has been placed on one end of a glass slide and then spread out in a thin even smear using another glass slide.

(2) Most laboratories prefer blood smears to be made from fresh capillary blood. Whole blood from a lavender top tube may also be used; however, fresh capillary blood provides a much better slide.

(3) The use of a transfer safety device, such as a DIFF-SAFE, allows a slide to be prepared from an EDTA tube without removing the stopper.

(4) The blood smear is performed immediately after wiping away the first drop of blood of a capillary puncture.

(5) Making a good blood smear is an art and takes practice to perfect. Blood smears that are improperly done have an uneven distribution of cells, which gives inaccurate test results.

(6) Making a blood smear (See Figure 6-3.)

   (a) Assemble the equipment and supplies.

   (b) Wash your hands; put on gloves.

   (c) Select two glass slides.

   (d) Place one medium-sized drop of blood (1 to 2 millimeters) on the end of each slide.

   (e) Use one of the slides as the first spreader slide.

   (f) Place the spreader in front of the drop of blood. Hold the spreader slide in your dominant hand at a 45-degree angle.

   (g) Slowly back the spreader slide into the drop of blood.

   (h) Lower the angle of the spreader slide to 30 degrees and quickly push the slide along the length of the stationary glass slide.

   (i) Evaluate the smear.

      (i) The smear should be at least half the slide's length; three-quarters of the slide's length is preferable.

      (ii) The thin end of the smear should be feathered, and, when the smear is held to the light, a rainbow should be seen. The feathered edge is only one cell thick and the most important area of the slide. It is the location where the differential is read.

      (iii) A differential is the number and type of cells, determined by microscopic examination of

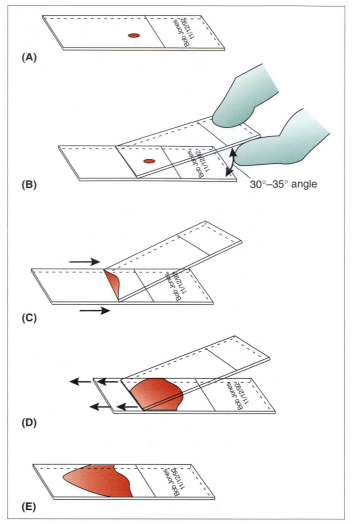

Figure 6-3

Making a Blood Smear: (A) Position labeled end to the right if you are right-handed or to the left if you are left-handed. Place a small drop of blood on the slide. (B) Grasp the slide with your nondominant hand to steady it. (C) Pull the spreader slide back into the drop of blood. Let the blood spread along the back side of the spreader slide. (D) Quickly, without jerking, push the spreader slide to the left. (E) Allow the blood smear to air-dry before it is stained.

a thin layer of blood on a glass slide.

      (iv) The smear should be free of any holes, lines, or jagged edges, and it must be centered on the slide.

   (j) Once the smear has been made on the first slide, repeat the procedure on the second slide.

   (k) When both slides have been made they are left to air dry, standing on end with the drop of blood end down. If the phlebohtomist is using frosted slides he/she may write the patient's name in pencil on the frosted slide. Otherwise, attach a paper label to the blood end of the slide. Do not use ink as it will be washed off during the staining process.

   d. Transport the slide to the laboratory.

IV. VENIPUNCTURE

A. Equipment and supplies

  1. Syringe

    a. A syringe should be used when drawing blood from fragile veins, when the pressure behind the vacuum in evacuated tubes could cause a patient's vein to collapse.

    b. Syringes come in a variety of sizes: 3 cc, 5 cc, 10 cc, 20 cc, and 60 cc.

     (1) The 10-cc syringe is most commonly used for routine venipuncture.

    c. A syringe may be used with either a butterfly infusion set or a hypodermic needle.

    d. If you are using a syringe to collect a venous blood sample, the specimen needs to be transferred to the appropriate evacuated tube for the test ordered.

     (1) The use of a conventional hypodermic needle and syringe to transfer venous blood to a blood collection tube or blood culture bottle is a dangerous procedure and an OSHA-prohibited practice [OSHA Standard 1910.1030(d)(2)(vii)(A)].

     (2) The specimen can safely be transferred using the BD Blood Transfer Device (a latex free, single-use device that reduces the risk of transfer-related injuries while maintaining the specimen integrity) or other similarly manufactured devices.

  2. Needles

    a. Two basic types of needles are used when performing venipuncture:

     (1) Multisample needles

      (a) Multisample needles are most commonly used with the evacuated tube system.

      (b) The needle has two sharp ends. One end is beveled and is used to penetrate the patient's skin. The other end, covered with a rubber sheath and generally shorter, is used to penetrate the evacuated tube.

      (c) The needle gauge is a standard for measuring the diameter of the lumen (inside) of a needle. The higher the gauge number is, the smaller the lumen of the needle. Needle sizes used may vary slightly.

      (d) A 20- to 21-gauge, 1- to 1½-inch needle is recommended and most commonly used.

     (2) Single-sample or hypodermic needles

      (a) Hypodermic needles are used when performing syringe draws.

      (b) The gauge and length of needle options are the same as multi-sample needles.

  3. Butterfly collection device, or butterfly infusion set

    a. The butterfly collection device is a ½- to ¾-inch stainless steel needle connected to a 5- to 12-inch length of tubing.

    b. It is called a butterfly because of its wing-shaped plastic extensions, which are used for gripping the needle.

    c. This system is the best choice when:

     (1) A patient's veins are small, as is often the case with children and the elderly.

     (2) Collecting large quantities of blood, such as for blood cultures, as recommended by the Center for Phlebotomy Education

    d. The main drawback to this method is the risk of hemolysis because of the small gauge of the needle. (The standard needle gauge for a butterfly needle is 23.)

  4. Tube holder, or adapter

    a. The tube holder/adapter is a plastic tube slightly larger than the evacuated tube.

    b. It is designed to hold the needle at one end and allow insertion of the evacuated tube onto the needle at the other.

  5. Tourniquets

    a. Tourniquets are available in a variety of styles.

     (1) Penrose drain

      (a) The tubing is 18–20 inches in length and ½ to 1 inch wide.

      (b) A penrose drain is the most common tourniquet available.

     (2) Rubber straps

     (3) Velcro tourniquets

(4) Blood pressure cuffs
    (a) Blood pressure cuffs are not recommended for routine use, because they can cause tissue damage and discomfort to the patient.
    (b) They should be used only for blood banking procedures.
  b. Tourniquets are designed to:
    (1) Temporarily reduce the flow of venous blood in the arm.
    (2) Distend veins to facilitate venipuncture for intravenous punctures.
  c. Tourniquets should not be left in place for longer than 1 minute because blood may become more concentrated when constricted. This is called hemoconcentration, which adversely affects test results.

6. Evacuated tubes
  a. These vacuum tubes are made of either glass or plastic and are available in a range of sizes from 2 to 15 milliliters.
  b. Vacuum
    (1) Evacuated tubes fill immediately with blood because of their precisely premeasured amount of vacuum.
    (2) The vacuum in a tube is lost if:
      (a) The cap is removed prior to the draw.
      (b) The tube is dropped.
      (c) The tube is pushed too far into the needle holder.
      (d) The needle is pulled slightly out of the vein during the draw.
  c. Color-coded cap system—Used to identify which additive, if any, has been added to the tube
  d. Order of draw
    (1) Color-coded evacuated tubes must be drawn in the correct order, called the order of draw.
    (2) The order of draw for evacuated tubes is shown in Figure 6-4.

7. Blood drawing trays
  a. Phlebotomists can easily carry their equipment between stations and hospital rooms if they use blood drawing trays.
  b. The trays should be made of a sturdy material with a handle and divided storage areas to keep equipment organized.
  c. The trays should always be kept clean and equipment and supplies restocked.

8. Blood drawing, or phlebotomy, chair

  a. Blood drawing chairs are used in outpatient labs, which are all equipped with a comfortable chair for the patient.
  b. The blood drawing chair has:
    (1) An arm support.
    (2) A restraint system to secure the patient in the chair should he or she have a syncopal episode.

B. Blood collection by means of the evacuated tube system
1. Patient identification and preparation—Critical
  a. Ask the patient to state his or her full name. A patient on medication may not be able to respond appropriately.
  b. Inpatient—If the patient is at the hospital:
    (1) Verify the information on the patient's identification bracelet against the laboratory orders and the information supplied by the patient.
    (2) If an identification bracelet is not present, the patient's nurse or physician must be asked to confirm the patient's identification.
    (3) The nurse's or physician's name is then documented on the requisition form.
  c. Outpatient—If the patient is an outpatient, CLSI standard requires the patient to verify identification by stating his or her:
    (1) Name.
    (2) Date of birth (DOB).
    (3) Address.

2. Diet restrictions—Verify that the patient has followed the required diet restrictions.
  a. Example: Nothing by mouth (NPO) after midnight, or fasting for 12 hours

3. Perform proper handwashing and don PPE.

4. Assemble the equipment and supplies, and perform the procedure.
  a. Set out the equipment and supplies required for the procedure.
    (1) Have a variety of needle sizes and types available within easy reach because needle selection should be made after locating the vein.
    (2) Vein size dictates needle size to assure that specimen integrity is not affected.
    (3) Once the size of needle has been determined, secure the needle on the tube adapter or assemble the syringe or butterfly infusion set.
  b. Open the antiseptic.

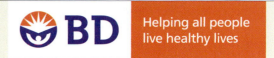

BD Vacutainer® Order of Draw for Multiple Tube Collections

Designed for Your Safety

Reflects change in NCCLS recommended Order of Draw (NCCLS H3-A5, Vol 23, No 32, 8.10.2)

* When using a winged blood collection set for venipuncture and a coagulation (citrate) tube is the first specimen tube to be drawn, a discard tube should be drawn first. The discard tube must be used to fill the blood collection set tubing's "dead space" with blood but the discard tube does not need to be completely filled. This important step will ensure maintenance of the proper blood-to-additive ratio of the blood specimen. The discard tube should be a nonadditive or coagulation tube.

Closure Color	Collection Tube	Mix by Inverting
BD Vacutainer® Blood Collection Tubes *(glass or plastic)*		
	• Blood Cultures - SPS	**8 to 10 times**
	• Citrate Tube*	**3 to 4 times**
or	• BD Vacutainer® SST™ Gel Separator Tube	**5 times**
	• Serum Tube *(glass or plastic)*	**5 times (plastic) none (glass)**
	• Heparin Tube	**8 to 10 times**
or	• BD Vacutainer® PST™ Gel Separator Tube With Heparin	**8 to 10 times**
or	• EDTA Tube	**8 to 10 times**
	• Fluoride (glucose) Tube	**8 to 10 times**

Note: Always follow your facility's protocol for order of draw

Handle all biologic samples and blood collection "sharps" (lancets, needles, luer adapters and blood collection sets) according to the policies and procedures of your facility. Obtain appropriate medical attention in the event of any exposure to biologic samples (for example, through a puncture injury) since they may transmit viral hepatitis, HIV (AIDS), or other infectious diseases. Utilize any built-in used needle protector if the blood collection device provides one. BD does not recommend reshielding used needles, but the policies and procedures of your facility may differ and must always be followed. Discard any blood collection "sharps" in biohazard containers approved for their disposal.

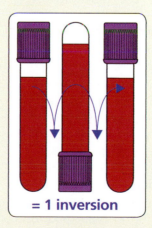

= 1 inversion

**BD Global
Technical Services
1.800.631.0174**

**BD Customer Service
1.888.237.2762
www.bd.com/vacutainer**

BD Diagnostics
Preanalytical Systems
1 Becton Drive
Franklin Lakes, NJ 07417
www.bd.com/vacutainer

Figure 6-4

Order of Draw. (Courtesy of BD Diagnostics)

c. Set out the required tubes in the correct order of draw.

d. Open the bandage.

e. Set out a small stack (5–6) of 2 × 2-inch gauze squares.

5. Reassure and calm the patient.

6. Position the patient either in a sitting position or lying down prior to the blood draw.

   a. Never draw a patient's blood while the patient is standing.

   b. If the patient is sitting, ensure that he or she can sit with the feet comfortably on the ground.

   c. Do not use a chair with rollers or allow a patient to sit in a chair that keeps the feet from comfortably reaching the ground. Place a box or book under the feet if necessary.

7. Gain the patient's cooperation: Be honest and efficient.

   a. Talk to your patient throughout the entire procedure.

   b. Involve your patient in the procedure.

   c. Do not surprise the patient with the stick. Always tell the patient that you are ready to insert the needle.

8. Seat the patient.

   a. Most laboratories have special blood drawing, or phlebotomy, chairs.

   b. Hospital inpatients are generally positioned in a supine position, as are outpatients who feel faint or who have a history of fainting during blood draws.

9. Special considerations for inpatients

   a. Bed rails

      (1) The bed rails are lowered on the side of the bed where the phlebotomist is working.

      (2) Avoid catching IV lines, catheter bags, or other tubing or equipment when lowering the bed rails.

      (3) The rails are raised when the draw is complete, for the safety of the patient.

   b. Eating or drinking during the draw

      (1) Patients are not permitted to eat or drink or have anything in their mouths, such as candy thermometers or lozenges, during a blood draw.

      (2) Patients could reflexively bite down or choke on anything in their mouths at the time of the draw.

10. Sequence of venipuncture procedure

    a. Site identification

(1) Most frequently venipuncture is performed in the antecubital area of the arm.

(2) In this area, the median cubital, cephalic, and basilica veins are located close to the surface.

b. Application of tourniquet

   (1) Proper tourniquet application should allow arterial blood flow to the area below the tourniquet but obstruct venous blood flow away from the area.

   (2) Procedure (See Figure 6-5.)

      (a) Select the appropriate tourniquet.

      (b) Inspect the patient's arms for the most likely vein.

      (c) Wrap the tourniquet around the patient's arm approximately 3–4 inches above the venipuncture site. To gauge this distance, place your little finger on the site, and measure up four fingers.

      (d) Bring both ends of the tourniquet around to the front of the patient's arm.

      (e) Pull the left end of the tourniquet taut and hold it steady.

      (f) Pull the right end tighter as you pull across the front of the patient's arm, crossing the right end over the top of the left end and grasping both sides of the tourniquet with the thumb and forefinger of one hand.

      (g) Pull the right loose end slightly down and create a loop.

      (h) Tuck the loop up under the area of the tourniquet that has been crossed.

      (i) The loose ends should be running up the patient's arm and away from the venipuncture site.

      (j) To release the tourniquet, gently tug on the right free end.

   (3) Additional tourniquet considerations

      (a) When applying a tourniquet to a patient with fragile skin that tears or bruises easily, apply the tourniquet on top of the patient's shirt or blouse; this reduces the friction applied directly to the skin. You may also wrap gauze around the area prior to application of the tourniquet.

      (b) The improper application or extended use (longer than 1 minute)

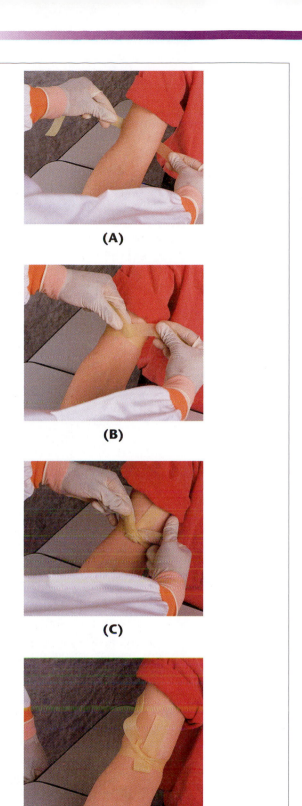

Figure 6-5

(A) Wrap the tourniquet around the arm 3 to 4 inches above the venipuncture site, keeping the tourniquet flat. (B) Stretch the tourniquet tight across the ends. (C) While holding the ends tight, tuck one portion of the tourniquet under the other. (D) Check that the tourniquet will not come loose. The ends of the tourniquet should be pointed upward and not hang into the venipuncture site.

of tourniquets during a venipuncture can cause hemoconcentration of the specimen. The sample renders inaccurate test results, and the specimen will be rejected.

(c) Asking your patient to make a fist helps make the vein more prominent.

(d) Do not request the patient to vigorously open and close the fist, because this action increases potassium and ionized calcium levels due to the muscle movement.

c. Locating the vein

(1) Do not rely on visually locating a vein.

(2) Using the tip of the index finger to palpate the vein is the most accurate method of locating a vein. Gently "bounce" your index finger across the antecubital area. Veins bounce back; arteries pulsate.

(3) Palpating veins allows you to identify the direction of the vein, how deep beneath the surface of the skin the vein is located, and the size of the vein.

(4) Do not slap or rub your finger across the patient's arm.

(5) Train yourself to locate veins while wearing gloves.

(6) *Do* select a vein that:

(a) Feels large and well anchored.

(b) Will not "roll" off to one side when pushed by the needle.

(7) *Do not* select a vein that:

(a) Feels hard or cordlike. (These veins may be sclerosed and are more difficult to penetrate with the needle. A thrombosed vein also feels hard and should not be selected.)

(b) Are located beneath scar tissue, burns, tattoos, or moles. Select another site.

(8) Once a vein is selected, keep a mental picture of its location.

(9) Hand veins

(a) If an antecubital site is not suitable on either arm, check the wrists and backs of each hand for a vein.

(b) If a suitable site cannot be located: Warm the arm or hand by wrapping a warm, moist towel (108° Fahrenheit or 42° Celsius) around the site (with the tourniquet off).

Leave it in place for 3 to 5 minutes. Reapply the tourniquet. Try to locate a vein again.

    (10) Ankle veins

        (a) When no other site can be located, ankle veins may be used.

        (b) To use ankle veins, written permission from the patient's physician is needed.

    (11) If a vein cannot be located, follow institutional protocols, which may include asking another phlebotomist, a nurse, or physician to perform the draw.

d. Releasing the tourniquet, cleansing the site, and reapplying the tourniquet

    (1) There are two options for cleansing the venipuncture site:

        (a) Alcohol wipes are most frequently used.

        (b) Povidone-iodine is used for blood cultures, when a patient is allergic to alcohol, or for collection of specimens for blood alcohol level testing.

    (2) Guidelines

        (a) Remove the alcohol prep or povidone-iodine prep from its package.

        (b) Cleanse the venipuncture site in a circular motion from the center to the periphery.

        (c) Allow the area to air dry for 30–60 seconds. Do not wipe with an unsterile gauze square. Do not fan or blow on the site to dry it faster.

        (d) Do not touch the site once it has been cleansed. If it is necessary to repalpate the vein, the site must be recleansed.

        (e) Being very careful not to touch the cleansed site, reapply the tourniquet.

        (f) *Remember:* A tourniquet must not be left in place for longer than 1 minute.

e. Performing an evacuated tube draw

    (1) Place the first evacuated tube in the tube adapter. Do not push it onto the needle.

    (2) Remove the needle cover.

        (a) Examine the needle for defects such as chips or burrs; replace it if needed.

        (b) Once the needle cover has been removed, the needle may not touch any surface prior to insertion into the patient's vein, or it must be replaced.

    (3) Prepare the needle, tube, and tube holder.

        (a) Hold the blood drawing equipment in your dominant hand.

        (b) Rest the blood drawing equipment on your fingertips, with your index and middle finger holding the tube adapter and your ring and little finger holding the evacuated tube.

        (c) Press up gently on the evacuated tube so that the tube is firmly against the top of the inside of the tube adapter. Your thumb will be resting on the top of the tube adapter. Using this method gives you a more secure hold when inserting the needle.

        (d) Do not push the tube onto the needle.

        (e) Some phlebotomists prefer not to put the evacuated tube into the adapter until after the needle has been inserted into the vein. Either method is acceptable.

    (4) With your nondominant hand, grasp the patient's arm approximately 1–2 inches below the venipuncture site.

    (5) Pull the skin taut with your thumb. This procedure:

        (a) Secures the vein and helps to keep it from rolling.

        (b) Eases the insertion of the needle into the patient's skin and decreases patient discomfort.

    (6) Insert the needle, bevel up, holding it at a 15- to 30-degree angle. Penetrate the skin and then the vein in one quick, smooth motion.

        (a) Adjust the angle to the angle of the patient's vein.

        (b) Position the needle to follow the line of the patient's vein.

        (c) As soon as you sense the needle is in the vein, stop advancing the needle and anchor the tube adapter.

        (d) The needle is generally inserted so that the entire bevel is in the vein.

    (7) Holding the equipment steady, push the evacuated tube onto the needle.

        (a) Grasp the flanges of the tube adapter with the index and middle finger.

(b) While gently pulling with these fingers, push the evacuated tube onto the needle with your thumb.

(c) Blood will begin to fill the tube immediately if the needle is in the vein.

(8) Keep the needle steady in the patient's arm.

(a) Keep the patient's arm and the tube in a downward position, with the tube filling from the bottom up.

(b) If the tube is in an upward position, it is possible a backward flow of blood will enter the evacuated tube. This process is called reflux.

(9) Due to the amount of vacuum pressure, most evacuated tubes fill approximately two-thirds of the way full.

(a) The vacuum inside the tube is exhausted at approximately the two-thirds point and blood flow stops.

(b) There are tubes that are considered full when filled only halfway. They are designed for specific lab tests requiring a smaller volume of blood or a greater concentration of the anticoagulant.

(10) Remove the tourniquet.

(a) If you are drawing only one tube of blood, loosen the tourniquet as soon as blood begins to fill the tube.

(b) If you are drawing more than one tube of blood, wait to remove the tourniquet until the last tube starts filling with blood; then remove the tourniquet.

(c) Remember the rule of not keeping the tourniquet on longer than 1 minute.

(d) If drawing on an elderly patient or a patient with fragile veins, keep the tourniquet in place until just prior to removing the needle. Removing the tourniquet earlier on these patients may cause the vein to collapse and the blood flow to stop.

(11) If the tube contains an additive, after removing the tube from the needle and tube adapter, gently invert the tube 5–8 times before setting it down.

(12) When the last tube is filled, remove the tube from the needle and the adapter before removing the needle from the patient's arm.

(13) As the needle is removed from the vein, simultaneously place a clean 2 × 2-inch gauze square directly over the site.

(a) *Do not* press down on the gauze square until the needle is safely removed from the patient's arm.

(b) Click the needle's safety shield into place.

(14) Apply direct pressure to the site with the gauze square for 3–5 minutes.

(a) *Do not* allow the patient to bend his or her arm. Bending the arm keeps the vein open, and blood leaks into the surrounding tissues, causing a hematoma.

(15) Dispose of the collection unit (needle, tube adapter). The best practice to prevent needlestick injuries following phlebotomy procedures is to:

(a) Use a SESIP (sharp with engineered sharps injury protection, i.e., a safety needle), attached to the blood tube holder.

(b) Immediately dispose of the entire unit after each patient's blood is drawn. (CLSI standards state that tube holders should not be reused.)

(16) Although requirements may vary from institution to institution, the tubes are typically labeled with the following information:

(a) Patient's name

(b) Patient number or hospital ID number

(c) Patient's room number (for an inpatient)

(d) Time and date of collection

(e) Phlebotomist's initials

(17) If special handling is required:

(a) Place the specimen in an ice "slurry" to keep it cool (e.g., ammonia).

(b) Place it in a heat block to keep the specimen warm (e.g., cold agglutinin).

(c) Wrap it in aluminum foil to protect it from light (e.g., bilirubin).

(18) Check on the patient.

(a) Make sure that the bleeding has stopped.

(b) Patients who are on anticoagulant therapy or have bleeding disorders must be monitored closely for a minimum of 30 minutes.

(19) Place a slight pressure dressing over the site.
  (a) Fold a 2 × 2-inch gauze square into fourths.
  (b) Place it over the site.
  (c) Secure with either tape or a self-adhesive bandage strip.
  (d) Instruct the patient to leave the bandage on for 5 to 10 minutes, at which time it may be removed.
  (e) Instruct patients not to carry or lift any heavy objects with the arm the venipuncture occurred on for approximately 1 hour.
  (f) Tell patients who have been fasting that it is okay to eat now.
(20) Dispose of all contaminated items in the biohazardous waste container.
  (a) Do not leave any supplies or equipment in the patient's room.
(21) Thank the patient.
(22) Remove your gloves and dispose of them in the appropriate biohazardous waste container.
(23) Wash your hands.
(24) Promptly transport the specimen to the laboratory for processing.
(25) Enter the specimen information into the computer system or logbook.
  (a) The venipuncture must be documented.
  (b) From a legal point of view, collections not documented have not been done.

C. Blood collection syringe method
  1. The pressure exerted by the evacuated tube method may be too great for the veins in some patients, such as children and the elderly.
  2. Using the syringe method, the phlebotomist can control the amount of pressure by pulling the plunger of the syringe back slowly.
  3. Procedure
    a. Patient identification, patient preparation, and site selection are the same as in the evacuated tube procedure.
    b. Prepare the syringe and needle by removing them from their sterile wrappers.
      (1) To comply with OSHA regulations, only needle-locking syringes are to be used with integrated safety devices.
    c. Pull the plunger of the syringe back to ensure that it moves freely in the barrel.
    d. Return the plunger to its original position.
    e. Attach the safety needle to the syringe unless the needle is preattached.
      (1) Make sure that the needle is securely locked into place.
      (2) Do not uncap the needle at this time.
    f. Apply the tourniquet, cleanse the site, remove the needle cap, inspect for defects, and enter the vein with the bevel up in the same manner as you would in the evacuated tube method.
      (1) When the needle is in the vein, blood appears in the hub of the needle. This is called flash.
      (2) You may remove the tourniquet at this point.
    g. Secure the syringe, in the same manner as in the evacuated tube procedure, by resting the supporting hand on the patient's arm.
    h. Slowly pull back on the plunger of the syringe until the barrel is filled with blood.
    i. Remove the needle in the same manner as in the evacuated tube method.
      (1) If one syringe does not provide enough blood for the requested tests, it is recommended that a butterfly infusion set be used rather than a hypodermic needle, because the length of tubing allows for the attachment of additional syringes without causing damage to the patient.

D. Blood collection with the butterfly infusion set
  1. The butterfly infusion set is used with patients who have small, fragile veins, such as:
    a. An elderly patient.
    b. An infant.
    c. A small child.
    d. An adult patient who has small antecubital, wrist, or hand veins.
  2. The butterfly infusion set, with an integrated safety device needle, is typically a 23-gauge ⅝-inch in length.
  3. It is recommended that pediatric-sized (2-milliliter) evacuated tubes be used with pediatric-sized tube adapters.
    a. The force of the vacuum in the 5-milliliter evacuated tube is often too great for fragile veins and causes them to collapse.
    b. In addition, the use of 5-milliliter tubes with a 23-gauge needle may cause hemolysis of the specimen. Hemolysis is caused when:
      (1) The needle is too small for the vein selected.
      (2) The vacuum in the tube is too strong for a small vein.

4. The procedure for using a butterfly infusion set is the same as for the syringe method, with a few exceptions.
   a. When assembling the equipment, the tubing attached to the needle is coiled. Uncoil the tubing and stretch it slightly to help keep it from recoiling during the draw.
   b. Attach the butterfly infusion set to the syringe or evacuated tube system. If you are using the evacuated tube method, rest the first tube in the adapter.
   c. If you are drawing from an antecubital vein, the draw continues from this point in the same manner as in an evacuated tube draw.
   d. When drawing blood from a hand or wrist vein, the following adjustments are made:
      (1) Apply the tourniquet above the wrist.
      (2) Ask the patient to make a fist or bend the fingers. It is helpful for the patient to grasp a ball or, if a ball is not available, an unopened package of 2 × 2-inch gauze squares.
      (3) The hand must be well supported. Use rolled towels or an armrest.
      (4) Select the vein, and cleanse the site.
         (a) For hand draws, use your thumb to pull the skin taut over the top of the patient's knuckles.
         (b) For wrist draws, pull the skin taut with your thumb just below the venipuncture site.
      (5) Prepare the collection unit (butterfly infusion set and tube adapter or syringe).
         (a) Hold the tube adapter/syringe and tubing in your dominant hand, or lay it next to the patient's hand.
         (b) With the bevel up, grasp the "wings" and fold them together with your thumb and index finger.
      (6) Perform the puncture.
         (a) Align the needle with the vein.
         (b) Using a 10- to 15-degree angle, enter the vein with a quick but steady motion.
         (c) Once the vein has been entered, you will see a "flash" of blood in the tubing.
         (d) When you do, you can pull the plunger back to fill a syringe or push the evacuated tube onto the needle in the tube adapter.
      (7) The tourniquet may be:
         (a) Removed once you have established blood flow into the syringe or evacuated tube.
         (b) Or left in place until the draw is complete as long as the draw is accomplished within the 1-minute window.
      (8) Keep the tube adapter and tube lower than the patient's arm pointing downward so that the tube fills from the bottom up.
      (9) When the last tube is filled:
         (a) Release the tube from the needle.
         (b) Place gauze over the venipuncture site.
         (c) Remove the needle activating the needle safety device.
         (d) Apply pressure in the same way as with a routine evacuated tube venipuncture.
      (10) If using a syringe:
         (a) Transfer the collected blood to the appropriate evacuated tubes, using a transfer safety device.
         (b) Mix with the additives, as described earlier.
      (11) Dispose of the butterfly infusion set.
         (a) Place the needle, attached tubing, and tube adapter as one unit into the sharps container.
         (b) If a syringe has been attached, dispose of the attached needle and tubing in the sharps container and attach the transfer safety device to the syringe.
         (c) Once the blood has been transferred to the appropriate evacuated tubes, dispose of the syringe and transfer safety device.

V. ARTERIAL BLOOD GAS (ABG) TEST

A. Purpose of test—To provide valuable information regarding the status of the patient's:
   1. Oxygenation.
   2. Ventilation.
   3. Acid-base balance.
      a. Acid-base balance is the mechanism by which the acidity and alkalinity of body fluids are kept in a state of equilibrium so that arterial blood is maintained at approximately a 7.35–7.45 pH level.

B. Arterial blood is used for blood gases because its composition is the same throughout the body.
  1. Venous blood has various compositions relative to the metabolic activities in surrounding tissues.
C. Training requirements
  1. If the ABG test is performed incorrectly, the patient can be seriously injured.
  2. Personnel performing ABGs must be specially trained and, as a rule, certified by their health care institution as having met the qualifications to perform this advanced procedure.
  3. CLSI has determined the criteria for meeting these qualifications to be:
     a. Didactic (theory) training.
     b. Observation of a demonstration of the technique.
     c. Performance of the procedure under the supervision of qualified personnel.
D. Equipment and supplies
  1. Safety equipment when collecting ABGs—PPE includes:
     a. Fluid-resistant lab coat, gown, or apron.
     b. Gloves.
     c. Face protection (arterial punctures have a high risk of splattering blood)
     d. Puncture-resistant sharps container.
  2. Antiseptic solution—Povidone-iodine (Betadine) solution or chlorhexidine
  3. Local anesthetic solution—0.5–1 percent lidocaine to numb the site.
  4. Hypodermic needles
     a. Size and length vary depending on the site location, but they are selected from the range of 20–25 gauge, ⅝–1½ inches in length.
     b. The most commonly used needles are:
        (1) 22-gauge, 1-inch for radial and brachial punctures.
        (2) 22-gauge, 1½ inch for femoral punctures.
        (3) A 25- to 26-gauge needle for the administration of an anesthetic.
     c. All needles must have integrated safety devices.
  5. Syringes
     a. ABGs are collected in 1- to 5-milliliter syringes, depending on the amount of blood require.
     b. ABG kits contain a special glass or plastic syringe that is prefilled with heparin and designed to fill spontaneously upon puncture of the artery.

     c. A 1- or 2-milliliter syringe is used for the administration of an anesthetic.
     d. Evacuated tubes should not be used for collection of ABGs because the tubes alter the partial pressure of the gas in the blood sample.
  6. A small block of latex or rubber or a similar device to insert the needle in immediately after collection, to prevent air from entering the syringe.
  7. Lithium (or sodium) heparin (1,000 units/milliliter solution)—To prevent the specimen from clotting
  8. Coolant—Plastic bag or cup with crushed ice and water. Must be 1–5 degrees Celsius (34–41 degrees Fahrenheit) to:
     a. Prevent gases from escaping into the atmosphere.
     b. Slow the metabolism of WBCs, which consume oxygen.
  9. Gauze—2 × 2-inch gauze squares to apply pressure over the puncture site
  10. Patient identification label
  11. Waterproof marker or pen
  12. Alcohol pad
  13. Adhesive bandage or tape
  14. Oxygen measuring device—For patients who are on oxygen-enriched gases instead of room air.
     a. The oxygen concentration is recorded on the laboratory requisition slip.
     b. This measurement is taken prior to the collection of the specimen.
  15. Thermometer
  16. Puncture resistant sharps container
  17. Prepackaged arterial blood gas kits—Supplied by several medical supply companies. Although ABG kits vary in content from manufacturer to manufacturer, the most standard kit contains:
     a. A 1-cc syringe.
     b. A 25-gauge × ⅝-inch preattached needle.
     c. A 23-gauge × 1-inch packaged needle.
     d. A vented tip cap.
     e. A needle stopper.
     f. Two gauze pads.
     g. A povidone-iodine preparation.
     h. An alcohol preparation.
     i. A patient identification label.
     j. An adhesive bandage.
     k. A Ziploc for ice.

E. Selection of the arterial puncture site
   1. Site considerations—The site should not be:
      a. Inflame
      b. In close proximity to a wound.
      c. On a limb with an AV shunt or fistul
   2. Preferred sites—The radial, brachial, and femoral arteries
      a. The radial artery
         (1) The radial is the most commonly selected.
         (2) Although the radial artery is smaller than the brachial or femoral artery, the risk of hematoma is considerably less.
         (3) It typically has the best collateral circulation (as determined by the Allen test).
            (a) Collateral circulation means that blood is supplied to the area by more than one artery.
            (b) Under normal circumstances, the hand and wrist (preferred sites) are supplied blood via the radial and ulnar artery.
            (c) If the radial artery is damaged during the arterial puncture, the ulnar artery continues to supply blood to the area.
      b. The brachial artery is the second choice.
         (1) It is larger and easier to palpate than the radial artery.
         (2) It also has sufficient collateral circulation but not as much as the radial artery.
      c. The femoral artery is the third choice.
         (1) It is used as a last resort when other sites cannot be used.
         (2) It is a large artery, located superficially in the groin area and can be easily palpated.
         (3) A physician or specifically trained emergency room personnel has to perform this procedure. A phlebotomist is not trained to perform it.
         (4) The risk of infection is increased when puncturing the femoral artery due to pubic hair.
   3. Additional sites
      a. Other sites are:
         (1) The umbilicus of the newborn.
         (2) The dorsalis pedis arteries of an adult patient.
      b. As with draws from the femoral artery, a physician or specifically trained emergency room personnel must perform this procedure. A phlebotomist is not trained to perform it.

F. Preparation
   1. Check the physician's order written on the lab requisition form.
   2. Identify the patient, explain the procedure, and obtain the patient's consent.
   3. Determine allergies (e.g., latex, alcohol, anesthetics) and current medications (e.g., anticoagulant therapy).
   4. Calm the patient, who must be in what is termed a steady state.
      a. This means the patient has been resting comfortably for a minimum of 30 minutes with no exercise, treatments, or respirator changes.
      b. A patient who is afraid of needles or the pain associated with arterial blood collection quickly moves out of a steady state.

G. Complications of arterial punctures
   1. Discomfort—Arterial punctures can cause the patient discomfort even with the use of anesthesia.
   2. Infection
      a. As with any other invasive procedure, infection is a risk.
      b. Proper antiseptic procedures minimize this risk.
   3. Hematoma—The chance of a hematoma is increased in arterial puncture because the blood in the arteries is under great pressure.
   4. Arteriospasm
      a. Arteriospasms may occur when the insertion of the needle into the artery causes irritation of the arterial muscle. The artery reflexively contracts.
      b. The condition is usually temporary, but it does make collection of a specimen difficult.
   5. Thrombus formation—Injury to the lining of the artery can cause a thrombus to form, which can obstruct the flow of blood, impairing circulation.

H. Errors and specimen rejection—An arterial blood sample can render inaccurate test results or be rejected by the laboratory for a number of reasons:
   1. Air bubbles in the specimen
   2. Inadequate amount of blood collected
   3. Improperly cooled specimen
   4. Venous sample collected instead of arterial sample
   5. Incorrect anticoagulant used
   6. Too much or not enough anticoagulant used

7. Specimen improperly mixed
8. Improper syringe used
9. Improper labeling of specimen
10. Too long a delay in transporting the specimen to the laboratory

VI. BLOOD CULTURES

A. Reasons for blood cultures
   1. A physician often orders blood cultures when:
      a. A patient has a fever of unknown origin (FUO).
      b. The physician suspects:
         (1) Bacteriemia (bacteria in the blood).
         (2) Or septicemia (the presence of pathogenic microorganisms in the blood).
   2. Blood cultures can provide the physician with information regarding:
      a. The presence of infection.
      b. The extent of the infection and the organism causing it.
      c. The antibiotics the organism is most susceptible to.

B. Considerations
   1. Timed procedure—The specimens are collected from a patient with an FUO at the height of the fever when the microorganisms are thought to be most plentiful in the blood.
   2. Antimicrobial therapy
      a. Specimen bottles
         (1) Blood cultures drawn to monitor antimicrobial therapy are drawn in special collection bottles, which contain a resin solution to inactivate the antimicrobial agent. This allows the bacteria to grow.
         (2) The collection bottles containing resin are called antibiotic removal device (ARD) bottles. The resin removes the antimicrobial agent from the blood.
         (3) Specimens collected in ARD bottles must be submitted to the laboratory as soon as possible for processing, because blood should not be exposed to the device for more than 2 hours.
      b. Specimen quantity
         (1) The amount of blood collected is critical for the optimal recovery of microorganisms. Up to 10 milliliters of blood is typical, but the amount can vary according to the recommendations of the manufacturer of the collection bottle.
         (2) The volume of blood and the ratio to culture medium volume are critical for growing organisms. The optimal ratio is 1:5.
         (3) Collections from infants and children are 1–5 milliliters.
      c. Blood cultures are often ordered in sets. The collection of sets can occur in two ways:
         (1) Both sets can be collected at the same time from different sites.
         (2) They can be collected 30 minutes apart from approximately the same site.
      d. Specimen quality
         (1) Particular attention must be paid to the preparation of the venipuncture site. Bacteria are normally present on the skin surface. For quality test results, bacteria must *not* be introduced into the specimen.
         (2) Before the collection of a specimen for blood culture analysis, the selected venipuncture site must be prepared by aseptic technique. (The cleansing procedure varies from one laboratory to another.)
            (a) Before cleansing the site, ask the patient about any allergy to iodine. If the patient has an iodine allergy, the only recourse is to cleanse thoroughly with 70 percent alcohol; some places may also use green soap.
            (b) The site is first painted with alcohol for 1 minute to remove the oils and dirt on the skin surface.
            (c) The site is then cleansed with a 2 percent tincture of iodine solution (or with 70 percent alcohol or green soap).
            (d) The cleansing is done with a circular motion, starting at the site of the puncture and moving outward in concentric circles.
            (e) The iodine is painted on the area, not flooded over the site.
            (f) Iodine is an effective antiseptic only if it is allowed to dry before the venipuncture is attempted.
            (g) Once the site has been prepared, *do not repalpate!* Repalpating the site contaminates it.
         (3) Due to the increased risk of contamination, blood cultures should not be

drawn through an indwelling intravenous or intra-arterial catheter unless it cannot be obtained by venipuncture or upon physician request.

    (a) You should "waste" 5 milliliters of blood.

    (b) Anticoagulants, such as citrate, oxalate, EDTA, and heparin, are toxic to some bacteria.

VII. PEDIATRIC COLLECTION

A. Unique challenges in collecting blood specimens from children

  1. Children's blood vessels are smaller and thus more difficult to visualize and palpate.

  2. Explaining the procedure to children may be difficult because they do not have the same skills for logical and emotional reasoning as adults.

B. Gaining cooperation

  1. Introduce yourself; be warm, friendly, and confident.

  2. Talk with the child and establish a positive rapport even before looking at the child's arm or touching equipment.

  3. Never tell a child that the procedure is not going to hurt. Even the most skilled phlebotomist may cause the patient some discomfort when inserting a needle.

  4. Involve a parent or guardian.

    a. If the adult prefers to stay with the child, ask the adult to assist by holding the child on the lap as a means of restraint.

    b. Have the adult distract the child during the procedure, offering encouragement and reassurance.

C. Older children

  1. Involve an older child in the procedure. Ask the child to be your helper by holding the adhesive bandage or gauze squares.

  2. If the child is an inpatient, if at all possible perform the procedure in a treatment room rather than in the child's bed. The child's bed should be a "safe" place, free from pain and anxiety, to promote the healing process.

D. Preparation—All supplies and equipment are gathered and assembled prior to interacting with the patient. Preparing for the procedure after initial interaction prolongs the procedure and may add to the child's anxiety.

E. Specimen quantity

  1. Draw the least amount of blood possible to perform the ordered tests, because children have a smaller ratio of blood to body mass and cannot maintain homeostasis if large quantities are removed.

  2. Removal of large quantities of blood over long periods of time can cause the child to become anemic.

  3. Removal of over 10 percent of an infant's blood volume can cause cardiac arrest.

F. Restraining the child

  1. Restraining the child is often the safest and least traumatic method of obtaining a specimen.

  2. Types of restraint

    a. Very young children and infants can be restrained by means of a papoose.

      (1) A papoose is a specially designed board with attached canvas flaps.

      (2) The child is positioned in the center of the device, and the flaps are wrapped around the infant and securely fastened, leaving the extremity being drawn exposed.

    b. Young children can easily be restrained by sitting them on an adult's lap.

    c. Older children can be restrained in a couple of ways:

      (1) The child can sit in the phlebotomy chair, with the adult standing behind the chair helping to steady the child's arm.

      (2) The child can be in the supine position, with an adult leaning over the child from the opposite side of the bed, grasping the child's arm being drawn on from behind, and holding the free arm close to the patient's body.

G. Supplies and equipment

  1. Because a child or infant's blood vessels are significantly smaller than those of an adult, you must use smaller tubes and needles for the collection process.

  2. Needles—For best results, use:

    a. The 23-gauge butterfly infusion set with a 2- to 3-milliliter evacuated tube.

    b. At an antecubital site.

  3. Tourniquets are available in pediatric sizes.

  4. Evacuated tubes

    a. A child's small veins are not able to withstand the same amount of vacuum from an evacuated tube as an adult's veins.

    b. With smaller tubes, the vacuum pressure is less, the puncture causes less damage, and there is less of a chance of the vessel collapsing.

H. Site selection
1. Antecubital veins are preferred.
2. However, the dorsal hand veins are excellent sites for drawing labs on children under the age of 2 and neonates.

VIII. BLOOD BANKING

A. Collection requirements
1. Almost every blood bank test requires a large plain red top evacuated tube or a large lavender top EDTA evacuated tube.
2. Identification of the patient and the labeling of the specimen must be completed with the utmost care. The laboratory will reject specimens that are mislabeled or incomplete.
   a. Blood bank specimens require the following information:
      (1) The patient's full name, including middle initial
      (2) The patient's hospital identification number or social security number (if an outpatient)
      (3) The patient's date of birth
      (4) The date and time of collection
      (5) The phlebotomist's initials
      (6) The room number and bed number (optional)
B. Type and crossmatch—One of the most common blood-banking tests
1. Purpose of test
   a. Blood type and crossmatch is performed to determine the compatibility of blood to be used for a transfusion.
   b. Every patient has a particular blood type and can receive blood only from a donor with a compatible blood type.
   c. If incompatible blood is transfused, it could prove fatal because of agglutination (clumping) or lysing of red blood cells.
   d. Therefore, whenever a blood transfusion might be required, a type and crossmatch must be completed using strict identification and labeling guidelines.
C. Blood donation programs
1. Collecting blood from a volunteer blood donor requires a properly trained health care individual, such as a certified phlebotomist, laboratory technologist, or nurse.
2. Blood donor collections are performed within a division of blood-banking procedures and may be a part of a regional blood bank or hospital.

3. All blood donor facilities must follow the guidelines of the American Association of Blood Banks (AABB).
D. Blood donor criteria
1. General criteria—The donor must:
   a. Be at least 17 years of age (some states permit younger persons to donate with the permission of a parent or guardian). Most blood banks do not have upper age limits.
   b. Weigh at least 110 pounds.
   c. Be in generally good health.
2. Physical and health history examinations
   a. All donors must pass the physical and health history examinations given prior to donation.
   b. Both exams are required every time a person donates, regardless of how many previous times they have donated.
   c. The physical includes:
      (1) Checking the blood pressure, pulse, and temperature.
      (2) Taking a few drops of blood from a capillary puncture to ensure that anemia is not present.
   d. Any abnormalities found as a result of the physical examination may be a cause for a deferral.
   e. The health history examination includes questions that are designed to protect the health of both the donor and the recipient.
      (1) To ensure that every donor is asked the same questions, the American Association of Blood Banks (AABB) recommends the use of a uniform donor history questionnaire.
      (2) However, donor centers often create their own questionnaires using the same general guidelines.
      (3) In addition to questions about transfusion-transmissible diseases, prospective donors are asked questions to determine whether donating blood might endanger their health.
   f. A prospective donor who responds positively to any of the questions is deferred or asked not to donate.
   g. All donor information is kept confidential.
   h. The donor is also required to sign a release giving permission for his or her blood to be used.
E. Blood collection
1. Once the prospective donor has successfully passed the physical and health history, the actual collection can take place.

2. The collection process takes approximately 20 minutes.

3. Procedure

   a. The donor sits in a recumbent position or lies down.

   b. Site selection—Typically the large antecubital vein, selected in the same manner as for routine venipuncture

   c. Cleansing the site (antecubital area)—In a two-step procedure, in much the same way as for blood cultures:

      (1) With alcohol.

      (2) With povidone-iodine.

   d. A blood pressure cuff or a tourniquet may be used. While typically a tourniquet is used for regular blood draws, a blood pressure cuff, pumped to 120 millimeters/inches of mercury, is used for blood donations.

   e. Equipment and supplies are gathered and assemble.

      (1) The collection unit is a sterile closed system consisting of:

         (a) A bag containing an anticoagulant to collect the blood.

         (b) A sterile needle connected to the bag by means of a length of tubing.

      (2) The needle most commonly used is 16 gauge and coated with an anticoagulant.

   f. The donor is asked to:

      (1) Make a fist around a small ball.

      (2) Periodically to squeeze his or her hand to help blood flow from the vein into the collection bag.

   g. Typically one unit of blood is collected, which is approximately the equivalent of 1 pint.

      (1) Because blood fills the bag by the pull of gravity, the bag must be placed lower than the patient's arm.

      (2) The bag is placed on a mixing device, or "rocker."

      (3) Only one puncture is allowed to fill a bag. If the bag does not fill completely and another puncture must be performed, the procedure must be repeated completely, using a new collection unit.

      (4) It takes approximately 7 minutes to fill a bag.

   h. After the collection is completed:

      (1) The blood pressure cuff is released.

      (2) The needle is removed.

      (3) An initial pressure dressing is applied over the puncture site until the bleeding stops.

      (4) A permanent pressure dressing is put on the puncture site prior to dismissing the donor.

      (5) The donor is returned to a full sitting position.

   i. The donor is checked.

      (1) The donor who feels faint or light-headed is returned to a recumbent position.

      (2) The donor who feels "fine" is offered light refreshment, such as juice and cookies, and escorted to an observation area to rest for a few minutes.

   j. The collected blood is sent to the laboratory for testing and component preparation.

F. Autologous blood donation

   1. Autologous transfusions are transfusions in which the blood donor and transfusion recipient are the same. In other words, a person donates blood for his or her own use.

      a. This may be done prior to elective surgeries or when a transfusion is anticipated.

      b. A person may donate one unit of blood each week for up to six weeks before surgery. Preoperative autologous donations may not be made within 72 hours of surgery.

      c. Blood can be stored in its liquid form for up to 42 days.

      d. Using one's own blood for transfusion eliminates numerous risks associated with donor transfusions, such as disease transmission and incompatibilities.

      e. If the blood is not required for transfusion, it may be used for the general population with the donor's permission.

G. Intraoperative blood collection

   1. In an intraoperative blood collection, blood lost by the patient during surgery is received and recycled throughout the surgery.

   2. Most intraoperative blood collection programs use machines in which shed blood is collected and the red blood cells are concentrated and washed prior to transfusion.

   3. This procedure is widely used for surgical procedures in which the anticipated blood loss is 20 percent or more of the patient's estimated blood volume and there will be no contamination of the area by bacteria or cancer cells.

      a. Examples

         (1) Cardiac

         (2) Vascular

(3) Orthopedic

(4) Urologic

(5) Trauma

(6) Gynecologic and transplant surgery

4. This procedure is generally not used in cancer surgery or surgery of the lower gastrointestinal tract.

IX. SPECIAL COLLECTIONS

A. Advanced training is required for the following blood collections. Many hospitals permit only the nursing staff to perform blood collection from indwelling catheters. However, it is important to be familiar with these procedures because you may be required to assist or have the opportunity for further on-site training.

B. Indwelling catheters

1. Indwelling catheters are also called vascular access devices (VADs).

   a. VADs consist mainly of tubing inserted into a main artery or vein.

   b. This main vein or artery is customarily the subclavian, which is located in the chest below the clavicle.

   c. VADs are generally inserted for:

      (1) Administering fluids and medications.

      (2) Monitoring pressures.

      (3) Drawing blood.

         (a) Example: A patient who is severely burned or terminally ill often has an indwelling catheter implanted to provide access for medications and blood draws.

2. Drawing blood specimens from VADs requires special techniques, special training, and experience.

3. Types of VADs

   a. Central venous catheters (CVC), or central venous lines, are inserted into a large vein, such as the subclavian, and advanced into the superior vena cava, proximal to the right atrium.

      (1) Several inches of tubing protrude from the exit site and are normally covered by a transparent dressing.

   b. Peripherally inserted central catheters (PICCs) are inserted into the peripheral venous system (veins of an extremity) and threaded into the central venous system (the main veins leading to the heart).

      (1) PICCs do not require surgical insertion.

      (2) They are commonly placed into the basilic or cephalic vein with the exit in the antecubital space.

      (3) PICCs tend to collapse on aspiration; drawing blood from a PICC is not recommended.

C. Implanted port

1. An implanted port is a small chamber that is attached to an indwelling line. It is surgically implanted under the skin.

2. The device can be located by palpating the skin.

3. A special noncoring needle is inserted into the self-sealing septum of the chamber.

4. The site is not normally covered with a bandage.

D. Arterial line

1. An arterial line is commonly located in the radial artery.

2. It is used to:

   a. Provide continuous monitoring of a patient's blood pressure.

   b. To collect arterial blood gases.

E. Heparin or saline locks (hep-lock)

1. Heparin or saline locks are special winged needle sets, or cannulas, that can be left in a patient's vein for up to 48 hours.

2. They are typically inserted into the lower arm above the wrist.

3. They are used to:

   a. Administer medication.

   b. Draw blood.

      (1) Because a hep-lock is periodically flushed with heparin or saline to keep it from clotting, a 5-milliliter tube is drawn and discarded prior to collecting a specimen when drawing blood from a hep-lock.

      (2) Coagulation studies are not to be drawn from a heparin or saline lock.

F. Arteriovenous (AV) shunts

1. AV shunts are artificially created connections between a vein and an artery.

2. They are typically created to provide access for dialysis.

3. Venipuncture or blood pressures are not to be performed on an arm with an AV shunt.

G. External AV shunt (cannula)

1. An external AV shunt, or cannula, is a temporary external connection between a vein and artery. The tubing of the cannula:

   a. Extends to the outside surface of the arm.

b. Is capped by a small rubber diaphragm, in which a needle can be inserted and blood drawn.

2. External AV shunts are used for:

a. Dialysis.

b. Drawing blood.

   (1) Drawing blood through a cannula:

       (a) Must be performed by specially trained professionals.

       (b) May be performed only with permission from the patient's physician.

H. Internal AV shunt (fistula)

1. An internal AV shunt, or fistula, is created by a surgical procedure, which permanently fuses a vein and artery together.

   a. The connection is made close to the surface of the skin.

   b. It can easily be seen and felt.

2. It is used for dialysis.

   a. It should never be used for phlebotomy.

   b. Blood specimens must be drawn from the patient's other arm or other acceptable location.

X. SPECIMEN IDENTIFICATION AND TUBE LABELING

A. General guidelines for tube labeling

1. Indelible ink must be used when writing on prefixed tube labels.

2. Specimens must be labeled immediately following collection.

3. Typically, most institutions require the following information:

   a. The patient's full name

   b. The patient's number or hospital identification number

   c. The patient's room number (if an inpatient)

   d. The time and date of collection

   e. The phlebotomist's initials

XI. FAILURE TO OBTAIN BLOOD AND OTHER CONSIDERATIONS

A. Incomplete draw, short draw, or complete failure

1. In an incomplete, partial, or short draw. the evacuated tube or syringe does not contain the required amount of blood to perform the requested tests.

2. There are several situations leading to incomplete (short) draws or to a complete failure to obtain a blood specimen:

a. Collapsed vein—A patient's vein can collapse because of:

   (1) The pressure caused by the vacuum of an evacuated tube.

   (2) The plunger of a syringe being pulled back too quickly or forcefully.

b. Damaged or occluded veins—Sclerosed or occluded veins are often the result of inflammation and disease or occur in patients who have had repeated punctures to veins.

c. Obesity

   (1) Obese patients commonly have antecubital veins that are difficult to either see or palpate. With the knowledge of where the veins are typically located and with practice the phlebotomist will be able to locate the vein and perform the venipuncture.

   (2) The phlebotomist should never perform a "blind stick" because it can:

       (a) Be dangerous to the patient.

       (b) Cause accidental arterial puncture or severe nerve damage.

   (3) An excellent alternative to locating antecubital veins on obese patients is to use the wrist or hand veins.

d. Incorrect tube position

   (1) Check to see that:

       (a) The tube has been properly seated onto the needle.

       (b) There is no loss of vacuum. If you suspect that the tube has lost its vacuum, insert another tube into the tube adapter and push it onto the needle.

e. Incorrect needle positioning

   (1) This may be caused by a number of things:

       (a) The needle is not inserted deeply enough.

       (b) The needle is inserted too deeply. If this is not corrected immediately, blood seeps into the tissues and causes a hematoma (an accumulation of blood at a venipuncture site, identified by swelling and discoloration, "bruising").

       (c) The needle bevel is against the wall of the vein.

       (d) The needle is alongside the vein.

       (e) You are unable to determine position of the needle.

3. Do not stick a patient more than twice. If a third attempt is necessary, it is to be performed by another phlebotomist.

4. Other considerations

a. Typically, blood may be drawn from a patient no more than three times a day.

b. The total volume of blood that may be drawn per day on a patient is based on the patient's weight.

c. It is acceptable to share basic information, such as the name of the test that has been ordered. Encourage the patient to direct further questions to the physician.

d. All competent patients have the right to refuse treatment.

   (1) Make every effort, using your best judgment, to persuade the patient to agree to the blood draw. However, do not harass the patient.

   (2) Note the refusal in the patient's chart and explain to the patient that the physician will be notified.

XII. OTHER CONSIDERATIONS REGARDING ROUTINE VENIPUNCTURE

A. Intravenous (IV) infusion

1. *Do not* stick above an IV infusion.

2. A typical protocol is that, if an IV is running in both arms and there is no other alternative except to use the IV site:

a. The phlebotomist may draw blood at least 2 inches below the IV site once permission has been given by the patient's physician.

b. Ask the nurse to turn off the IV for a minimum of 2 minutes prior to the draw.

c. Apply the tourniquet below the IV site.

d. Use a vein other than the one the IV is attached to.

e. Discard the first 5 milliliters of blood, then draw the sample to be used for testing.

B. Effects of stress and exercise

1. Stress and exercise can increase the test values for:

a. Lactate dehydrogenase (LDH).

b. Aspartate aminotransferase (AST).

c. Platelet count.

d. Creatine kinase (CK) levels.

2. Outpatients should remain sitting for 15 minutes before you attempt a venipuncture for certain procedures. Sitting allows the body to recover from stress and/or exercise prior to collection of the specimen.

C. Swelling at the puncture site—If during the venipuncture process the site begins to swell:

1. Immediately release the tourniquet and remove the needle.

2. Apply firm direct pressure, using several gauze squares on the site for 8–10 minutes.

3. Elevate the patient's arm while continuing to apply pressure.

4. An ice pack may be applied to the area as well.

XIII. SPECIMEN INTEGRITY—QUALITY ASSURANCE

A. Proper handling of the specimen:

1. Begins the moment the blood is drawn into the evacuated tube or syringe and continues throughout the collection process.

2. Includes transporting the specimen to the laboratory and processing the specimen in the laboratory.

B. General guidelines

1. Handling routine specimens—Although procedures and techniques may vary from institution to institution, the following are general guidelines:

a. Inversion of blood tubes must be done immediately after the blood draw; additive tubes must be gently inverted 8–10 times.

b. Blood specimens should be transported carefully to prevent tube breakage. Tubes should be transported stopper up, which helps to prevent hemolysis and aids in clot formation.

c. Specimens that are being sent via mail must be specifically packaged. Medical specimens transported by the U.S. Post Office or by private carrier, such as Federal Express or UPS, must be labeled with biohazardous labels affixed to the outside of all bags.

2. Specimens requiring special handling

a. Specimens requiring protection from light

   (1) Several tests are affected by the presence of light, which can cause falsely low values. Bilirubin is the most common.

   (2) To protect a specimen from light, wrap it in aluminum foil.

   (3) Specifically designed amber-colored microcollection containers are available for collection of bilirubin specimens from infants.

b. Specimens requiring chilling after collection

   (1) Examples:

      (a) Blood gases

(b) Ammonia

(c) Lactic acid

(d) Rennin

(e) Prothrombin time

(f) Partial thromboplastin time

(g) Glucagon

(2) Chilling a specimen after collection slows down the metabolic processes, which continue after the draw.

c. Specimens required to be kept warm

(1) Some specimens need to be kept at or near body temperature (37.5 degrees Celsius, 98.6 degrees Fahrenheit).

(a) Examples:

(i) Cold agglutinins

(ii) Cryoglobulin

(iii) Cryofibrinogen

(2) Warming can be accomplished by transporting the specimen in a commercially manufactured, 37.5-degree–Celsius heat block. For manually activated clotting times, the tube must be kept warm during the procedure as well as before the procedure.

d. Timing requirements

(1) All specimens must be transported to the lab in a timely manner.

(2) Routine specimens are to arrive at the laboratory within 45 minutes of collection and are to be centrifuged within 1 hour.

(3) Some tests require specific timing.

(a) NACCLS sets the maximum time limit for separating serum and plasma from the cells at 2 hours from time of collection.

(b) If specimens have been drawn in serum separator tubes (SSTs) or plasma separator tubes (PSTs), they only need to be centrifuged. Once centrifuged, the separator gel prevents glycolysis for up to 24 hours.

(c) Potassium and Cortisol specimens must reach the laboratory within a 45-minute window.

(4) Exceptions to the guidelines

(a) Lavender top tubes (EDTA), drawn for hematology studies, are never centrifuged. EDTA specimens are stable for 24 hours.

(b) Blood smears made from EDTA tubes must be completed within

1 hour of collection to preserve the integrity of specimen.

(c) Specimens drawn for glucose determination in tubes containing sodium fluoride, a glycolytic inhibitor, are stable for 24 hours at room temperature and for up to 48 hours when refrigerated.

XIV. PROCESSING A BLOOD SPECIMEN

A. Receipt in the laboratory

1. Once a specimen is received, it is:

a. Logged in.

b. Prioritized.

c. Prepared for testing.

2. Specimens requiring centrifugation are spun down, and the serum or plasma is pipetted off and transferred into aliquot tubes.

B. Centrifugation

1. A centrifuge is a machine that spins the blood at high revolutions per minute (rpm).

2. The spinning creates a force that causes the formed elements (red blood cells, white blood cells, and platelets) to separate from the serum or plasma. The formed elements are heavier than the serum or plasma and travel to the bottom of the tube.

3. Requirements

a. The specimen must be allowed to clot prior to being centrifuged.

b. The tubes must remain stoppered during this procedure to prevent:

(1) Blood from splashing out of the tube.

(2) The specimen from evaporating.

(3) The pH of the specimen from changing.

(4) The specimen forming an aerosol.

c. If stoppers are removed to add a separator device, they must be restoppered prior to centrifugation.

d. OSHA requires wearing protective apparel during the processing of specimens. Protective apparel includes:

(1) A buttoned lab coat.

(2) Gloves.

(3) Protective face gear.

e. The centrifuge must be balanced.

(1) It is important that the machine be balanced by placing equal tubes and volumes of specimens opposite each other.

(2) An unbalanced machine spins unevenly and causes the evacuated glass specimen tubes to break, creating aerosols.

f. Specimens requiring centrifugation fall into one of two categories: plasma or serum.
   (1) Plasma specimens are collected in tubes containing an anticoagulant specific for the requested test.
   (2) Serum specimens are collected in tubes that do not contain an anticoagulant and must be left to clot prior to centrifuging.
       (a) The specimen must be allowed to clot at room temperature for a minimum of 20 minutes and a maximum 45 minutes.
g. The lid of the centrifuge:
   (1) Must be closed and latched in place during the spinning of the specimens.
   (2) Opened only after the centrifuge comes to a complete stop.
h. Centrifuge specimens only once. Repeating centrifugation causes:
   (1) Hemolysis.
   (2) Inaccurate test results.
i. If a tube breaks during centrifugation:
   (1) Clean up the broken glass using wet paper towels, wearing a pair of heavy-duty utility gloves.
   (2) Disinfect the centrifuge, following the facility's blood spill cleaning protocols.
   (3) Dispose of broken glass in the appropriate sharps container.

C. Stopper removal
   1. When the stopper has to be removed:
      a. Use a stopper removal device.
      b. If a stopper device is not available:
         (1) Remove the stopper manually using a 4 × 4-inch gauze square placed over the stopper. This prevents any aerosol that might be released.
         (2) Pull the stopper straight up; do not "pop" it off.

D. Separation of plasma and serum: When testing on plasma or serum is required it must be transferred into an aliquot tube.

XV. SPECIMEN REJECTION

A. The following basic specimen rejection guidelines are common to most facilities.
   1. Discrepancies between requisition forms and labeled tubes
   2. Unlabeled tube
   3. Hemolyzed specimen
   4. Specimen collected in the wrong tube

5. Expired tube
6. Insufficient specimen for the test ordered (labeled QNS, quantity not sufficient)
7. Specimens collected at the wrong time intervals

B. The phlebotomist must collect new specimens as quickly as possible.

C. Causes of specimen contamination
   1. Inadvertent contamination of a specimen can occur by using the wrong antiseptic to cleanse the puncture site.
      a. Example: Cleansing a site with alcohol can contaminate a blood alcohol level test.
   2. Using povidone-iodine to clean a site can:
      a. Contaminate the specimen.
      b. Cause erroneously high levels of potassium, uric acid, and phosphate.
   3. Not allowing an antiseptic to completely air-dry prior to collection can also contaminate specimens used for blood cultures.
   4. Contamination of blood cultures can occur if the site of blood culture bottles has not been properly cleaned prior to collection.
   5. Powder from gloves can contaminate blood slides and skin puncture specimens.

XVI. PRIORITIZING PATIENTS

A. The phlebotomist is required to continuously make decisions regarding the order in which patients are drawn. The following are areas of consideration when making these decisions.

B. Timed specimens
   1. When tests are ordered to be done at a particular time, the phlebotomist must collect the specimens at the time ordered.
   2. Examples:
      a. Glucose levels are the most commonly ordered timed test.
      b. Other timed tests include:
         (1) Drug therapy levels.
         (2) Collecting blood for rennin activity.
         (3) Hormone levels such as cortisol and aldosterone.

C. Fasting specimens
   1. Fasting levels for glucose, cholesterol, and triglycerides are important in the diagnosis and monitoring of a patient's progress.

D. Stat specimens
   1. The term "stat" means immediately.
   2. It indicates that a patient's condition is critical and must be treated or responded to as a medical emergency.

3. The phlebotomist must draw the blood quickly and efficiently and ensure that the specimen is delivered to the laboratory stat.

XVII. COMPLICATIONS OF BLOOD COLLECTION

A. Accidental artery puncture
   1. You know you have accidentally punctured an artery if the blood entering the tube is:
      a. Bright red.
      b. Pulsing into the tube.
   2. If an accidental artery puncture occurs:
      a. Immediately remove the tourniquet and withdraw the needle from the site.
      b. Activate the needle safety device.
      c. Apply direct pressure using 2×2-inch gauze squares for a minimum of 5 minutes and/or until the bleeding stops.
B. Allergic response
   1. Types of possible allergies
      a. Latex
         (1) Examples:
            (a) Latex gloves
            (b) Latex tourniquet tubing
      b. Bandage adhesive
      c. Antiseptics
         (1) Examples:
            (a) Alcohol
            (b) Povidone-iodine
   2. As a precaution, ask every patient if he or she is allergic to latex, adhesive, or antiseptics.
   3. Alternatives
      a. Nonlatex gloves and tourniquets can be used in place of latex ones.
      b. Paper tape and 2×2-inch gauze squares are used in place of adhesive bandages.
      c. Patients allergic to isopropyl alcohol can have the skin cleansed with povidone-iodine or hexachloridine.
         (1) If the patient is allergic to povidone-iodine (Betadine), alcohol can be used.
         (2) For a blood culture or blood alcohol level collection, povidone-iodine or green soap should be used.
   4. Unknown allergies—If the patient is unaware of previous allergic responses and a reaction occurs during the collection procedure:
      a. *Either* complete the procedure as quickly as possible.
      b. *Or,* if an extreme reaction occurs, stop the procedure immediately.

c. Wash the affected area with a nonallergenic soap and running water.
      d. Report the reaction to the nurse and/or physician immediately.
   5. Severity of response
      a. Mild response
         (1) Most allergic responses are generally mild in nature and present as redness or as a rash of the surrounding tissue. They are unpleasant and the tissues are itchy.
         (2) Ointments prescribed by a physician, applied topically, cause the rash to subside and soothe the itching.
      b. Severe response
         (1) If the rash is severe, a systemic medication can be prescribed for the patient.
         (2) In extremely severe cases, the allergic response can lead to anaphylactic shock.
   6. Anaphylactic shock
      a. The patient in anaphylactic shock presents with:
         (1) Acute respiratory distress.
         (2) Hypotension.
         (3) Edema.
         (4) Hives.
         (5) Tachycardia.
         (6) Pale, cool skin.
         (7) Convulsions.
         (8) Cyanosis.
      b. If not treated immediately, anaphylactic shock can cause unconsciousness.
C. Collapsed vein
   1. Fragile veins—The veins of elderly and/or frail patients are often too fragile to withstand the force of the vacuum in the evacuated tube.
   2. Incorrect equipment or use of equipment—The phlebotomist can cause the patient's vein to collapse by:
      a. Using an evacuated tube that is too large for the patient's vein.
      b. Exerting too much force when drawing back the plunger of a syringe.
   3. Improperly applied tourniquet—A tourniquet can also cause a vein to collapse if it is:
      a. Tied too tightly.
      b. Positioned too close to the venipuncture site.
   4. Patient history—If a patient tells you that his or her veins "always collapse," pay attention.
      a. This is a good indication that alternative collection methods should be used, such as:

(1) Using smaller evacuated tubes (pediatric).

(2) Using a butterfly draw or syringe.

b. Whichever method is used, pull the blood slowly into the tube.

D. Excessive bleeding at the site

1. Occasionally a patient continues to bleed because he or she is on anticoagulant therapy or a hemophiliac.

a. Anticoagulant therapy.

(1) Anticoagulant is an agent that prevents or delays blood coagulation (clumping).

b. A hemophiliac.

(1) A hemophiliac is a person afflicted with a hereditary blood disease marked by:

(a) Greatly prolonged blood coagulation time.

(b) Consequent failure of the blood to clot and abnormal bleeding.

(c) Sometimes joint swelling.

2. If bleeding has not stopped after a few minutes:

a. Apply direct pressure over the site.

b. Raise the patient's arm above heart level.

3. If the bleeding has not stopped after 5 minutes:

a. Notify the nurse and/or physician.

b. Do *not* leave the patient unattended at *any* time during this situation, until the nurse or physician assumes responsibility.

E. Fainting (syncope) and seizures

1. Fainting

a. Fainting, or syncope, is a:

(1) Transient loss of consciousness resulting from an inadequate flow of blood to the brain due to:

(a) Breath holding.

(b) Vasovagal response.

(2) Common complication of blood collection.

b. Signs and symptoms

(1) The feeling starts with:

(a) Increased nervousness.

(b) Increased respirations.

(c) A slow and weak pulse.

(d) Decreased blood pressure.

(e) Pallor and mild sweating.

(f) Possibly nausea and vomiting.

(2) The feeling may progress to:

(a) Periods of unconsciousness.

(b) In extreme cases, seizures.

c. Detection

(1) Several million Americans fear needles so intensely that being stuck with one for an injection or a blood test can trigger fainting, convulsions, and, in 23 reported cases, death.

(2) Listen to the patient. Patients may tell you in advance that they faint every time their blood is drawn.

d. Response to fainting during a blood draw—If the patient says he or she feels faint or starts to faint during the procedure:

(1) Remove the tourniquet and withdraw the needle as quickly as possible.

(2) Talk to the patient to divert attention. This helps the patient to stay alert and to retain consciousness.

(3) Ask the patient to lower his or her head between the knees, and help the patient do this.

(4) Ask the patient to breathe slowly and deeply.

(5) Physically support the patient to prevent further injury.

(6) Loosen tight clothing, such as collars or ties.

(7) Apply a cold compress or washcloth to the forehead and back of the neck.

(8) If necessary, use an ammonia inhalant to bring the patient "back around."

(a) Note: Alcohol wipes work just as well as ammonia inhalants and are generally quicker to get to.

(9) Alert the nurse and/or physician as quickly as possible.

(10) Monitor the patient's vital signs, until he or she returns to normal or a nurse or physician assumes responsibility.

2. Seizures

a. Frequency—Seizures are rare.

b. Responses to a seizure—If a patient has a seizure during a blood draw:

(1) Immediately remove the tourniquet and withdraw the needle.

(2) Apply pressure over the site without restricting the patient.

(3) Notify the nurse and/or physician.

(4) Protect the patient's head, and move items out of the way that might cause injury.

(5) *Never* place anything in a patient's mouth or leave the patient unattended.

c. Once the patient has stopped seizing, it is typically recommended that:
   (1) The patient stay in the area for minimum of 15–30 minutes.
   (2) The patient should be instructed not to operate a vehicle unless released to do so by the physician.
      (a) Note: Patients with seizure disorders may have restrictions placed on their licensure to drive automobiles or to operate machinery or equipment. This regulation varies from state to state. However, most states require a release from a physician stating that the individual is capable of the activity before reinstating the license.

F. Hematoma
   1. A hematoma is:
      a. An accumulation of blood at the venipuncture site.
      b. Caused by blood leaking into the tissues around the site.
      c. Identified by swelling and discoloration (bruising).
      d. Often painful and can cause damage to underlying tissues.
   2. Causes
      a. Inadequate pressure applied to the venipuncture site for an inadequate amount of time
      b. Excessive probing to locate a vein
      c. Partial penetration of the needle into the vein, allowing blood to seep into the tissue
      d. Penetration of the needle all the way through the vein, allowing blood to seep into the tissue
      e. Failure to remove the tourniquet before the needle is withdrawn
      f. Too large a needle used for the vein size
   3. Responses—If a hematoma starts to occur during the venipuncture procedure:
      a. Immediately release the tourniquet and withdraw the needle.
      b. Apply direct pressure over the site for a minimum of 5 minutes.
      c. Do not allow the patient to bend the arm at the elbow to apply pressure; this causes further bruising.
      d. Possibly apply an ice pack to the site to reduce pain and swelling.
         (1) Do not apply a cold pack directly on the patient's skin.

         (2) The patient should be instructed on the appropriate method to use the ice pack at home. (Apply an ice pack for twenty minutes then remove for 20 minutes.)

G. Nerve damage
   1. Frequency—Rare but it can occur
   2. Cause—Generally due to excessive probing to locate a vein
      a. To eliminate the risk of hitting a nerve, avoid excessive probing for the vein.
   3. Detection
      a. You know you have hit a nerve because the patient will report a very painful burning sensation.
      b. Hitting a nerve is painful and can cause permanent damage.

H. Uncooperative patient
   1. An uncooperative patient can occur for a variety of reasons.
      a. Examples:
         A young child who does not understand the procedure and is afraid of being hurt.
         A very ill patient who is tired of being "poked and prodded."
         An extremely anxious patient in the emergency room.
   2. Responses
      a. Remain calm.
      b. Consider restraints only as last resort to obtain a specimen.
      c. When a collection is performed on a restrained patient, always request the assistance of a second person.
   3. Refusal of procedure
      a. When patients are ill and have been through numerous procedures, they may be very resistant and refuse to allow you to perform the procedure.
      b. Patients have the right to refuse treatment.
      c. If a patient refuses a procedure, refer the situation to the patient's nurse or physician or to your supervisor.

PRACTICE

1. Puncturing the calcaneous bone of an infant may not only be painful but can cause _____.
   a. osteomyelitis
   b. osteoblastomas
   c. anemia
   d. hemorrhaging

2. Which one of the following is *not* a reason a hematoma may occur?
   a. Excessive probing is used to locate a vein.
   b. The needle is only partially in the vein.
   c. Tourniquet is not removed before the needle is withdrawn.
   d. Too small a needle is used.

3. If a patient is allergic to isopropyl alcohol, use _____ instead as an antiseptic.
   a. sodium chloride
   b. green soap
   c. povidone-iodines
   d. Zephiran Chloride

4. A _____ is an accumulation of blood at a venipuncture site caused by blood leaking into the tissue.
   a. hemotoma
   b. hematoma
   c. hemitoma
   d. hemertoma

5. A patient should remove a bandage _____ minutes after a venipuncture.
   a. 2–3
   b. 4–6
   c. 5–10
   d. 10–20

6. Sodium citrate is the additive in the _____ top evacuated tube.
   a. royal blue
   b. light blue
   c. light gray
   d. green-black

7. A _____ top evacuated tube is drawn for the collection of blood cultures.
   a. red
   b. light blue
   c. brown
   d. yellow

8. A _____ top evacuated tube must not be inverted.
   a. red
   b. lavender
   c. yellow
   d. black

9. _____ is a type of nonallergenic tape that can be used if a patient is allergic to adhesive.
   a. Paper tape
   b. Transpore tape
   c. Surgical tape
   d. Scotch tape

10. The _____ fingertip is the only one that should not be used for capillary puncture.
    a. 1st
    b. 3rd
    c. 4th
    d. 5th

11. If an elderly patient tells you his or her veins are fragile, you should _____.
    a. use a pediatric evacuated tube set
    b. use a butterfly infusion set
    c. use a syringe and a small-gauge needle
    d. any of the above

12. Anaphylactic shock is an immediate allergic reaction characterized by which one of the following?
    a. Acute respiratory distress, hypertension edema, and a rash
    b. Acute respiratory distress, fast pulse rate, edema but no rash
    c. Acute respiratory distress, hypotension, edema, and a rash
    d. Acute gastric distress, hypertension, flatulence, bloating

13. _____ is a hereditary blood disease marked by greatly prolonged blood coagulation time with a failure of the blood to clot and abnormal bleeding.
    a. Anaphylactic shock
    b. Hemophilia
    c. CHF
    d. Erythroblastosis

14. If an artery is accidentally punctured, the phlebotomist should apply pressure for a minimum of ____ minutes.
    a. 2
    b. 5
    c. 10
    d. 20

15. Alcohol pads or alcohol wipes should contain a _____ percent isopropyl alcohol solution.
    a. 50
    b. 60
    c. 70
    d. 100

16. A tourniquet may stay on the patient for only _____ minutes.
    a. 1–2
    b. 2–3
    c. 3–4
    d. 4–5

17. When selecting veins for venipuncture, try to avoid veins that are hard or cordlike because they may be _____.
    a. fragile
    b. sclerosed
    c. occluded
    d. tendons

18. If an antecubital vein cannot be located on either arm, check the wrists and hands. If a suitable site cannot be located, try _____.
    a. elevating the area
    b. warming the area with moist heat
    c. chilling the area with moist cold
    d. all of the above

19. The point of the needle that has been cut on a slant for ease of entry is called the _____.
    a. bevel
    b. periphery
    c. edge
    d. phlange

20. What is the typical gauge and length of the needle of a butterfly infusion set?
    a. 21 gauge, 1 inch
    b. 22 gauge, 1 inch
    c. 23 gauge, 5/8 inch
    d. 22 gauge, 5/8 inch

21. Which one of the following does *not* cause hemolysis?
    a. Using a needle with too small a bore
    b. Using too large an evacuated tube for a butterfly infusion set
    c. Forcing blood from a syringe into an evacuated tube
    d. All of the above cause hemolysis.

22. When you are using a butterfly infusion set, the needle should be inserted into the vein at a _____ degree angle.
    a. 5- to 10-
    b. 10- to 15-
    c. 15- to 20-
    d. 40- to 45-

23. Sclerosed or _____ veins are often the result of inflammation and disease, or they occur in patients who have had repeated punctures to veins.
    a. occluded
    b. ischemic
    c. strictured
    d. hemolysis

24. The phlebotomist, if there are no other options, may draw blood at least _____ inches below an IV site once permission has been given by the patient's physician.
    a. 1
    b. 2
    c. 3
    d. 4

25. If drawing blood from a venipuncture site with an IV, ask the nurse to turn the IV off for a minimum of _____ minutes prior to the draw.
    a. 1
    b. 2
    c. 4
    d. 5

26. Immediately after a blood draw, additive tubes must be gently inverted _____ times.
    a. 3–4
    b. 4–5
    c. 5–8
    d. 8–10

27. _____ top evacuated tubes drawn for blood banking are never inverted.
    a. Light blue
    b. Lavender
    c. Red
    d. Gray

28. _____ are small, sterile, single-use instruments used to puncture the capillaries of the skin.
    a. Microhematocrit tubes
    b. Lancets
    c. Hypodermic needles
    d. None of the above

29. A(n) _____ should be used when drawing blood from fragile veins.
    a. lancet
    b. microhematocrit tube
    c. syringe
    d. evacuated tube

30. When you are using the evacuated tube system, the needle should be inserted into the site at a _____ degree angle.
    a. 10- to 20-
    b. 15- to 30-
    c. 20- to 40-
    d. 25- to 45-

31. When using the _____ method of drawing, the phlebotomist can control the amount of pressure placed on the vein.
    a. butterfly
    b. capillary
    c. dyringe
    d. evacuated tube

32. When you are performing a venipuncture, the patient can be in any position *except* _____.
    a. laying down
    b. sitting in a phlebotomy chair
    c. standing
    d. position does not matter.

33. The _____ is the most frequent area used to perform venipuncture.
    a. antecubital area
    b. forearm
    c. hand
    d. top of the foot

34. When palpating the vein, use the tip of the _____ finger.
    a. index
    b. little
    c. middle
    d. ring

35. Direct pressure to the venipuncture site should be applied for _____ minutes.
    a. 1–2
    b. 2–4
    c. 3–5
    d. 4–5

36. Microhematocrit tubes are also known as _____.
    a. blood tubes
    b. capillary tubes
    c. micro tubes
    d. microcollect tubes

37. Microhematocit tubes without any anticoagulant have a _____ band at one end.
    a. blue
    b. red
    c. green
    d. yellow

38. Microcollection containers are often referred to as _____ because of their size and shape.
    a. bullets
    b. "beebees"
    c. torpedoes
    d. salvos

39. The most common size syringe used for a routine venipuncture is a _____cc (cubic centimeter) syringe.
    a. 3-
    b. 5
    c. 10-
    d. 20-

40. _____ should be drawn in a lavender top evacuated tube.
    a. Coagulation studies
    b. Complete blood count
    c. Sedimentation rate
    d. Toxicology profiles

41. A(n)_____ test provides physicians with information about the respiratory status and acid-base balance of a patient.
    a. arterial blood gases
    b. hematocrit
    c. hemoglobin
    d. glucose

42. A capillary puncture should be made _____ to the fingerprint.
    a. horizontal
    b. perpendicular
    c. going with
    d. any of the above

43. When you are performing a _____, a small incision is made in the patient's forearm, and the blood is blotted at 30-second intervals.
    a. bleeding time
    b. hematocrit
    c. protime
    d. sedimentaion rate

44. _____ is a common complication of blood collection and a transient loss of consciousness resulting from an inadequate blood flow to the brain.
    a. Hematoma
    b. Shock
    c. Syncope
    d. Seizure

45. Needle phobias can be so intense that the patient may experience _____.
    a. convulsions
    b. death
    c. fainting
    d. all of the above

46. If the patient experiences a hematoma, the phlebotomist should apply an ice pack to the site and instruct the patient to apply an ice pack for _____ minutes on, _____ minutes off when returning home.
    a. 5s, 10
    b. 10, 10
    c. 15, 20
    d. 20, 20

47. "Hitting" a(n) _____ during venipuncture can cause permanent damage.
    a. artery
    b. capillary
    c. nerve
    d. vein

48. It may be necessary to restrain a(n) _____ patient in order to collect a blood specimen.
    a. severely ill patient
    b. drug-overdosed
    c. uncooperative adult
    d. all of the above

49. As a matter of routine the phlebotomist should ask all patients if they are allergic to antiseptics, adhesives, and _____ as a means of preventing allergic reactions.
   a. cotton
   b. nylon
   c. latex
   d. all of the above

50. Ointments prescribed by a physician and applied _____ can reduce an allergic rash reaction.
   a. topically
   b. sublingually
   c. subcutaneously
   d. none of the above

51. Toxicology profiles may be performed on blood from a _____ top evacuated tube.
   a. black
   b. royal blue
   c. lavender
   d. red

52. A puncture of a vein for any reason is called _____.
   a. ABG
   b. capillary stick
   c. glucose test
   d. venipuncture

53. Do not ask a patient to vigorously open and close the fist prior to a venipuncture, because this can contribute to _____, causing inaccurate test results.
   a. interstitial fluid leakage
   b. hemoconcentration
   c. sclerosis
   d. decreased glucose levels

54. If an antecubital vein cannot be located on either arm, check the wrists and hands. If a suitable site cannot be located, what other location may be drawn on with permission from the patient's physician?
   a. Feet and ankle veins
   b. Popliteal veins
   c. Clavicle veins
   d. Axillary veins

55. _____ top evacuated tubes are drawn for hematology studies and are *never* centrifuged.
   a. Light blue
   b. Lavender
   c. Red
   d. Gray

56. Cleanse the venipuncture site in a _____ motion.
   a. circular
   b. scrubbing
   c. swiping
   d. none of the above

57. A _____ top evacuated tube must be a full draw or rejection occurs.
   a. black
   b. brown
   c. light blue
   d. red-gray

58. If the evacuated tube is not filling with blood, the phlebotomist should check that the _____.
   a. tube is seated properly into the needle
   b. tube has not lost its vacuum
   c. needle is in the correct position
   d. all the above

59. Before performing any procedure on an inpatient, the phlebotomist should _____.
   a. ask the patient to see his or her social security number
   b. look at the patient's identification bracelet
   c. ask the patient for a driver license
   d. ask a friend the patient's name

60. The first thing a phlebotomist should do when meeting a patient for the first time is _____.
   a. find out the patient's name
   b. introduce yourself and identify yourself as a phlebotomist
   c. skip the introductions because you'll have a white lab coat on
   d. wait till the patient is asleep and then draw the blood

61. If an injury prevents the phlebotomist from using a patient's fingertips for a capillary puncture, all of the following can be used *except* _____.
   a. ears
   b. heels
   c. toes
   d. wrists

62. VADs are inserted for all of the following reasons *except* _____.
   a. monitoring the patient's acid-base balance
   b. administering fluids and medications
   c. monitoring pressures
   d. drawing blood

63. When you are performing an arterial blood gas collection, the site with the highest risk of infection is the _____ artery.
   a. radial
   b. brachial
   c. femoral
   d. umbilical

64. _____ should not be used for the collection of ABGs because they alter the partial pressure of the gas in the blood sample.
   a. Syringes
   b. Butterfly infusion sets
   c. Twenty-two-gauge needles
   d. Evacuated tubes

65. A patient must be in a "steady state" for a minimum of _____ minutes before collection of ABGs.
   a. 2
   b. 15
   c. 30
   d. 60

66. When collecting a specimen for bilirubin testing, you must protect the specimen from _____.
   a. cold
   b. heat
   c. light
   d. all the above

67. _____ are designed to temporarily reduce the flow of venous blood in the arm.
   a. Blood pressure cuffs
   b. Rubber bands
   c. Tourniquets
   d. All of the above

68. _____ is an example of a PPE.
   a. Face gear
   b. Scrubs
   c. Alcohol preps
   d. Temperature probes

69. Because of the danger of aspiration and suffocation, a bandage should not be used on a patient who is less than _____ year(s) old.
   a. 1
   b. 2
   c. 3
   d. 4

70. NCCLS guidelines state that an infant's heel puncture should not exceed _____ millimeters in depth.
   a. 1.2
   b. 1.8
   c. 2.1
   d. 2.4

71. When performing a capillary puncture, position the patient seated or lying down, with the _____ side of the hand facing up.
   a. dorsal
   b. palmar
   c. ventral
   d. plantar

72. Perform a capillary puncture using a quick _____ motion.
   a. darting
   b. pushing
   c. scooping
   d. sliding

73. In the correct order of evacuated tube filling from a syringe draw, the first tube is _____.
   a. green
   b. light blue
   c. gray
   d. yellow

74. When an artery has been effectively entered, a _____ of blood appears in the hub of the needle.
   a. bubble
   b. flash
   c. speck
   d. copious amount

75. The most critical factor in collecting blood culture specimens is _____ of the patient's skin.
   a. antisepsis
   b. sterilization
   c. tautness
   d. color

76. One of the most common blood-banking tests performed is a _____.
   a. type and crossmatch
   b. hematocrit
   c. ESR
   d. CBC

77. A(n) _____ is a temporary connection between a vein and artery used for dialysis and for drawing blood.
   a. PICC
   b. external AV shunt
   c. arterial line
   d. CVC

78. Transferring blood from a syringe to a(n) _____ poses a greater risk to the phlebotomist for accidental needle sticks than collection from an evacuation tube.
   a. evacuated tube
   b. slide
   c. capillary tube
   d. aliquot tube

79. The phlebotomist must wash his or her hands thoroughly for a minimum of _____ minutes before invasive procedures.
   a. 2
   b. 3
   c. 4
   d. 5

80. When you are performing a finger stick, the activity to be done first should be _____.
   a. explain the procedure to the patient
   b. dispose of the lancet
   c. identify the patient
   d. assemble and prepare equipment and supplies

81. Alcohol wipes should *not* be used for draws when testing a patient's _____.
   a. blood alcohol level
   b. hematocrit
   c. glucose
   d. proteins

82. A reflectively contracted artery during an ABG can be caused by a(n) _____.
   a. angiospasm
   b. arteriospasm
   c. venospasm
   d. venispasm

83. _____ protect the phlebotomist from aerosol exposure.
   a. Gloves
   b. Goggles
   c. Lab coats
   d. Shoe booties

84. The risk of using a small-gauge needle includes all of the following *except* _____.
   a. long draw time
   b. hemolysis
   c. hard-to-draw large quantities
   d. vasoconstriction

85. _____ supplies blood to an area by more than one artery.
   a. Arterial circulation
   b. Coronary circulation
   c. Collateral circulation
   d. Venous circulation

86. A(n) _____ is a specific amount of blood, approximately 1 pint, supplied by a volunteer as part of a blood bank procedure.
   a. allotted amount
   b. donor unit
   c. specimen unit
   d. volunteer unit

87. A(n) ____ is a catheter inserted into the peripheral venous system and then threaded into the central venous system.
   a. arterial line
   b. central venous catheter
   c. PICC
   d. VAD

88. Coagulation studies cannot be drawn from a(n) _____.
   a. arterial line
   b. heparin lock
   c. PICC
   d. VAD

89. The withdrawal of large quantities of blood over a long period of time can cause a pediatric patient to become _____.
   a. anemic
   b. apprehensive of needles
   c. homostatic
   d. none of the above

90. Removal of over _____ percent of an infant's blood can cause cardiac arrest.
   a. 2
   b. 5
   c. 10
   d. 12

91. _____ is an OSHA-required item, such as the gloves that a phlebotomist is required to wear when in contact with body fluids.
   a. PAD
   b. PPE
   c. PAE
   d. PAF

92. Hypodermic needles are typically _____ needles, used when performing syringe draws.
   a. multisample
   b. single-sample
   c. reusable
   d. small

93. The most common multisample needle length used is _____ inches.
   a. 1/2–1
   b. 1–1½
   c. 1–2
   d. 1½–2

94. The most common gauge multisample needle used by a phlebotomist is _____.
   a. 15–20
   b. 18–20
   c. 20–21
   d. 20–25

95. When lead determinations are being made the _____ top evacuated tube is drawn.
   a. blue
   b. brown
   c. green-gray
   d. royal blue

96. A _____ needle is most commonly used with the evacuated tube system because it has two sharp ends, one beveled and the other covered with a rubber sheath.
   a. simple-sample
   b. single-sample
   c. multisample
   d. multigauged

97. _____ is fluid between the tissues, surrounding a cell.
    a. Arterial blood
    b. Capillary blood
    c. Interstitial fluid
    d. Venous blood

98. Capillary blood flow can be greatly increased when the site is _____.
    a. cool
    b. cold
    c. warm
    d. hot

99. _____ can be applied to the finger during a capillary puncture to ensure a steady flow of blood.
    a. Firm pressure
    b. Massaging
    c. Milking
    d. All the above

100. All of the following are considered "tools of the trade" for the phlebotomist except _____.
    a. gloves
    b. utility tray
    c. goggles
    d. antiseptics

101. A butterfly infusion set contains a needle that is _____ inches long and is made of stainless steel.
    a. 1/8–3/4
    b. 1/4–1/2
    c. 1/2–3/4
    d. 1/8–1/2

102. A _____ is used to seal the open end of micro-hematocrit tubes.
    a. plastic stopper
    b. paraffin wax disk
    c. clay sealer tray
    d. white glue

103. Never _____ a needle from the tube adapter or syringe prior to disposal.
    a. unscrew
    b. bend
    c. recap
    d. all of the above

104. Of the following categories, which group will likely require the use of a lancet for blood specimen collection?
    a. 15-year-old female
    b. 87-year-old male
    c. 37-year-old male
    d. 29-year-old female

105. Which evacuated tube has the special requirement of inversion for proper mixing?
    a. Royal blue
    b. Green-gray
    c. Red-gray
    d. Both a and c

106. Which item is not commonly found in a well stocked blood drawing tray?
    a. Hemostats
    b. Glass slides
    c. Povidone-iodine swabs
    d. Microhematocrit tubes

107. Puncturing the bone during a heel stick on an infant can cause_____.
    a. osteomyelitis
    b. osteomialitis
    c. osteomylitis
    d. osteomyalitis

108. The infant's leg should be held securely with the phlebotomist's _____ hand and arm, while the_____ hand uses a pediatric lancet to perform a capillary heel stick.
    a. predominant, nondominant
    b. dominant, nondominant
    c. strongest, weakest
    d. nondominant, dominant

109. The standard for measuring the diameter of the _____ of a needle is called the needle gauge.
    a. dialogue
    b. lumen
    c. bevel
    d. lunar

110. Medical supply manufacturers have produced some innovative new products to accommodate the new _____ regulations.
    a. HIPAA
    b. NCCLS
    c. CDC
    d. OSHA

111. Wrap the tourniquet around the patient's arm approximately _____ inches above the venipuncture site.
    a. 2–4
    b. 3–4
    c. 1–3
    d. 3–5

112. The loose ends of a tourniquet should be _____ the patient's arm, away from the puncture site.
    a. running up
    b. running down
    c. to the right of the vein
    d. to the left of the vein

113. Outpatients should remain sitting for _____ minutes before attempting a venipuncture for certain procedures.
   a. 30
   b. 10
   c. 15
   d. 20

114. If a patient tells you he or she feels faint or starts to faint during a phlebotomy procedure, you should first _____.
   a. apply a cold compress to the back of the patient's neck
   b. lower the patient's head between the knees
   c. remove the tourniquet and withdraw the needle
   d. call 911

115. If a patient has had a seizure, he or she should stay in the area for at least _____ and should be instructed not to operate a vehicle for at least _____.
   a. 30 minutes, 1 hour
   b. 15 minutes, 30 minutes
   c. 15 minutes, 45 minutes
   d. 45 minutes, 1 hour

116. _____ occurs when an improperly placed needle results in blood escaping from a vein.
   a. Hematoma
   b. Hemostasis
   c. Hemotoma
   d. Hemophilia

117. A child's blood vessel is smaller and is harder to _____.
   a. visualize
   b. auscultate
   c. palpate
   d. both a and c

118. _____ has determined the criteria for meeting the qualifications required for those who are to perform ABGs.
   a. CDC
   b. OSHA
   c. NCCLS
   d. CLIA

119. Blood smears that are improperly prepared will have a(n) _____ distribution of cells, which will give inaccurate test results.
   a. uneven
   b. smooth
   c. feathered
   d. exact

120. Which of the following is *not* a syringe size commonly used in the laboratory?
   a. 0.5 cc
   b. 5.0 cc
   c. 10.0 cc
   d. 60.0 cc

121. Which one of the following types of needles is *not* typically used when performing a venipuncture on an outpatient?
   a. Multisample needles
   b. Single-sample needles
   c. Hypodermic needles
   d. 18-gauge IV catheter needle

122. The phlebotomist may use up to a _____ inch blood collection needle when using the Saf-T Clik needle adaptor.
   a. 1-
   b. 1½-
   c. 1/2-
   d. 2-

123. A _____ is used to distend veins to facilitate venipuncture for intravenous injections.
   a. tourniquet
   b. plastic belt
   c. clenching of the fist
   d. none of the above

124. The Penrose drain tubing, used as a tourniquet, is typically _____ inches in length and 1/2 to 1 inch wide.
   a. 18 to 20
   b. 15 to 18
   c. 15 to 17
   d. 20 to 22

125. All of the following tubes are required to have a full draw *except* a _____ top evacuated tube.
   a. light blue
   b. lavender
   c. yellow sterile
   d. All of the above are required.

126. Nitrile gloves are _____.
   a. reusable
   b. hard to tear
   c. relatively inexpensive
   d. all of the above

127. Evacuated tubes are made of either glass or plastic and are available in a range of sizes of _____ milliliters.
   a. 2–13
   b. 3–15
   c. 1–13
   d. 2–15

128. All of the following are needed to perform an arterial puncture *except* _____.
   a. alcohol prep
   b. 0.5–1 percent lidocaine
   c. lancet
   d. plastic bag with ice

129. Which one of the following colored top evacuated tubes contains EDTA as an additive?
   a. Light blue
   b. Green-gray
   c. Royal blue
   d. Gray

130. When is it more appropriate to perform a venipuncture than a capillary puncture?
   a. When drawing on infants
   b. When a substantial vein can be located
   c. When a patient has fragile veins
   d. When a patient is overly apprehensive

131. When handling routine specimens after the blood draw, additive tubes must be _____.
   a. chilled immediately
   b. placed in a warming tray
   c. gently inverted
   d. quickly shaken

132. What is the best way to ensure that the centrifuge is balanced prior to spinning down your specimen for a STAT test?
   a. Wait for more specimens before running the centrifuge.
   b. Place an empty tube filled with equal amounts of water opposite your specimen.
   c. The centrifuge does not need to balanced if you are spinning down only one tube.
   d. None of the above applies.

133. When you are operating a centrifuge, the tubes must remain stoppered to prevent all of the following *except* ____.
   a. alteration of the specimens pH
   b. formation of an aerosol
   c. formation of condensation
   d. splashing of the specimen

134. To obtain a serum specimen, a _____ top evacuated tube must be used.
   a. green-gray
   b. red-gray
   c. brown
   d. gray

135. _____ is released into the blood during the process of a capillary puncture and contaminates the blood sample.
   a. Intersitial fluid
   b. Interstial fluid
   c. Interstitial fluid
   d. Interstitual fluid

136. _____ levels are higher than total proteins in capillary blood specimens.
   a. Potassium
   b. Calcium
   c. Iron
   d. Glucose

137. _____ is an inflammation of the bone marrow caused by a pathogenic organism.
   a. Osteochondiritis
   b. Osteomyelitis
   c. Osteocondritis
   d. Osteomylitis

138. Which one of the following is *not* a needed piece of equipment when performing a finger stick?
   a. Multisample needle
   b. Biohazardous waste container
   c. Pen
   d. Gloves

139. The blood smear is performed immediately after wiping away the _____ drop of blood from a capillary puncture.
   a. 1st
   b. 2nd
   c. 3rd
   d. There is no need to wipe any drops away.

140. "Antecubital" means _____.
   a. behind the elbow
   b. in front of the elbow
   c. beneath the elbow
   d. above the elbow

141. Of the following, which items may *not* be used when testing for blood alcohol levels?
   a. Green soap
   b. Water
   c. Iodine preparations
   d. Both a and b

142. During the centrifuge process, specimens are spun down for _____ minutes.
   a. 3
   b. 6
   c. 5
   d. 7

143. A _____gauge butterfly infusion set with a 2- to 3-milliliter evacuated tube provides the best results for blood specimen collection from an infant.
   a. 21-
   b. 23-
   c. 25-
   d. 27-

144. A patient's blood may be drawn, on average, _____ time(s) per day.
  a. one
  b. two
  c. three
  d. four

145. Cytogenics testing is drawn in a _____ top evacuated tube.
  a. gray
  b. black
  c. green-black
  d. green

146. Arterial blood is used for blood gases because its composition _____.
  a. is the same throughout the body
  b. is different throughout the body
  c. has metabolic activities
  d. none of the above

147. The _____ guidelines state which areas may be punctured and how deep the puncture may be on an infant heel stick.
  a. NCCLS
  b. CDC
  c. OSHA
  d. NIOSH

148. Patients must not be permitted to do which one of the following during the blood draw?
  a. Eat
  b. Sleep
  c. Talk
  d. None of the above

149. Pulling the skin taut when inserting the needle for venipuncture accomplishes which of the following?
  a. Secures the vein for ease of insertion
  b. Increases the pressure of blood flow
  c. Aids in helping the vein roll away from the needle
  d. All of the above

150. It is recommended that pediatric-sized _____ milliliter evacuated tubes be used with pediatric-sized tube adapters.
  a. 2-
  b. 4-
  c. 1-
  d. 3-

151. Arterial punctures can be performed in various sites; one such site is the _____.
  a. dorsalys pedas
  b. doralis pedes
  c. dorsalis pedis
  d. dorsilys pedis

152. ABGs are typically collected in _____ milliliter syringes depending on the amount of blood required.
  a. 1- to 3-
  b. 2- to 5-
  c. 3- to 5-
  d. 1- to 5-

153. Which one of the following is a step in the collection of an ABG?
  a. Cleansing of the site with povidone-iodine
  b. Cleansing the site with 70 percent isopropyl alcohol
  c. Recapping of the needle
  d. 5 minutes of exercise by the patient

154. PT tests are drawn using a _____ top evacuated tube.
  a. red
  b. royal blue
  c. light blue
  d. none of the above

155. What type of specimen is required when using a gray top evacuated tube?
  a. Serum
  b. Sodium
  c. Whole blood
  d. Plasma

156. A yellow top sterile evacuated tube is drawn after a _____ top evacuated tube.
  a. light blue
  b. green-gray
  c. red
  d. none of the above

157. In a capillary blood draw, a _____ stick ensures a better blood flow.
  a. sweeping
  b. deep
  c. slow
  d. both a and b

158. A phlebotomist may perform venipuncture on a patient with _____ directly above their veins.
  a. tattoos
  b. burns
  c. moles
  d. freckles

159. The Allen test determines _____.
  a. collateral circulation
  b. placement of the radial artery
  c. placement of the ulnar artery
  d. none of the above

160. Instruct patients not to carry or lift anything heavy with the arm the venipuncture occurred on for approximately _____ minutes.
    a. 90
    b. 30
    c. 60
    d. 45

161. After a venipuncture is performed, the bleeding should stop within _____ minutes or the physician must be notified.
    a. 7
    b. 3
    c. 5
    d. 6

162. The most commonly used needle is a _____ gauge, _____inch for radial and brachial punctures.
    a. 23-, 1-
    b. 22-, 1-
    c. 22-, 1½
    d. 23-, 1½-

163. The chance of a _____ is increased in an arterial puncture.
    a. hemostasis
    b. hematoma
    c. hemolysis
    d. hemolisys

164. Which one of the following is a step in the collection of an ABG?
    a. Rinsing the syringe with isopropyl alcohol
    b. Positioning the patient in the true anatomical position
    c. Having the patient extend his or her wrist
    d. Assessing collateral circulation

165. Clot activators and polymer gels are a special requirement for which color top evacuated tube?
    a. Red-gray
    b. Green-black
    c. Red-green
    d. All of the above

166. Which color top evacuated tube is affected by volume requirements?
    a. Red
    b. Yellow-black
    c. Green-gray
    d. Red-green

167. When collecting a capillary specimen on an infant, which of the following applies?
    a. Chill the heel to increase blood flow to the area.
    b. Never mix the specimens from microcollection containers.
    c. Label specimens with the patient's name and other appropriate information.
    d. Immediately place a bandage over the puncture site after completion of the puncture.

168. In the order of draw, a gray top evacuated tube is drawn before a _____ top evacuated tube.
    a. brown
    b. light blue
    c. green
    d. lavender

169. Which of the following procedures best describes how to position a tourniquet when a patient's skin is fragile or tears easily?
    a. Place the tourniquet on top of a thick hand towel.
    b. Place the tourniquet on top of the patient's shirt.
    c. Place the tourniquet over a paper tape brace.
    d. Do not use a tourniquet.

170. Dorsal hand veins are excellent sites for drawing labs on _____.
    a. teenagers
    b. neonates
    c. children over the age of 2
    d. adults

171. A venipuncture needle is generally inserted so that the _____.
    a. entire bevel is directly into the patient's vein
    b. entire bevel is slightly under the skin to prevent a hematoma
    c. bevel is partially in the vein to allow for quicker filling of the evacuated tube
    d. bevel is partially inserted through the vein into the underlying muscle

172. If the venipuncture needle has been inserted through the vein, blood seeps into the tissues causing a _____.
    a. hematoma
    b. hemolysis
    c. hemoconcentration
    d. hemostasis

173. When performing an ABG, a local anesthetic solution of _____ percent lidocaine is used to numb the site.
    a. 0.25–0.5
    b. 0.75–1
    c. 0.5–1
    d. 0.5–0.75

174. A lithium heparin solution of _____ units/milliliter is used to prevent the specimen needed for an ABG from clotting.
    a. 500
    b. 1,000
    c. 1,500
    d. 750

175. Lithium iodoacetate is an additive found in a _____ top evacuated tube.
   a. green
   b. gray
   c. green-gray
   d. light blue

176. Blood cultures are often ordered in sets that may be performed at the same time from two different sites or can be collected _____ apart.
   a. 30 minutes
   b. 20 minutes
   c. 1 hour
   d. 45 minutes

177. The total volume of blood drawn each day on a patient is determined by _____.
   a. age
   b. weight
   c. height
   d. gender

178. When warming an area for a capillary blood collection, a warm moist towel must be no hotter than _____ degrees Fahrenheit.
   a. 106
   b. 98
   c. 100
   d. 108

179. In sustaining the order of draw, a _____ top evacuated tube must be drawn before a lavender top evacuated tube.
   a. gray
   b. light blue
   c. brown
   d. red-green

180. The best way to learn to palpate veins is _____.
   a. with gloves on
   b. without gloves on
   c. by rubbing your finger across the patient's forearm
   d. after cleansing the site

181. There is a considerably less risk of creating a hematoma if ABGs are drawn from the _____ artery.
   a. femoral
   b. radial
   c. brachial
   d. ulnar

182. Patients that are on anticoagulant therapy or have bleeding disorders must be monitored closely for a minimum of _____ minutes after a blood draw.
   a. 15
   b. 30
   c. 20
   d. 45

183. When collecting specimens for a blood culture, inadvertent contamination can occur by _____.
   a. not allowing the antiseptic to dry
   b. using the wrong antiseptic
   c. not properly cleaning the site or blood culture bottles
   d. all of the above

184. Hypodermic needles for an ABG are _____ inches in length.
   a. 5/8–1½
   b. 1–1½
   c. 1¼–2
   d. 7/8–1

185. A(n) _____ concentration is taken prior to the collection of a specimen for an ABG.
   a. carbon dioxide
   b. oxygen
   c. carbon monoxide
   d. hemo

186. Mottled evacuated tube top colors indicate that the tube contains _____.
   a. lithium heparin
   b. sodium citrate
   c. gel barriers
   d. potassium oxalate

187. To prepare the syringe for an ABG puncture, the phlebotomist first needs to draw _____ milliliter of heparin in a syringe.
   a. 0.2
   b. 0.5
   c. 0.6
   d. 0.3

188. Tubes that contain anticoagulants should be no less than _____ percent full.
   a. 50
   b. 75
   c. 90
   d. 25

189. Of the following, which is the 4th step when collecting a capillary specimen?
   a. Washing hands
   b. Identifying the patient
   c. Explaining the procedure
   d. Gathering the supplies and equipment

190. Most standard ABG kits contain which of the following?
   a. A butterfly infusions set
   b. Patient ID labels
   c. Hot packs
   d. Both a and c

191. The improper application or use of tourniquets during a venipuncture can cause _____.
   a. hemoconcentration
   b. homeostasis
   c. hemostasis
   d. hemopoesis

192. An acid-base balance maintains arterial blood at approximately a _____ pH level.
    a. 7.25–7.35
    b. 7.75–7.25
    c. 7.35–7.45
    d. 7.45–7.55

193. For a syringe draw, insert the needle while holding it at a _____ degree angle.
    a. 15- to 20-
    b. 15- to 30-
    c. 20- to 30-
    d. none of the above

194. A _____ stick requires approximation of the anatomic location of the vein.
    a. palpated
    b. blind
    c. visual
    d. all of the above

195. The following are all included in the PPE and supplies required for ABGs except _____.
    a. gloves
    b. face masks
    c. goggles
    d. 10 percent bleach solution

196. The needle gauge used to administer an anesthetic for an ABG is _____.
    a. 17 or 18
    b. 20 or 21
    c. 22 or 23
    d. 25 or 26

197. A _____ top evacuated tube requires a whole blood specimen.
    a. yellow sterile
    b. black
    c. lavender
    d. all of the above

198. Bacteria in the blood is called _____.
    a. sepsis
    b. septicemia
    c. bacteriemia
    d. viralemia

199. If during the venipuncture process the site begins to swell, immediately remove the needle, release the tourniquet, and apply firm pressure with gauze pads on the site for _____ minutes.
    a. 7–9
    b. 7–10
    c. 6–9
    d. 8–10

200. A _____ top evacuated tube is drawn after a black top evacuated tube.
    a. gray
    b. red-green
    c. green-gray
    d. red-gray

201. A phlebotomist should clean the site of a capillary stick with a _____ percent isopropyl alcohol pad.
    a. 60
    b. 70
    c. 80
    d. 50

202. If a suitable vein cannot be found after checking arms, wrists, and back of hands, the phlebotomist should then ask the physician for permission to use which site?
    a. Feet veins
    b. Pelvic veins
    c. Ankle veins
    d. None of the above

203. The _____ artery has sufficient collateral circulation and is the second choice for an arterial draw.
    a. femoral
    b. radial
    c. ulnar
    d. brachial

204. Which one of the following steps should be performed last in an evacuated tube system of venipuncture?
    a. Cleaning the puncture site
    b. Withdrawing the needle
    c. Washing hands, donning gloves
    d. Removing the tourniquet

205. If a hematoma develops during a venipuncture, release the tourniquet, withdraw the needle immediately, and apply pressure for _____ minutes.
    a. 3
    b. 5
    c. 6
    d. 2

206. The most common needle size for a femoral arterial draw is a _____ gauge and _____ inches in length.
    a. 23, 1¼
    b. 23, 1½
    c. 22, 1¼
    d. 22, 1½

207. Of the following, which step is 1st in the collection of an ABG?
    a. Obtaining the patient's respiratory rate
    b. Opening the ABG kit
    c. Preparing the anesthetic
    d. Preparing the syringe

208. The black top evacuated tube contains 3.8 percent buffered _____.
    a. EDTA
    b. sodium citrate
    c. sodium bicarbonate
    d. heparin

209. To anesthetize for an ABG, insert the needle containing anesthesia at a _____ degree angle.
    a. 10-
    b. 25-
    c. 20-
    d. 15-

210. A _____ top evacuated tube has no special requirements.
    a. royal blue
    b. light blue
    c. black
    d. brown

211. A _____ top evacuated tube must be drawn after a royal blue top evacuated tube.
    a. yellow sterile
    b. lavender
    c. green
    d. yellow-black

212. While performing a venipuncture, do *not* _____.
    a. allow the patient to stand
    b. tell the patient it hurts
    c. use a chair without rollers
    d. talk to your patient

213. When applying a tourniquet do *not* _____.
    a. place the tourniquet 1–2 inches above the draw site
    b. place the tourniquet 3–4 inches above the draw site
    c. remove the tourniquet after 1 minute
    d. remove the tourniquet before withdrawing the needle

214. Which artery has the best collateral circulation?
    a. Brachial
    b. Femoral
    c. Radial
    d. Ulnar

215. When drawing on an elderly patient, the tourniquet must be _____.
    a. in place until just prior to the removal of the needle
    b. removed after insertion of the needle
    c. removed after the first tube is filled
    d. none of the above

216. When plasma or serum is required for testing, it must be transferred to a(n) _____.
    a. gray top evacuated tube
    b. brown top evacuated tube
    c. red top evacuated tube
    d. aliquot tube

217. The gauge of the hypodermic needles needed for an ABG varies from _____ to _____ depending on the location of the draw.
    a. 20, 23
    b. 20, 24
    c. 20, 25
    d. 23, 25

218. The collection syringe for an ABG must be placed in a coolant that can maintain a temperature of _____ degrees Celsius.
    a. 1–5
    b. 2–3
    c. 1–4
    d. 3–5

219. The additive in a green top evacuated tube is _____.
    a. Na heparin
    b. potassium oxalate
    c. ammonium heparin
    d. sodium fluoride

220. Glucose determinations are drawn on a _____ top evacuated tube.
    a. green
    b. gray
    c. brown
    d. none of the above

221. Blood cultures drawn for antimicrobial susceptibility testing are drawn in special collection bottles known as _____ bottles.
    a. RDA
    b. ARD
    c. DAR
    d. ADR

222. After cleaning the venipuncture site, allow the site to dry for a minimum of _____ seconds before performing venipuncture.
    a. 30–60
    b. 2–4
    c. 60–90
    d. 10–12

223. When you are collecting ABGs, the _____ artery is used only as a last resort, and the venipucture is typically performed by a physician.
    a. ulnar
    b. femoral
    c. radial
    d. brachial

224. Which of the following steps in an evacuated tube system of venipuncture is performed last?
    a. Applying the tourniquet
    b. Cleaning the site
    c. Allowing the site to air-dry
    d. Assembling equipment

225. "QNS" means _____.
    a. quality not satisfactory
    b. quality not sufficient
    c. quantity not sufficient
    d. quantity not satisfactory

226. To administer an anesthetic for an ABG a _____ gauge needle is used.
    a. 23- to 25-
    b. 25- to 26-
    c. 22- to 26-
    d. 23- to 26-

227. When preparing a syringe for an ABG, check for free movement of the barrel; then attach a _____ gauge needle to draw heparin with.
    a. 22-
    b. 23-
    c. 20-
    d. 25-

228. Serology testing is drawn on a _____ top evacuated tube.
    a. yellow sterile
    b. light blue
    c. red
    d. black

229. A _____ top evacuated tube contains the additive Na heparin.
    a. brown
    b. gray
    c. green
    d. royal blue

230. After an ABG has been collected, a patient on anticoagulation therapy must have pressure applied to the site for _____ minutes.
    a. 15
    b. 20
    c. 30
    d. 40

231. If the radial artery is damaged during arterial puncture, the _____ artery supplies blood to the area.
    a. femoral
    b. ulnar
    c. brachial
    d. all of the above

232. The blood-borne pathogens standards, set by _____, prohibit contaminated sharps from being bent, recapped, or removed.
    a. NIOSH
    b. CDC
    c. OSHA
    d. NACCLS

233. In the order of draw, a _____ top evacuated tube is the last to be drawn.
    a. black
    b. green-black
    c. red-green
    d. green-gray

234. In the order of draw sequence, a _____ top evacuated tube is the 6th tube to be drawn.
    a. royal blue
    b. gray
    c. lavender
    d. brown

235. Objects such as clothing, towels, and utensils that possibly harbor a disease agent and are capable of transmitting it are known as _____.
    a. carriers
    b. susceptible hosts
    c. fomites
    d. pathogens

236. The phlebotomist most commonly uses a gauze pad that is a _____ inch square.
    a. 2 × 2-
    b. 3 × 3-
    c. 4 × 4-
    d. none of the above

237. Microcollection tubes provide for all of the following *except* _____.
    a. centrifugation of the capillary specimen
    b. easy measuring
    c. chilling
    d. storing

238. Any needle smaller than a _____ gauge causes the red blood cells to lyse.
    a. 20
    b. 21
    c. 22
    d. 23

239. The point of a needle that has been cut on a slant for ease of entry is called a _____.
   a. lumen
   b. bevel
   c. luminary
   d. slant

240. Tube holders/adapters are _____.
   a. not available in adult sizes
   b. available in pediatric sizes
   c. not disposable
   d. not to be thrown into a sharps container

241. The equipment needed for a finger stick includes all of the following *except* _____.
   a. microcollection container
   b. biohazardous waste container
   c. tourniquet
   d. bandages

242. After the spreader slide has been backed into the drop of blood, it should be lowered to a _____ degree angle in order to quickly push the slide along the length of the stationary glass slide.
   a. 45-
   b. 30-
   c. 25-
   d. 15-

243. Which of the following is *not* a superficial vein of the arm?
   a. Basilic
   b. Cephalic
   c. Median cubital
   d. Radial

244. _____ is a relative increase in the number of red blood cells resulting from a decrease in the volume of plasma.
   a. Hemolysis
   b. Hemoconcentration
   c. Hemostasis
   d. Hematoma

245. Which of the following is *not* a method for temporarily marking a vein for venipuncture?
   a. Leaving a small dot of ink with a pen
   b. Leaving your finger over the vein
   c. Referencing the vein with a mole
   d. Positioning the corner of a clean alcohol prep pad in direct line with the vein

246. The _____ technique is not recommended because it increases the risk of an accidental needle stick.
   a. two-hand
   b. two-finger
   c. switching hand
   d. push/pull

247. Evacuated tubes are labeled with which of the following?
   a. Hospital ID number
   b. Patient's room number
   c. Tracking labels
   d. All of the above

248. Which multidraw needle is required equipment for an evacuated tube system venipuncture?
   a. 20 gauge
   b. 18 gauge
   c. 22 gauge
   d. 24 gauge

249. Using a _____ milliliter tube with a _____ gauge needle may cause hemolysis during a butterfly infusion set draw.
   a. 7-, 22-
   b. 5-, 23-
   c. 7-, 23-
   d. 5-, 22-

250. On a butterfly infusion set draw, the tourniquet may be left in place until the draw is complete, as long as the draw is accomplished within a _____ minute window.
   a. 1-
   b. 2-
   c. 3-
   d. 4-

251. Which of the following information needs to be included when you are labeling a tube of blood?
   a. Patient's initials
   b. Patient's social security number
   c. Phlebotomist's initials
   d. Patient's age

252. Specimens must be allowed to clot at room temperature for a minimum of _____ minutes before centrifuging.
   a. 10
   b. 15
   c. 20
   d. 30

253. The most commonly performed test requiring protection from light is a _____ test.
   a. glucose
   b. bilirubin
   c. cold agglutinins
   d. clotting factor

254. Specimens that require centrifuging are spun down, and the serum or plasma is pipetted off and transferred into a(n) _____ tube.
   a. spectrometer
   b. evacuated
   c. aliquot
   d. urine transfer

255. When making blood smears, which of the following statements is correct?
    a. The smear should be less than half the length of the slide.
    b. Once the slide has been made, you should blow on it to dry it quickly.
    c. The feathered edge is the most important area of the slide.
    d. Mark on the slide only with black ink.

256. If the physician has ordered a patient to be NPO, you must verify that he or she has *not* _____.
    a. vomited since midnight
    b. eaten or drunk anything since midnight
    c. had a bowel movement for 24 hours
    d. eaten anything that contained sugar in the last 24 hours

257. _____ requires wearing protective apparel during the processing of a specimen.
    a. CLIA
    b. CDC
    c. JCAHO
    d. OSHA

258. When removing the stopper from a tube, be sure to pull it _____.
    a. away from you
    b. toward you
    c. side to side
    d. straight up

259. A _____ specimen must be chilled after collection.
    a. liver enzyme
    b. blood gases
    c. thyroid panel
    d. CBC

260. All of the following cause an arterial blood sample to render inaccurate test results or to be rejected by the laboratory *except* _____.
    a. improper chilling of the specimen
    b. incorrect anticoagulant
    c. lack of air bubbles in the specimen
    d. air bubbles in the specimen

261. Destruction of the membrane of red blood cells and the liberation of hemoglobin, which diffuses into the surrounding fluid, is called _____.
    a. hemalisis
    b. hemalysis
    c. hemolysis
    d. hemilysis

262. Which one of the following tests is performed first?
    a. blood glucose
    b. blood smear slide
    c. hematocrit
    d. hemoglobin

263. _____ causes a blood specimen to be rejected by the laboratory.
    a. Use of PPE
    b. Using a butterfly collection system
    c. Inversion of blood tubes after collection of the specimen
    d. Improper labeling of tubes

264. _____ may also contain the same additives as evacuated tubes, and they are color coded in the same manner.
    a. Aliquot tubes
    b. Hematocrit tubes
    c. Microcollection containers
    d. Centrifuge balance tubes

265. An incomplete, or _____, draw refers to an evacuated tube or syringe that does not contain the required amount of blood to perform the requested tests.
    a. irregular
    b. long
    c. mini
    d. short

266. Although it may vary from laboratory to laboratory, the typical number of times a phlebotomist should attempt a draw on one patient before asking someone else to try is _____.
    a. 1
    b. 2
    c. 3
    d. 5

267. The return, or a backward flow, of blood in the evacuated tube is called _____.
    a. backflow
    b. reflow
    c. reflux
    d. flash

268. The _____ allows a slide to be prepared from an EDTA tube without removing the stopper.
    a. DIFF-SAFE
    b. EZ Drop
    c. Tube Eaze
    d. Slide-Safe

269. _____ is an excellent method for collecting blood specimens when only a small amount of blood is needed.
    a. Venipuncture
    b. Capillary puncture
    c. IV
    d. Butterfly

270. Specimens must be labeled immediately _____.
    a. after the patient leaves
    b. before transporting to the lab
    c. following the collection
    d. when through with rounds

271. Collection tubes should be transported stopper
_____.
    a. down
    b. horizontal
    c. upward
    d. off

272. When a specimen is received at the lab, all of the
following occur *except* _____.
    a. logging in
    b. prioritizing
    c. preparing for testing
    d. freezing

273. All of the following are reasons that blood specimens are rejected by the lab *except* _____.
    a. hemolyzed specimens
    b. QNS specimens
    c. labeled specimens
    d. improper tube selection

274. If the laboratory rejects a specimen, the phlebotomist must _____.
    a. collect the right specimens the next time the
    patient is drawn
    b. let another phlebotomist draw the patient
    c. collect a new specimen as quickly as possible
    d. wait exactly 24 hours and collect the speci-
    men again

275. _____ can contaminate blood slides and skin
punctures.
    a. Using alcohol to clean the site
    b. Allowing the antiseptic to dry
    c. The puncture site selected
    d. Powder from gloves

276. _____ specimens must be collected immediately.
    a. Fasting
    b. Timed
    c. Stat
    d. QNS

277. _____ sets the maximum time limit for separating serum and plasma from the cells at 2 hours
from time of collection.
    a. CLIA
    b. OSHA
    c. NACCLS
    d. Each lab sets own time frame.

278. A type of specimen requiring a near–body temperature (37.5 degrees Celsius, 98.6 degrees
Fahrenheit) even during transport is a _____.
    a. bilirubin
    b. cold agglutinins
    c. glucose
    d. thyroid-stimulating hormone

279. A(n) _____ is a machine used to separate substances of different densities.
    a. autoclave
    b. centrifuge
    c. hemacytometer
    d. incubator

280. Blood smears should be free of _____.
    a. jagged edges
    b. red blood cells
    c. bare slide surface
    d. white blood cells

281. Arterial blood specimens kept at 1–5 degrees
Celsius are accurate for _____ hours.
    a. 1–2
    b. 1.5–2
    c. 2–3
    d. 3–4

282. An order of draw is used to guarantee specimen
_____.
    a. integrity
    b. intensity
    c. sedimentation
    d. color

283. The _____ count is read on the feathered edge
of a blood slide.
    a. leukopenia
    b. differential
    c. RBC
    d. ESR

284. Routine specimens must arrive at the laboratory
within _____ minutes of collection.
    a. 20
    b. 35
    c. 45
    d. 60

285. Specimens can be centrifuged _____.
    a. once
    b. twice
    c. three times
    d. never

286. To clean a centrifuge of a broken evacuated glass
tube, you should *never* _____.
    a. use a wet paper towel
    b. wear heavy-duty utility gloves
    c. disinfect the area by following the facility's
    blood spill protocols
    d. sweep the tiny shards of glass into a gloved
    hand and dispose of them in a sharps con-
    tainer

287. Routine specimens must be centrifuged within
_____ minutes of collection.
    a. 45
    b. 60
    c. 90
    d. 120

288. Lavender top tubes are stable for 24 hours, but blood smears must be completed within _____ minutes of collection.
    a. 20
    b. 30
    c. 45
    d. 60

289. Potassium and cortisol specimens must reach the laboratory within a _____ minute window.
    a. 20-
    b. 30-
    c. 45-
    d. 60-

290. Once a specimen drawn in an SST is centrifuged, the separator gel prevents glycolysis for up to _____ hours.
    a. 8
    b. 12
    c. 24
    d. 36

291. A _____ specimen is collected for evaluation of microbial analysis or cytology studies.
    a. catheterized
    b. pediatric
    c. suprapubic
    d. midstream

292. Specimens drawn for glucose determination in tubes containing sodium fluoride, a glycolytic inhibitor, are stable for _____ hours at room temperature and for up to _____ hours when refrigerated.
    a. 24, 48
    b. 12, 24
    c. 24, 36
    d. 12, 36

293. _____ a specimen after collection slows down the metabolic processes, which would continue after the draw.
    a. Warming
    b. Chilling
    c. Inverting
    d. Centrifuging

294. For manually activated clotting times, the tube must be kept _____ during the procedure as well as before it.
    a. cold
    b. frozen
    c. warm
    d. hot

295. Proper handling of the specimen begins when the phlebotomist _____.
    a. receives the order
    b. prepares the equipment
    c. draws the specimen
    d. transports the specimen to the lab

296. To maintain specimen integrity, the phlebotomist must follow all of the following general guidelines *except* _____.
    a. transporting the specimen to the laboratory
    b. maintaining the temperature of the specimen
    c. selecting the time of collection
    d. processing the requisitions

297. Specimens requiring centrifugation are in one of two categories: _____ and _____.
    a. sodium, serum
    b. plasma, serum
    c. whole blood, serum
    d. plasma, whole blood

298. Repeating centrifugation causes _____ and inaccurate test results.
    a. hemolysis
    b. hemostasis
    c. hemoconcentration
    d. hyperkalemia

299. Specially designed _____ microcollection containers are available for the collection of bilirubin specimens from infants.
    a. black
    b. ecru
    c. amber
    d. brown

300. Tests requiring plasma specimens are collected in tubes containing _____, specific for the requested test.
    a. coagulants
    b. sodium heparin
    c. sodium citrate
    d. anticoagulants

CRITICAL THINKING

1. You are a phlebotomist for the blood bank, and it is your turn to work the front desk. Jillian, a patient of Dr. Hill, is having surgery in three weeks, and her physician has explained to her that she may need several units of blood during the surgery. The medical assistant at Dr. Hill's office mentioned that it might be possible for her to donate her own blood prior to surgery, and she has come to the blood bank today to find out what is required and if she can do this.
   • What will you tell her about this process?
   • What is this type of donation called?
   • What information will be needed for Jillian's specimens?

2. John, a firefighter, and his firehouse coworkers are in the clinic today for their semiannual physicals. Your responsibility is to collect a red top and lavender top evacuated tube from each firefighter. As

each of the firefighters has blood drawn, there is the expected heckling and joking with one another about who is going to pass out. The main heckler is next, and you immediately notice his sweaty brow as you verify his information and ask him to take a seat in the phlebotomy chair. You start to put together your needle and tube holder, all the while talking to him. You find a vein and ask, "How long have you been a firefighter?" You tie the tourniquet and say, "When was the last time you rescued a cat from a tree?" You uncap the needle, and, as you look up to see if he is smiling, he is dripping sweat, his eyes roll back, and without further warning he slumps forward and starts to slide out of the chair and onto the floor.

- What do you do next?

3. Suzie Allan, a 9-year-old mentally challenged young girl has been sent to the lab to have a stat lab test drawn. Suzie is sitting on her mother's lap in the draw chair, and she becomes agitated as you start to assemble your equipment and supplies. She tries to negotiate with her mom about coming back later. Suzie's mom tells her she has to have the test done now so the doctor can make her feel better. You try to establish a rapport with Suzie, telling her that it isn't going to hurt and that, if she is good, you will give her stickers when she is done. You convince her to let you look at the veins in her arm. The veins are rather small, but you think you might be able to collect the required specimen. You know you probably are going to have only one chance. You have assembled all the equipment, washed your hands, and donned your gloves. As you start to tie the tourniquet, Suzie becomes more and more agitated, arching her back and pulling away from you.

- Because this collection has been ordered stat what should you do?
- What error did you initially make with Suzie?

MODULE 7

Point-of-Care Testing, Other Laboratory Tests, and Nonblood Specimens

I. POINT-OF-CARE TESTING (POCT)

A. Point-of-care testing is performed by the phlebotomist at the location of the patient: at the patient's bedside, in the emergency room, or in ambulatory settings.

B. Types—Point-of-care tests
1. Hematocrit
2. Hemoglobin
3. Blood glucose level
4. Glucose tolerance test
5. Cholesterol
6. Coagulation monitoring (activated coagulation time, prothrombin time, activated partial thromboplastin time)
7. Bleeding time
8. Chemistry panels (blood gases, potassium, calcium, pH, sodium, blood urea nitrogen)
9. Pregnancy test
10. Strep test
11. Chemstrip urinalysis

C. Types—Each point-of-care test will be discussed under its own heading.

II. HEMATOCRIT

A. Purpose
1. The hematocrit measures the volume of the patient's red blood cells as a percentage of whole blood in relationship to the plasma.
2. Hematocrits are ordered by the physician to aid in the diagnosis and monitoring of:
   a. Anemia.
   b. Polycythemia.

B. Specimen collection, equipment, and processing
1. The specimen is collected in a plastic microhematocrit tube.
   a. Capillary puncture—If the blood specimen is collected from a capillary puncture, the specimen is collected in a heparinized microhematocrit tube, labeled by a red band around the top of the tube.
   b. Venipuncture—If the specimen is collected by venipuncture, it can be collected in a "plain" EDTA evacuated tube (containing no anticoagulant) and transferred to a microhematocrit tube, identified by a blue band toward one end.
2. Filling the microhematocrit tubes
   a. Two microhematocrit tubes are always collected.
   b. The tubes are filled a minimum of three-quarters of the way full.
   c. The tubes must be free of air bubbles.
   d. One end of the tubes is sealed with clay.
3. Centrifugation
   a. The microhematocrit tubes are placed in the centrifuge with the clay end out.
   b. The centrifuge must be balanced.
      (1) If only one patient's specimens are being "spun down," the two tubes are placed opposite each other in the centrifuge.
      (2) If specimens for more than one patient are being spun down, you must document which slots the tubes were placed in for each patient to avoid assigning the wrong test results.
   c. Specimens are spun down for 5 minutes.

C. Determining test results

1. Hematocrit reference value range—Normal results are within the following ranges:

   a. Newborns—51–61 percent

   b. 1 month—35–49 percent

   c. 6 months—30–40 percent

   d. 1 year—32–38 percent

   e. 6 years—34–42 percent

   f. Adult males—42–52 percent

   g. Adult females—36–48 percent

2. Using reader charts

   a. Procedure

      (1) Place the reader chart next to the spun-down tube.

      (2) Line up the top of the clay at the —0— Line on the chart and the top of the plasma line is lined up with the top line of the chart.

      (3) The result is determined by reading the line at which the red blood cells and buffy coat (white blood cells) separate.

      (4) Both tubes are read in this manner.

      (5) Take an average of the two tubes (add the two results and divide by two), and record it as the test result.

   b. Availability of charts

      (1) Some microhematocrit centrifuges are equipped with built-in charts.

      (2) Separate laminated microhematocrit reader charts are also available for those centrifuges containing no chart.

III. HEMOGLOBIN (hgb)

A. Purpose

1. Hemoglobin is the iron-containing protein pigment of the red blood cells that aids in:

   a. The transportation of oxygen to the cells of the body.

   b. The return of carbon dioxide to the lungs as a waste product to be expelled.

2. Tests for hemoglobin levels are performed to aid in the diagnosis of anemia.

B. HemoCue procedure—Clinical Laboratory Improvement Act (CLIA) waived POCT versus hemoglobinometer procedure.

1. The test may be performed on venous, arterial, or capillary blood.

2. The specimen is placed in the HemoCue microcuvette, and the microcuvette is inserted into the HemoCue machine.

3. Results are registered in the LED readout window of the machine and recorded.

4. The microcuvette is properly disposed of in a sharps container.

IV. BLOOD GLUCOSE LEVEL

A. Purpose

1. Blood glucose level tests are performed to:

   a. Aid in the diagnosis and management of diabetes mellitus in which patients are hyperglycemic.

      (1) Hyperglycemia pertains to the condition in which the blood sugar (glucose) is increased, as in diabetes mellitus.

   b. Monitor hypoglycemia.

      (1) Hypoglycemia pertains to a condition in which the blood sugar (glucose) is abnormally low, as in hyperinsulinism.

B. Types

1. Blood glucose tests may be ordered stat or as a timed specimen.

   a. For timed specimens, glucose levels not performed at the designated times may lead to a misinterpretation of the results.

2. Two types of timed requests are:

   a. Fasting blood sugar (FBS).

      (1) The patient is required to restrict dietary intake for 12 hours prior to the collection of a specimen for testing for glucose levels in the blood.

   b. 2-hour postprandial (PP).

      (1) Collection of this specimen occurs 2 hours after the ingestion of the patient's last meal.

C. Equipment and supplies

1. The handheld device is designed so that patients may use it at home.

2. Reagent strips are required by most glucose analyzers.

   a. Reagent strips must be kept in the airtight container in which they are packaged.

   b. The container may be opened only long enough to remove the reagent strip.

   c. Each reagent strip container is coded.

      (1) The analyzer must be set to match the code of the container for all reagent strips in the container.

      (2) This applies to the units that patients use at home and must be part of the patient education process.

D. Specimen collection and analysis

1. After a capillary puncture, the first drop of blood is wiped away and the next drop of blood is placed on the reagent strip.

2. Depending on the requirements of the analyzer used, the strip:
   a. *Either* has already been inserted into the analyzer.
   b. *Or* is now inserted into the analyzer.
3. The analyzer determines the results and displays them on the LCD readout screen.
   a. Note: Some glucose analyzers use microcuvettes instead of reagent strips. The procedure is basically the same, except that blood from the microcuvette, rather than a drop of blood, is placed on the reagent strip.

V. GLUCOSE TOLERANCE TEST (GTT)

A. Purpose—To evaluate the metabolism of glucose
B. Procedure
   1. A glucose tolerance test involves multiple collections of blood and urine over time.
   2. The test is similar to the 2-hour postprandial testing procedure, but rather than ingesting a high-carbohydrate meal, the patient is given a commercially prepared glucose drink, which consists of;
      a. Approximately 75 to 100 grams of glucose liquid for adults.
      b. About 1 gram per kilogram of a child's weight.
   3. Verification of test requirements
      a. Verify that the patient has fasted for the specified amount of time.
      b. Determine whether the patient has taken any of the various medications and substances that can interfere with the accuracy of the GTT.
         (1) Medication and substances that can interfere with the accuracy of the GTT are:
             (a) Salicylates.
             (b) Diuretics.
             (c) Alcohol.
             (d) Blood pressure medications.
             (e) Corticosteroids.
             (f) Anticonvulsive medications.
             (g) Estrogen or birth control pills.
      c. If the patient has not been fasting or has taken any of the medications listed below, the patient's physician must be notified to obtain instructions on how to proceed.
      d. Typically the test is rescheduled.
   4. The GTT procedure:
      a. Varies from institution to institution.

   b. Is specifically outlined in the facility's procedure manual, so that testing is performed consistently within the facility.
   c. Can vary in duration from 3 to 6 hours, with specimens being collected each half hour or hour.
5. Some facilities require a urine specimen be collected at the same time as the blood specimen and a urine glucose reagent test performed.
6. Timing is critical.
   a. Specimens not collected at a specific time may cause misinterpretation of results.
   b. It is normal for a patient's blood glucose level to be elevated after the ingestion of a high-carbohydrate meal, with glucose levels not returning to the normal parameters for approximately 2 hours.
   c. If a GTT specimen is collected prior to the 2-hour window, an elevated glucose level is recorded and misinterpreted by the physician.
7. Glucose tolerance testing can be performed:
   a. On the same handheld devices as a fasting blood glucose or 2-hour postprandial test.
   b. On more advanced devices.
      (1) Example: The OneTouch II Hospital Blood Glucose System automatically stores QC (quality control) data. The data is then linked via a laptop computer to the hospital's mainframe computer system, where the patient/client's permanent record is created and can be printed.

C. Determining results
   1. Glucose levels fluctuate normally throughout the day.
   2. In a person with a healthy carbohydrate metabolism, blood glucose levels return to the normal ranges of 65–110 milligrams/deciliter within 2 hours after ingesting high levels of carbohydrates or the glucose preparation.
   3. In a diabetic patient, due to the inability to metabolize glucose, values remain elevated over a longer than normal period of time.

VI. CHOLESTEROL

A. Function of cholesterol
   1. The medical community and the public have become increasingly concerned with HDL and LDL levels since the correlation between elevated cholesterol levels and heart disease has been established.

2. Cholesterol serves important functions:
   a. Approximately 80 percent of cholesterol is used to manufacture bile acids, allowing the body to digest lipids and fats.
   b. Cholesterol also plays a role in the production of hormones, such as testosterone, progesterone, and estrogen.
   c. It also can be found in the skin in large amounts. Cholesterol located in the skin assists in keeping the skin waterproof and aids in preventing evaporation of water from the body.

B. Diet and cholesterol levels
   1. Diet
      a. Certain foods are very high in cholesterol and therefore contribute to an increase in the cholesterol levels of individuals consuming large amounts of these foods.
      b. Examples:
         (1) Egg yolks
         (2) Dairy products
         (3) Red meat
   2. Effects of increased cholesterol levels
      a. With increased cholesterol levels, fats can be deposited in the inner lining of the arteries, creating a condition known as atherosclerosis.
      b. As the fat is deposited, it narrows the lumen of the artery, causing the edges to be rough.
         (1) This can result in blood clot formation. Blood clots may break off and cause a heart attack or stroke.
         (2) The artery may become so narrow that blood cannot circulate through it, cutting off blood supply to vital organs.

C. Purpose of test
   1. Overall cholesterol level has some diagnostic value; however, high-density lipoprotein (HDL) and low-density lipoprotein (LDL) levels have much more diagnostic value.
   2. HDL cholesterol:
      a. Functions to transport the fat from the tissues to the liver to be metabolized into bile acids.
      b. Therefore it is labeled the "good" cholesterol.
   3. LDL cholesterol:
      a. Transports the cholesterol to the tissues, such as the lining of the arteries, where it is deposited as plaque.
      b. It has earned the name "bad" cholesterol.

D. CLIA-waived POCT cholesterol kits.
   1. The majority of these kits involve the use of a reagent strip embedded with chemicals.

2. The chemicals react like the urine reagent strips in that the reaction to the chemicals makes the reagent strip change color.
3. Waived cholesterol kits
   a. Kits in use
      (1) AccuChek uses a reagent strip which changes colors to identify the levels.
      (2) The Cholestech LDX Analyzer has gained in popularity because it's able to determine blood not only cholesterol levels, but also HDL and LDL levels with a high degree of accuracy.
         (a) A cuvette, or cassette, is inserted into the analyzer in much the same way as in glucose testing.
         (b) The Cholestech LDX Analyzer is factory-calibrated and the cassette is encoded with a magnetic strip, which is read by the analyzer, as each cassette is tested.
         (c) Quantitative controls are included in each kit.
   b. Requirements
      (1) Many of the kits must be stored in the refrigerator and warmed to room temperature before use.
      (2) To prevent possible errors in cholesterol testing:
         (a) A fasting specimen is preferred.
         (b) If using capillary blood, it must be free-flowing
         (c) If using venipuncture blood, do not use tubes containing fluoride, oxalate, citrate, or EDTA as anticoagulants.
      (3) Maximum and minimum values are determined for accuracy. For each type of cholesterol test, determine the limitations of the device used.
      (4) Various substances can interfere with cholesterol testing. Read the accompanying literature of the test kit to determine what, if any, substance(s) interfere with the test results.
      (5) Do not touch the reagent pads or pipette tips with fingers, gloved or ungloved.
      (6) Quality control (QC) measures must be performed with each run of client samples.
      (7) Mix QC materials thoroughly by gentle inversion before testing.
      (8) Do not use test kits or controls beyond the expiration dates.

(9) Capillary samples must be inserted into the cassette within 4 minutes of collection.

VII. COAGULATION MONITORING

A. Purpose
1. Coagulation tests provide information concerning the ability of the patient's blood to clot.
2. Hemostasis is a critical factor when patients are:
   a. Being considered for surgical procedures.
   b. Treated for trauma.
   c. Receiving coagulation therapy for clotting disorders.
3. The ability to provide coagulation results quickly is imperative in settings such as:
   a. The emergency room.
   b. Intensive care units.
   c. Operating rooms and with dialysis patients.
4. Coagulation testing has a two-level quality control verification process in addition to a temperature control verification device. Coagulation studies must occur at 37.5 degrees Celsius (98.6 degrees Fahrenheit) to assure accuracy of results.

B. Equipment and supplies
1. There are several different types of hand-held instruments used for coagulation monitoring.
   a. Some devices use only a single drop of whole blood obtained from a capillary puncture.
   b. Others use citrated blood obtained by venipuncture.
   c. Most devices provide results in 5 minutes.
2. Coagulation monitoring includes ACT, PT, and PTT or APPT.
   a. Activated coagulation time (ACT)
      (1) ACT analyzes the activity of the intrinsic coagulation factors and is used to monitor heparin therapy.
         (a) Heparin is an anticoagulant that is administered intravenously to minimize and control clotting.
         (b) Heparin therapy must be closely monitored.
      (2) Procedure
         (a) A discard tube (red top) and a special gray top tube will be drawn. The ACT analysis is performed by collecting a small volume of blood in the discard tube, then transferring it to the prewarmed special gray top tube, containing a coagulation activator, such as siliceous earth, silica, or celite.
         (b) Assemble routine venipuncture equipment with the addition of a heat block or incubator and a stopwatch or timer.
         (c) Perform a routine venipuncture. Draw a 4-milliliter discard tube.
         (d) Draw blood into the prewarmed tube containing the clot activator. Start the timer as soon as blood flows into the tube.
         (e) When the vacuum in the tube is exhausted, mix the tube thoroughly and place it in the heat block for 60 seconds. *Note*: Even though the gray top tube looks like all other evacuated tubes, it contains less vacuum. Draw only a small volume of blood, approximately 2 cc.
         (f) After 60 seconds, rock the tube gently back and forth and visually inspect the blood for the first visible sign of a clot.
         (g) If no clot is apparent, place the tube back into the heat block for 5 seconds. After 5 seconds, remove it from the block and inspect it again.
         (h) Repeat the procedure every 5 seconds until the first visible clot is observed. At the first sign of a clot, stop the timer and record the time.
      (3) Inaccurate results—A number of situations can cause erroneous results.
         (a) Neglecting to start the timer as soon as the blood enters the tube; values are decreased.
         (b) A traumatic draw or an inadequate sample causes decreased values.
         (c) If the tube is not mixed thoroughly, the values increase.
         (d) Anticoagulant drugs, antibiotics, steroids, and barbiturates can also lead to erroneous results.
      (4) An automated version of the ACT test is available, the Hemochron system. With this system, the machine does the mixing and timing automatically. A special tube with a black plastic cap, provided by the manufacturer, must be used.
   b. Prothrombin time (PT)
      (1) Purposes—The PT procedure may be performed alone to:
         (a) Monitor oral anticoagulation therapy (Coumadin).

(b) In conjunction with a PTT, give an accurate picture of the patient's total clotting abnormalities.

(2) Role of prothrombin

   (a) Oral anticoagulants affect the synthesis of prothrombin, one of the 12 clotting factors produced by the liver.

   (b) Clotting occurs naturally when trauma or injury to tissue releases tissue thromboplastin.

   (c) Tissue thromboplastin, when combined with blood, activates the clotting mechanism.

   (d) Prothrombin then converts to thrombin, which causes fibrinogen to form the fibrin matrix in the clot.

(3) POCT using the Hemochron Jr. device

   (a) The device uses whole blood.

   (b) The PT normal values are 17 to 22 seconds.

   (c) If performed on plasma collected in sodium citrate tubes, the normal values are slightly less (11 to 13 seconds).

   (d) Some devices compensate for using whole blood versus plasma. If using one of these devices, the normal value range for whole blood is similar to plasma values.

c. Partial thromboplastin time (PTT) and/or activated partial thromboplastin time (APPT)

   (1) Purpose—Either the PTT or the APPT is used to evaluate doses of heparin therapy.

   (2) Procedure and results—Similar for both tests

      (a) The term "activated" in the second test indicates that the activation of a clotting factor has occurred to make the test more reproducible and sensitive.

      (b) Values from whole blood differ from plasma values, as with the PT procedure.

      (c) Normal values for the PTT or APPT using plasma may be between 24 and 34 seconds.

      (d) Whole blood values of 93 to 127 seconds are normal using the Hemochron Jr.

   (3) Testing devices

      (a) The CoaguChek and Hemochron Jr. are POCT devices that analyze coagulation values. Both devices are easy to operate and portable.

      (b) Hemochron Jr. requires that approximately 50 units/liter of whole blood be placed into a plastic cartridge.

      (c) CoaguChek requires less blood and uses programmed credit card–like cartridges that automatically calibrate the device and correct for changes in the lot number of reagents. This technology uses a laser photometer to detect the formation of a clot.

VIII. BLEEDING TIME

A. Purpose

   1. The bleeding time test detects platelet function disorders by testing platelet plug formation in the capillaries.

   2. Bleeding times are sometimes performed prior to surgeries to detect problems with hemostasis.

B. Prolonged bleeding time

   1. Prolonged bleeding can occur because of abnormal platelet function.

   2. The ingestion of aspirin, other salicylate-containing medications, or a number of other medications within 2 weeks prior to the test may result in a prolonged bleeding time.

C. Type of puncture

   1. A bleeding time test is performed using a standardized puncture performed in the earlobe, finger, or inner surface of the forearm.

   2. Beginning in 1910 bleeding times were routinely performed on the earlobe, as described by Duke. Physicians rarely request the use of the earlobe today.

   3. In 1941 Ivy modified the Duke bleeding time by requiring the incision be performed on the volar surface of the forearm, using a blood pressure cuff to maintain a constant pressure. A thin incision was made with a sterile lancet.

   4. Today most labs use a modified version, controlling the width and depth of the incision by using an automated incision device, such as the Surgicutt.

IX. CHEMISTRY PANELS

A. Purpose

   1. Chemistry panels are groups of tests, such as blood gases and electrolytes, that are commonly ordered as stat tests.

a. The body must maintain these analytes in very narrow ranges.

b. If they are out of range, they must be corrected quickly or the imbalance can lead to death.

2. When ordered in the ER or critical care situations, results must be accurate and supplied immediately.

B. Chemistry panel devices

1. A number of devices are available to perform POCT chemistry panels:

   a. i-STAT

   b. IRMA

   c. AVL OPTI

   d. NOVA Stat Profile Analyzer

   e. Gem Premier

2. Use of equipment

a. The machines initially calibrate upon start-up.

b. Once the calibration is completed, a blood sample is injected into the device's sensors.

c. After the procedure, which takes less than 2 minutes, the cartridge is removed from the device and discarded in a biohazardous waste container.

d. The results are displayed on the readout screen of the device and a printout can be generated.

C. Types—Values for blood gas values (pH, pCO_2, pO_2, and BUN), electrolytes, glucose, and Hct values

1. Arterial blood gases

a. Arterial blood gases include:

(1) pH—Measurement of the bodies acid-base balance

   (a) Indicates the patient's metabolic and respiratory status.

   (b) The normal range for arterial blood pH is 7.35 to 7.45.

   (c) Below 7.35 is referred to as acidosis, and a pH level above 7.45 is considered to be alkalosis.

(2) Partial pressure of carbon dioxide (pCO_2) measurement of the patient's ability to exchange air between the blood and lungs.

   (a) pCO_2 measures the pressure exerted by dissolved CO_2 and is proportional to the pCO_2 in the alveoli.

   (b) Rate and depth of respiration maintain CO_2 levels.

   (c) An increase in pCO_2 is associated with hypoventilation, while a decrease in levels is associated with hyperventilation.

(3) Partial pressure of oxygen (pO_2)—Measurement of the pressure exerted by dissolved O_2 in the plasma

   (a) pO_2 indicates the lung's ability to diffuse O_2 through the alveoli into the blood.

   (b) pO_2 levels are used to determine the effectiveness of oxygen therapy.

b. Importance

(1) Analysis of the blood for these gases is important in helping to evaluate the extent of the deviation of acids and bases from the normal.

(2) Before appropriate therapy can be instituted, information obtained from those values is analyzed with respect to other laboratory results and clinical conditions.

2. Electrolytes—The most common electrolytes measured by POCT:

a. Sodium (Na+)

(1) Sodium functions in maintaining osmotic pressure and acid-base balance.

(2) It also aids in the transmission of nerve impulses.

(3) It is the most plentiful electrolyte in serum or plasma.

b. Potassium (K+)

(1) Location

   (a) Potassium is primarily found in the cells of the tissue.

   (b) It is released into the blood plasma only when cells are damaged, and it can be falsely increased if a blood specimen is hemolyzed.

(2) Functions—Potassium plays a major role in:

   (a) Nerve conduction.

   (b) Muscle function.

   (c) Acid-base balance.

   (d) Osmotic pressure.

   (e) Cardiac output (helps to control the rate and force of heart contraction).

(3) A lack of potassium is called hypokalemia; increased potassium is called hyperkalemia.

c. Chloride (C1−):

(1) Location—In the extracellular spaces, as sodium chloride (NaCl)

(2) Functions—Maintains cellular integrity by affecting osmotic pressure and acid-base water balance.

(3) Importance—Must be replaced along with potassium when treating a patient for hypokalemia

d. Bicarbonate ion (HCO_3-)—Aids in:

(1) Transporting carbon dioxide (CO_2) to the lungs.

(2) Regulating blood pH.

e. Ionized calcium (iCA++)

(1) Location

(a) Approximately 45 percent of the blood's calcium is ionized calcium.

(b) The remaining calcium is bound to proteins and other body substance.

(2) Functions—Used by the body for critical functions, such as:

(a) Muscular contraction.

(b) Cardiac function.

(c) Transmission of nerve impulses.

(d) Blood clotting.

(3) Only ionized calcium can aid in the above functions.

3. Blood urea nitrogen (BUN) level

a. Purpose—To provide a rough estimate of the patient's kidney function.

b. Significance

(1) Nitrogenous waste in the blood, in the form of urea, is the metabolic product of the breakdown of amino acids used for energy production.

(2) The normal concentration is 8 to 18 milligrams/deciliter.

(3) An increase in the blood urea nitrogen level usually indicates decreased renal function.

X. PREGNANCY TEST

A. Purpose

1. Pregnancy tests determine the levels of human chorionic gonadotropin (hCG or HCG).

2. Human chorionic gonadotropin:

a. Is present in increasingly higher levels during pregnancy, in both urine and blood.

b. Peaks between the 50th and 80th day of gestation.

c. Then starts to decrease.

B. Determining results

1. The first morning specimen has the highest concentration of hCG and is the optimum specimen to test.

2. Reasons for false results

a. hCG may not be present in sufficient amounts for the first 1 to 2 weeks after conception; so it is possible to have false negative test results during this time period.

b. hCG has been found to increase in other conditions, such as choriocarcinoma or malignant tumors of the ovaries or testes.

c. Various medications may also interfere with the test by producing false positive and negative results.

d. Detergents, protein, hematuria, and excessive bacterial contamination may invalidate test results.

C. Test kits—One-step tests are:

3. QuickVue One-Step HCG-Urine test

4. CARDS OS

D. Quality control—A positive and negative control test should be performed with each patient's specimen, making sure to accurately document each controls result.

XI. RAPID STREP TEST

A. Purpose

1. A rapid strep test is performed to determine the presence of a group A beta streptococcal infection. Typically performed when a patient has a sore throat or tonsillitis and strep is suspected as the causative agent.

2. Strep A can be detected by bacterial culture or by a rapid slide or tube test.

a. Time is the number one advantage to performing a rapid strep test versus a bacterial culture. If a bacterial culture is performed, the results will not be available for 24 to 48 hours.

b. If the test results from a rapid strep test are positive, antibiotic therapy can be started right away. If the results are questionable, a bacterial culture and sensitivity can be performed to confirm results.

B. Specimen collection

1. There are several CLIA-waived throat culture collection and testing kits available.

2. Follow the manufacturer's directions included with the kit.

XII. CHEMSTRIP URINALYSIS

A. Purpose

1. The value of these tests in clinical diagnosis can be immeasurable.

2. The physical and chemical analysis of urine involves simple observation and color comparisons.
B. Physical characteristics—Include color, appearance (clarity or transparency), odor, and foam
   1. Color
      a. Urine color can vary from almost completely colorless to black, with a range of colors in between.
      b. Observe the color in the collection cup or in the centrifuge tube.
         (1) The color may vary by degrees from one to the other.
         (2) Observe according to testing involved.
      c. The color of a normal urine specimen is directly related to the concentration of the specimen's solutes. Concentration may vary depending on the time of day.
         (1) First morning specimens are often darker in color because the urine has been collecting in the bladder overnight and has a higher concentration of solutes.
         (2) Random midday specimens may appear lighter in color because they have been diluted due to fluid intake.
      d. Normal versus abnormal color
         (1) Normal urine color is described as yellow, gold, amber, or straw, and may be further clarified by pale, light, or dark (i.e., pale yellow or dark amber).
         (2) The normal colors of urine are due to three urinary pigments:
            (a) Urochrome (yellow)
            (b) Uroerythrin (red)
            (c) Urobilin (orange/yellow)
         (3) Abnormal urine colors come in a wide variety. Some are clinically significant, while others are simply due to the ingestion of certain foods or medications.
   2. Appearance/transparency—Includes turbidity, sediment, and clarity
      a. The specimen must be:
         (1) Well mixed prior to examination so that any sediment that has settled in the bottom of the container is evenly distributed throughout the specimen.
         (2) Observed in a clear container so that there is no distortion.
      b. Terms used to describe the transparency of the urine specimen
         (1) Clear
         (2) Hazy

         (3) Cloudy
         (4) Turbid
         (5) Milky
      c. Results
         (1) A normal freshly voided specimen appears clear.
         (2) Urine may appear hazy, cloudy, turbid, or milky due to the presence of:
            (a) Epithelial cells.
            (b) White blood cells
            (c) Red blood cells.
            (d) Crystals.
            (e) Fats.
            (f) Protein.
            (g) Bacteria.
            (h) Other contaminants, such as toilet tissue, medications (e.g., antibiotics), talcum powder, or radiographic material.
         (3) Other considerations: A urine specimen may be cloudy due to crystals and cells that will centrifuge out; bacteria will not.
         (4) Some of these substances are normal constituents of urine in small amounts.
            (a) Example: Bacteria and epithelial cells are pathological only in larger quantities.
      d. Chemical testing of specimens (with reagent strips) may help to differentiate an increase in some of these substances, but for a definitive clarification a microscopic examination must be performed.
         (1) Microscopic urine readings are not CLIA-waived tests.
   3. Odor and foam
      a. Urine specimens are no longer wafted to odor, because doing so presents a health risk to the health professional.
      b. Strong urine odors are hard to ignore.
         (1) Aromatic—A freshly voided specimen
         (2) Fruity or sweet—May be due to acetone in diabetic acidosis, starvation, or dieting
         (3) Foul or putrid—Urine may not be freshly voided or may be associated with the growth of bacteria
         (4) Rotten egg—Decomposition of urine containing cystine or pus
         (5) Ammonia—Particularly during decomposition of urine upon standing (alkaline fermentation) or retention in the

urinary bladder, possibly related to some bacterial infections

    (6) Foam

        (a) The appearance of a "lasting" white foam suggests the presence of increased protein and perhaps renal disease.

        (b) The presence of a deeply pigmented yellow foam on yellow-brown or yellow-green urine may indicate the presence of bilirubin or biliverdin. Proceed with caution because this may indicate hepatitis.

        (c) Note: Wear appropriate PPE when handling urine specimens.

C. Chemical analysis

  1. The reagent strip, used in what is sometimes called the dipstick method, may be used to evaluate:

    a. pH.

    b. Protein.

    c. Glucose.

    d. Ketones.

    e. Blood.

    f. Bilirubin.

    g. Urobilinogen.

    h. Nitrite.

    i. Leukocytes.

    j. Specific gravity.

  2. Reagent strips are thin white plastic strips with a number of absorbent pads attached, one for each analysis. Each pad is impregnated with all the necessary reagents for a color change.

    a. After the strip has been dipped into the urine, the color is then compared at a specific time to a color chart on the product bottle.

    b. The number of tests on the strip can vary.

    c. Some tests are available individually.

  3. Types of strips—Multistix and the Chemstrip are two brands of reagent strips that are very similar and dominate the medical market.

  4. Procedure

    a. Preparation

      (1) Remove the strip(s) from the bottle, which must be stored in a cool, dry, and dark place and never refrigerated.

      (2) Never remove more than the number of strips to be used immediately. Replace the lid and keep it tightly closed.

      (3) Make sure the urine specimen has been well mixed.

      (4) Completely immerse the strip into the urine specimen, and wipe the excess specimen off the strip against the rim of the tube or specimen container. The strip may also be blotted with an absorbent paper.

      (5) Keep the strip in a horizontal position, so as not to allow the mixing of reagents from one pad to another.

      (6) Begin timing at the time of immersion.

      (7) Each pad's timing requirement is listed on the color comparison chart on the side of the bottle. Note the results of each reagent pad at the exact time indicated.

        (a) Note: For some tests, the reaction continues to change after the designated time. Therefore accurate timing is critical.

    b. Reading the reagent pads

      (1) pH—Measure of the acidity or alkalinity of the specimen.

        (a) The measurement of the urine pH may identify a respiratory, metabolic acid-base balance disorder, a urinary tract infection, or renal calculi formation.

        (b) Urinary pH varies from 5 to 9, with 7 being considered neutral.

        (c) Acidity is less than 7 and alkaline is greater than 7.

        (d) If urine from the protein pad is allowed to run over the pH reagent pad, an alkaline specimen can produce an acid result.

      (2) Protein

        (a) Albumin is the primary protein found in urine, and the reagent strip test detects only its presence; other types of proteins are not detected.

        (b) In normal urine there is no (or very little) protein.

        (c) The normal range is reported as negative to trace amounts.

        (d) If there is damage to the Bowman's capsule, as might occur in renal disease, the large protein molecules may pass into excreted urine. This is called proteinuria.

      (3) Glucose

        (a) Glucose is a metabolic threshold substance that spills over into the urine when the blood concentration surpasses approximately 170 milligrams/deciliter (the amount required for body function).

(b) The value of determining the presence of glucose in the urine, glucosuria, is for the diagnosis and management of diabetes mellitus.

(c) The reagent strip for glucosuria is enzymatic and a specific test; in other words, it is positive only if glucose is present.

(d) The color changes vary with the concentration of glucose. The color chart ranges from negative to 2,000 milligrams/deciliter, or 0.1 to 2.0 percent.

(4) Ketones

(a) Ketones, or ketone bodies, are normal end products of fat metabolism.

(b) Ketones may be toxic to the brain and are most often elevated in patients with diabetes but may be present in patients with severe vomiting, dieting, and starvation.

(c) The muscles of the body normally utilize ketones, but when the supply of carbohydrates is jeopardized or depleted, as in extreme dieting, the body increases the metabolism of fat for energy and ketonuria is the result.

(5) Blood

(a) Blood is detected in the urine as either intact red blood cells (hematuria) or as hemoglobin from lysed cells (hemoglobinuria).

(b) Blood can be present as part of a pathological process, or it can be nonpathological.

Nonpathological blood could be caused by contamination of the specimen from menstrual blood.

If pathological blood is present due to kidney damage, it suggests damage of the glomerular membrane or bleeding along the urinary tract.

(c) Myoglobin, a muscle form of hemoglobin, will also give a positive reaction.

(6) Bilirubin

(a) Bilirubin is a normal end product of the breakdown of hemoglobin, as a part of red blood cells' destruction.

(b) It is normally present in the blood but not in the urine.

(c) In the urine, it is a significant indicator of liver disease, such as hepatitis and cirrhosis, disease of the gallbladder, and cancer.

(7) Urobilinogen

(a) Urobilinogen is a product of disintegration of bilirubin after it passes from the bile ducts into the intestines.

(b) The bilirubin reaction and the urobilinogen reaction, when studied together, give the physician valuable diagnostic information.

(c) Urobilinogen then continues to be transformed by bacteria into urobilin. Urobilin is one of the normal urinary chromogens, a strong urinary pigment.

Urobilin is also responsible for the normal color of feces, but it is not detectable by the reagent strip test.

(d) It is abnormal to have a negative urinary urobilinogen value unless the bile duct is obstructed.

(8) Nitrite test

(a) The nitrite test is performed, like the leukocyte test, to screen for urinary tract infections (UTIs).

(b) It is an indirect method to detect significant bacteria in the urine, detecting the presence of nitrites rather than bacteria.

(c) The leukocyte test helps to further determine the presence of a UTI.

(9) Leukocytes (white blood cells)

(a) The presence of leukocytes (white blood cells) in urine is often associated with bacterial urinary tract infections.

(b) A positive nitrite test, in conjunction with a positive leukocyte test, is often indicative of a urinary tract infection.

(c) The reagent pad changes to shades of purple, in direct relationship with the numbers of leukocytes present.

(d) Besides the nitrite and leukocyte tests, other chemical results that clinically support the UTI findings are a urinary pH that is alkaline, positive blood, and positive protein reactions.

(10) Specific gravity

(a) The specific gravity of urine evaluates the kidneys' ability to concentrate and dilute.

(b) The reagent pad color changes are easy to interpret.

XIII. OTHER LABORATORY TESTS

A. Toxicology specimens—Blood alcohol and forensic specimens

1. Purposes

   a. Occasionally, for forensic or legal reasons, law enforcement officials request a blood, urine, or other body fluid specimen. The most commonly requested tests are blood alcohol levels, drug levels, and specimens for DNA analysis.

   b. A patient's blood alcohol (ethanol or ETOH) level may be ordered by the patient's physician to monitor alcohol intake.

   c. The police department may request blood alcohol levels be drawn for legal reasons.

2. Forensic specimens

   a. For forensic specimens, you must follow a special protocol, referred to as a chain of custody.

   b. Chain of custody:

      (1) Requires detailed documentation.

      (2) Entails accountability for the specimen at all times, from the time it is collected until the results are reported.

      (3) If the documentation is incomplete or inaccurate, specimen integrity may be called into question and any legal action may be impaired.

   b. Requirements

      (1) A chain of custody form is used to identify the specimen and the person or persons who obtained the specimen.

         (a) Particular attention must be paid to the date, time, and place of the collection.

         (b) The person from whom the specimen was obtained and the signature of the person obtaining the collection must both be on the form in the appropriate places.

(c) Identification of the person and the collection of the specimen must both be performed in the presence of a witness, frequently a police officer.

(d) Special seals and containers are required for the specimen.

(e) The phlebotomist who performs the collection of a specimen may be summoned to appear and testify in court as to the collection of the specimen.

(2) Cleansing the site

   (a) Because they may affect the results of the alcohol content determination, do not use in skin preparation: 70 percent isopropyl alcohol wipes. Iodine preparations, which also contain alcohol.

   (b) A nonalcohol-containing alternative, such as green soap and water, is used instead.

(3) Container

   (a) A gray top, sodium fluoride evacuated tube is required for specimen collection.

   (b) The tube may or may not have an anticoagulant, depending on the need for serum or plasma.

   (c) Alcohol is volatile and easily evaporates; completely fill the tube until the vacuum is depleted.

   (d) The stopper should not be removed until absolutely necessary for testing.

3. Drug testing specimens

   a. Drug testing always has legal implications. As with forensic and blood alcohol testing, drug testing requires special chain-of-custody protocols.

   b. Drug testing requires special donor preparation and collection procedures, as defined by the National Institute on Drug Abuse (NIDA).

   c. Donor preparation requirements

      (1) Positive identification of the donor, in the form of a picture identification, is required.

      (2) The test purpose and procedure must be explained.

      (3) The donor has to be advised of his or her legal rights.

         (a) The donor has the right to refuse the test if it is for preemployment.

(b) The company requesting the test is advised of the donor's refusal.

(c) Normally, a consent form has been previously signed by the donor, with the company requesting the test.

d. Every organization requesting drug testing must have an outline, following NIDAs guidelines, of the exact procedures to follow in its policies and procedures manual.

e. Other requirements

(1) On-site or off-site collections must designate a secure area for drug testing, according to NIDA standards.

(2) The lavatory must be specially prepared.

(a) Access to water must be eliminated.

(b) Faucets must be taped off.

(c) Toilet tank lids must be taped shut.

(d) A special tape is used that tears easily but that, once applied, cannot be pulled free from the surface. If removed or torn, it leaves a telltale sign that it has been tampered with.

(e) A blue dye is placed in the toilet water and must be replaced for subsequent collections.

(f) The lavatory must be inspected for hidden urine samples or other substances that could affect the test. Cabinets under the sink must be inspected and taped shut. Waste receptacles, paper towel dispensers, and the area under the toilet bowl must be investigated.

(3) Once the facility is prepared and the donor identified:

(a) Open the drug testing collection kit in front of the patient.

(b) Ask the donor to fill in the required areas on the chain of custody form.

(c) The donor will be asked to provide proof of any prescription medications if there is a positive result.

f. Specimen collection

(1) A witness may be present in the lavatory during the collection of the specimen to ensure that the required patient provides the sample.

(2) Drug testing collection kits provide a collection container with a temperature strip attached, to ensure the specimen is freshly voided.

(3) The temperature of the specimen is written on the chain of custody form.

(4) A split sample may be requested for confirmation or parallel testing. In this case the sample that is collected in the collection cup is poured into two separate containers.

g. The collection container

(1) The specimen from the collection cup is poured into the container(s) while the patient witnesses the procedure.

(2) Evidence seals are attached to the chain of custody form, and the specimen ID number from the chain of custody form is stamped on the evidence seal.

(3) Once the specimen is in the transportation container, remove the evidence seal from the form and place it over the lid so that it covers both sides of the container.

(4) The donor and the collector both initial the seal, and the collector writes the date and time of collection in the appropriate space.

(5) The specimen is then placed in a tamperproof bag and sealed in the presence of the donor.

(6) The form is completed and signed by the donor.

(7) The collector signs the form, indicates the date, time, and collection site.

h. The specimen is delivered to the laboratory for testing.

(1) All laboratory personnel and anyone else (including delivery personnel) who handle the specimen document their involvement by signing the chain of custody form until the results are reported.

i. Most common drugs detected in drug screens

(1) Alcohol

(2) Amphetamines—Meth, speed, crystal meth, ice

(3) Barbiturates—Seconal, phenobarbital

(4) Benzodiazepines—Valium, Libruim, Xanax

(5) Cocaine—Crack

(6) Cannabinoids—Marijuana

(7) Methadone—Dolophine

(8) Opiates—Heroin, morphine, codeine

(9) Phencyclidine—PCP, angel dust

(10) Propoxyphene—Darvon, Darvocet

B. Therapeutic drug monitoring (TDM)
  1. Purpose
    a. Prescription drug effects may vary depending on the dosage. Exact dosages are required to produce the desired effect; so physicians order therapeutic drug monitoring to manage individual patient drug treatment.
    b. This allows the physician to:
      (1) Establish drug dosages.
      (2) Maintain dosages at beneficial levels.
      (3) Avoid drug toxicity.
  2. Peak and trough levels—Require monitoring and evaluation at peak and trough levels for the physician to determine a safe and effective dose
    a. Peak levels
      (1) Are collected when the highest serum concentration of the drug is anticipated, typically 30 to 60 minutes after administration.
      (2) Screen for drug intoxication.
      (3) And/or help in monitoring whether the blood level is within the therapeutic range for that day.
    b. Trough levels:
      (1) Are when the serum concentration of the drug is at its lowest point, usually just prior to administration of the next scheduled dose.
      (2) Are monitored to ensure that levels of the drug stay within the range of therapeutic effectiveness.

C. Paternity testing
  1. Purpose—To determine the probability that a specific individual fathered a child.
    a. Typically paternity testing eliminates the possibility of paternity, rather than proving it.
    b. Paternity testing can be requested by physicians, lawyers, child support enforcement bureaus, or by individuals.
  2. Nature of test—Based on:
    a. ABO and Rh typing.
    b. Other proteins on the surface of the red blood cells.
  3. Note: This procedure is rapidly being replaced by DNA testing.
  4. Requirements
    a. Paternity testing requires chain of custody procedures.
    b. It may require fingerprinting of the individual.
    c. The mother, child, and alleged father are all tested.

D. Skin tests
  1. Types and purposes
    a. The TB test, also called a PPD test, is the test for tuberculosis and is the most common type of skin test.
    b. The Schick test is for diphtheria.
    c. The Dick test is for susceptibility to scarlet fever
    d. The Coccidioidomycosis (cocci) test is for an infectious fungus disease.
    e. The Histoplasmosis (histo) test is for past or present infection by the fungus *Histoplasma capsulatum.*
  2. Procedure
    a. Skin testing involves the injection of minute amounts of allergens or disease-producing microorganisms that stimulate an antibody reaction.
    b. The substance is injected intradermally, using a TB syringe or 1-cc syringe with a 26- to 27-gauge, 1/2-inch needle.
    c. The syringe is held at a 15- to 20-degree angle, and the needle is inserted under the skin just past the bevel of the needle.

E. Fecal occult blood test
  1. Purpose—The detection of occult blood in a patient's stool (feces) is an important diagnostic tool in the early detection of:
    a. Colorectal cancer.
    b. Other digestive disorders, including gastric ulcers and colitis.
  2. Nature of the test
    a. The test is performed using specially designed, CLIA-waived fecal blood test kits, containing a small cardboard card on which feces are smeared.
      (1) Examples:
        (a) HemaCheck
        (b) Hemoccult SENSA Fecal Occult Blood Test
    b. The primary reaction is caused by a color reaction, which occurs due to the mixture of hemoglobin and gum guaiac.
      (1) Some of the kits use a filter paper that has been impregnated with gum guaiac.
      (2) Other kits add it as a reagent.
      (3) All kits use visual color comparison to determine results.
  3. Procedure—The two parts to this procedure (patient preparation and specimen collection) are equally important.
    a. Patient preparation

(1) Diet—Patients must:
  (a) Not eat red meat, turnips, or horse-radish for at least 2 days prior to testing and throughout the duration of the test
  (b) Discontinue the use of aspirin and iron intake for at least 1 week prior to the test.
  (c) Discontinue taking Vitamin C and anti-inflammatory drugs.
  (d) Eat only small amounts of chicken, tuna fish, peanuts, popcorn, or bran cereal.
  (e) Eat a high-bulk diet of breads and cereals, plenty of vegetables (such as lettuce, spinach, and corn), and plenty of fruits (such as prunes, grapes, plums, and apples) for a minimum of 1 week prior to the collection.

b. Specimen collection—The following procedure is commonly repeated for 3 consecutive days. The patient must:
  (1) Be instructed in the appropriate collection techniques, especially if the collection is to take place at home.
  (2) Be provided with three collection kits, each containing a wooden applicator stick and a cardboard test apparatus.
  (3) Completely fill out the required information on the cover of the cardboard kit, especially the date and time of collection.
  (4) Be instructed on how to collect the specimen properly:
    (a) Flush the toilet before beginning and collect the specimen in a clean container.
    (b) Take care so that water from the toilet is not collected with the specimen. There are a variety of way to accomplish this:
      Specially designed toilet "hats" can be fit over the toilet bowl under the seat.
      Saran Wrap can be fit over the bowl in much the same manner as the toilet hat.
      A paper plate may also be used.
    (c) Once the specimen is collected, smear a sample on the paper side of one cardboard kit.
    (d) Take a sample from a completely different part of the specimen and smear it on the other test area.
    (e) The wooden stick is then discarded. (If the specimen is collected in a medical facility, the stick must be discarded in a biohazard container.)
    (f) The cardboard slide pack is sealed and either mailed or delivered to the lab. If it is mailed, all postal regulations for biohazardous substances must be followed.

c. Testing the specimen—When the specimen arrives in the laboratory:
  (1) Use the appropriate barrier precautions.
  (2) Open the back of the slide pack and apply the color developer supplied in the kit.
    (a) Note: Handle the reagents with care; some are flammable and poisonous.
  (3) Determining results
    (a) Any blue color change is a positive reaction.
    (b) Always compare the reaction to the picture of positive and negative reactions that accompanies the kit.
    (c) Follow the manufacturer's guidelines in quality control testing.
    (d) Document the results.
    (e) Dispose of the cardboard kits in a biohazardous waste container.

4. Possible sources of error
  a. Noncompliance with dietary restriction or collection procedures
  b. Expired kits
  c. Not completing the test within 2 days of collection of the specimen.
    (1) Patients who mail the hemoccult kit to the laboratory must be reasonably sure that the test will reach the laboratory within the 2-day window.
  d. Not reading results within the required time (30–60 seconds).

XIV. NONBLOOD SPECIMEN COLLECTION

A. Collection of nonblood specimens
  1. Nonblood specimen requests—Include:
    a. Throat cultures.
    b. Urine specimens.

c. Fecal specimens.

d. Semen specimens.

e. Gastric secretions.

f. Amniotic fluid collections.

g. Cerebrospinal fluid or nasopharyngeal culture collections.

2. Other nonblood specimens are collected by a nurse or physician.

3. You may also be required to perform CLIA-waived point-of-care testing on collected specimens.

B. Requirements

1. Labeling

a. All nonblood specimens must be labeled with the same patient identification information as blood specimens.

b. Most laboratories require that the type of specimen and the source of the specimen be included on the label.

2. Handling

a. Use the same standard precautions as handling blood specimens.

b. Nonblood specimens may be of a body fluid or contain a body fluid that may present risk of contamination.

C. Types of nonblood specimens

1. Throat cultures—Ordered by physicians to aid in the diagnosis of streptococcal infections (strep throat)

2. Fecal (stool) specimens—Examined to aid in the evaluation of gastrointestinal disorders and conditions

a. Specimens are evaluated for the presence of:

(1) Intestinal parasites and their eggs (ova and parasite, O&P).

(2) Occult (hidden) blood (guaiac test).

(3) Fat.

(4) Urobilinogen content.

b. They can also be cultured to determine the presence of:

(1) Enteric bacteria, such as *Salmonella*, *Shigella*, *Staphylococcus aureus*.

(2) Enteric viruses.

c. Collection

(1) Fecal specimens are collected in clean, dry containers and must be kept at body temperature, especially those to be used for parasite testing.

(2) Special containers, containing a preservative, for O&P collections are provided to the patient.

(3) Patients requested to provide a 24-, 48-, or 72-hour stool collection for the determinations of fat and urobilinogen content are provided with large gallon containers resembling paint cans. These types of specimens must be kept refrigerated throughout the collection period.

(4) Guaiac test cards

(a) Used to determine occult blood, these are given to outpatients to collect stool specimens at home.

(c) The patient is typically instructed to eat a meat-free diet for 3 days prior to collecting the specimen.

(d) Patients are then instructed to collect specimens for 3 consecutive days.

(e) Cards can be either mailed or delivered to the lab after the collection.

3. Semen specimens

a. Purpose—A patient may be requested to provide a semen sample for:

(1) The determination of fertility.

(2) The effectiveness of a sterilization procedure (vasectomy).

(3) The criminal investigation of sexual assault.

b. Collection

(1) The specimen may be collected in a sterile urine container.

(2) Semen specimens are never to be collected in a condom. Condoms often contain spermicides, which will kill living sperm, rendering the test invalid.

(3) Semen specimens are to be kept warm and delivered to the lab immediately.

4. Gastrointestinal secretions, amniotic fluid, cerebrospinal fluid, and nasopharyngeal specimens

a. Collection

(1) These procedures are performed by a physician.

(2) The phlebotomist's role in the collection of these specimens is to label the specimen and transport it to the laboratory.

b. Gastrointestinal analysis

(1) Purpose—This test is performed to determine the function of gastric secretions in terms of acid production.

(2) Collection—The secretions are aspirated by passing a tube through the

mouth or nose, down the throat, and into the stomach.

5. Amniotic fluid
   a. Purpose—A physician performs this procedure to determine fetal abnormalities that can be detected through chromosomal analysis and chemical tests at approximately 16 weeks gestation.
   b. Amniotic fluid:
      (1) Surrounds a fetus in utero.
      (2) Is normally a clear pale yellow fluid.
   c. Collection
      (1) The fluid is aspirated by inserting a needle through the abdominal wall of the mother into the uterus.
      (2) The specimen is to be protected from light and extremes in temperature fluctuations, and it must be delivered to the laboratory ASAP.

6. Cerebrospinal fluid (CSF)
   a. Purpose—Tests might include:
      (1) Total protein level.
      (2) Glucose level.
      (3) Cell count.
      (4) Microbiological evaluations.
      (5) Chloride levels.
   b. Cerebrospinal fluid is a clear colorless liquid that circulates in the cavities of the brain and spinal cord.
      (1) The constituents of CSF closely resemble those of blood plasma.
   c. Collection—The physician must insert a needle into the lumbar spine.
      (1) The fluid is generally collected in three sterile containers, numbered in the order in which they are collected. Because the first tube is usually contaminated with blood, the second and third tubes are the specimens used for analysis.
      (3) CSF must be transported immediately to the laboratory.

7. Nasopharyngeal (NP) cultures
   a. Purpose—Collected to determine the presence of microorganisms that cause:
      (1) Diphtheria.
      (2) Meningitis.
      (3) Pertussis.
      (4) Influenza.
      (5) Pneumonia.
   b. Collection-
      (1) NP specimens are collected using a sterile Dacron or cotton-tipped flexible wire swab, which is inserted into the nasopharynx and gently rotated.
      (2) Once removed from the NP cavity, the swab is placed in transport media and taken to the lab.

8. Urine
   a. Purpose
      (1) Urine specimens provide the physician with a valuable diagnostic tool.
      (2) The physician can make several determinations of the patient's health status, based on this nonblood specimen, from urinary tract infections through metabolic disorders such as diabetes.
   b. Collection
      (1) Inpatients—Nursing staff typically collects specimens from inpatients.
      (2) Outpatients—The phlebotomist is required to instruct outpatients in the procedure for urine collection.
         (a) Generally, give instructions verbally but also give the patient written instructions, preferably with illustrations. The instructions may be printed on a chart posted in the laboratory's bathroom facilities.
         (b) Present this information in a concise and tactful manner because the discussion has the potential to be embarrassing for the patient.
      (3) Correct urine collection procedures are essential to the integrity of the specimen. The properties of the specimen can be greatly altered if the collection process is not followed as ordered.
   c. Types of specimens—Types of urine specimens refer to the *time* the specimen is collected (i.e., random, fasting, first morning).
      (1) Random
         (a) Collected at any time
         (b) Used for routine urinalysis (UA) and for screening tests
      (2) First morning
         (a) The specimen is collected immediately after the patient wakes, either first thing in the morning or after approximately 8 hours of sleep.
         (b) This specimen is often favored because the urine is at its highest concentration because it has been "incubating" in the bladder while the patient has been sleeping. It has a higher concentration of analytes, with a higher specific gravity.

(c) First morning specimens are requested for routine urinalysis, confirmation of random test results, or when higher concentrations of analytes are required, such as for pregnancy testing, protein, nitrites, and microscope evaluations.

(3) Timed collections (e.g., 2-hour, 4-hour, 24-hour)

    (a) Some tests require that the patient void at specific time intervals, such as when an excretion rate of an analyte is to be measured.

    (b) Example: Tolerance testing, such as the glucose tolerance test (GTT) requires the patient to provide urine specimens at regular intervals that corresponds to blood collection intervals, such as fasting half hour, 1 hour, etc.

    (c) The timing of these collections is critical for accurate determination of disorders. The specimens must be collected as closely as possible to the required time, and each specimen has to be labeled clearly with the time of the collection and the type of specimen (e.g., clean catch, fasting, half hour).

(4) 24-hour collections

    (a) Purpose—This timed collection is requested when a quantitative analysis of analyte is needed for analysis.

    (b) Collection—All urine voided within a 24-hour period is collected in a urine specimen container or toilet hat and is then transferred into a specially designed 24-hour collection container.

        The patient starts by voiding the first morning specimen of the first day into the toilet as usual, noting the time and date on the specimen container.

        Every specimen thereafter, including the first morning specimen of the second day (if it is in the 24-hour period), is collected.

    (c) Specimen handling

        (i) The patient must avoid contaminating the specimen with fecal matter by urinating first, transferring the urine into the collection container, and then proceeding with a bowel movement.

        (ii) Generally the specimen is refrigerated unless it is being collected for urate testing. Refrigeration can be accomplished by placing the collection container in an ice chest. Urine specimens must *not* be placed in a refrigerator used to contain food.

        (iii) Specimens not refrigerated require the use of a preservative that can be added to the specimen collection container.

        (iv) Special containers are used for the collection of 24-hour collections. Patients are provided with a special device that fits over the toilet, resembles an upside down hat, and makes collection much easier for the patient when quantities are required. The toilet hat has graduation markings that can measure output amounts as well.

        (v) Along with the required patient identification information, the specimen must be labeled as a 24-hour collection, the time the collection started and the date, and, if applicable, the preservative that was added.

(5) Fractional, or double void, specimen

    (a) Purpose—Used to compare concentrations of an analyte, such as glucose and ketones.

    (b) Collection

        (i) The patient first collects a urine specimen, emptying the bladder completely. The time is recorded and the specimen is tested for the analyte.

        (ii) The patient is then requested to drink approximately 200 milliliters of water and then wait a required amount of time (typically a half hour), while the urine has time to accumulate in the bladder.

        (iii) The patient then collects another urine specimen, which is tested for the analyte, and the results are compared.

    (c) Most tolerance tests are fractional specimens.

d. Collection methods—The collection method refers to how the specimen is collected (i.e., clean catch, midstream, regular voided.

(1) Regular void
   (a) There is no special patient preparation.
   (b) The urine is simply collected in a clean widemouthed container.

(2) Midstream
   (a) This method is used to ensure that the urinary opening is free from contaminates, such as genital secretions, pubic hair, and bacteria.
   (b) The patient is instructed to void the initial flow into the toilet, stop the flow momentarily, collect the specimen, and void the remainder of the urine into the toilet.

(3) Midstream clean catch:
   (a) A clean catch specimen allows for a specimen that is free of contaminates from the external genitalia, requested when microbial analysis or culture and sensitivity testing is to be done.
   (b) This specimen is collected in a sterile container.
   (c) Special cleaning procedures must be explained to the patient by the phlebotomist or given in writing. The procedure varies between male and female patients.

(4) Clean catch collection procedure—Female
   (a) Stand in a squatting position over the toilet.
   (b) Open 3 prepackaged towelettes, or prepare three sterile 2 × 2-inch gauze pad with soapy water.
   (c) Separate the folds of the skin around the urinary opening.
   (d) With one towelette, cleanse from front to back, wiping once down the right side. With the second towelette, follow the same procedure front to back on the left side. With the third towelette wipe from front to back down the center.
   (e) Void the first portion of urine into the toilet (midstream).
   (f) Collect the specimen into the sterile urine container.
   (g) Finish voiding in the toilet.

(5) Clean catch collection procedure—Male
   (a) Stand in front of the toilet.
   (b) Open 3 prepackaged towelettes, or prepare three sterile 2 × 2-inch gauze pad with soapy water.
   (c) Cleanse the end of the penis beginning at the urethral opening and working away from it. (patients who are not circumcised must retract the foreskin prior to cleaning).
   (d) Repeat the cleansing process twice more with additional towelettes or sterile 2 × 2-inch gauze pad with soapy water.
   (e) Void the first portion of urine into the toilet (midstream).
   (f) Collect the specimen into the sterile urine container.
   (g) Finish voiding in the toilet.

(5) Catheterization
   (a) A catheterized specimen is collected by inserting a sterile catheter through the patient's urethra into the bladder.
   (b) This specimen is collected when a patient either is having trouble voiding or is already catheterized, or when analysis must be done on the urine directly from the bladder, which is free from urethral and external genitalia contaminates.

(6) Suprapubic
   (a) Purpose—This type of specimen is:
   Collected for evaluation of microbial analysis or cytology studies.
   Sometimes performed on infants and small children to obtain an uncontaminated sample.
   (b) Collection
      (i) A suprapubic specimen is collected in a sterile syringe by inserting the needle directly into the bladder and aspirating urine.
      (ii) This procedure is done by a physician, typically with the use of a local anesthetic.
      (iii) The urine, once collected, is transferred into a sterile container or tube.

(7) Pediatric specimens
   (a) Purpose—Young children and infants present a unique challenge when a urine specimen is requested.

(b) Collection—A specially designed plastic urine collection bag with hypoallergenic skin adhesive is used.

The patient's genital area is cleaned and dried; the bag is then placed around the vagina of a female or over the penis of a male. A diaper is then placed over the collection bag.

The patient is checked every 15 minutes until an adequate specimen has been collected.

The bag is removed, sealed, labeled, and sent to the laboratory as soon as possible.

(c) Twenty-four-hour specimens can be collected in the same manner by using a bag with a tube attached that allows for periodic drainage of the specimen into a collection container.

(d) Pediatric patients may also require a straight catheterization to collect the specimen.

PRACTICE

1. The reference value range for blood glucose is _____ milligrams/deciliter.
   a. 90–140
   b. 60–105
   c. 75–100
   d. 110–140

2. If a GTT specimen is collected prior to the 2-hour waiting period, the resulting values are _____.
   a. misinterpreted
   b. unchanged
   c. clotted
   d. adjusted

3. Coagulation studies must occur at _____ to ensure the accuracy of results.
   a. 37.5 degrees F
   b. 37 degrees C
   c. 98.6 degrees F
   d. 37.5 degrees C

4. Activated coagulation time (ACT) is used to monitor _____ therapy.
   a. warfarin
   b. insulin
   c. antibiotic
   d. heparin

5. Coumadin therapy can be monitored by performing a(n) _____.
   a. activated coagulation time
   b. plasma compensation
   c. heat determination
   d. prothrombin test

6. Prothrombin time (PT) normal values are _____ seconds.
   a. 17–24
   b. 17–26
   c. 17–22
   d. 17–20

7. Which of the following is *not* an electrolyte?
   a. Potassium
   b. Glucose
   c. Sodium
   d. Chloride

8. An increase of _____ is often present in bacterial urinary tract infections.
   a. leukocytes
   b. erythrocytes
   c. thrombocytes
   d. glucose

9. When evaluating a patient's kidney function, the doctor may order a _____ level.
   a. BUN
   b. glucose
   c. prothrombin time
   d. blood gases

10. Drug testing procedures must be followed exactly, and the procedures for donor preparation and collection of the specimen are defined by _____.
    a. CDC
    b. CLIA
    c. NCCLS
    d. NIDA

11. A _____ is ordered by a physician to determine a safe and effective drug dosage.
    a. PTT
    b. P&T
    c. TMD
    d. TDM

12. _____ testing is based on ABO and Rh typing, as well as other proteins on the surface of red blood cells.
    a. PPD
    b. Paternity
    c. Hematocrit
    d. Tuberculosis

13. Pregnancy tests determine the level of _____ in both blood and urine.
    a. Hct
    b. Hgb
    c. hCG
    d. STD

14. _____ functions in the manufacturing of bile acids and in the production of hormones; when located in the skin, it also helps to keep it waterproof.
    a. Bilirubin
    b. Cholesterol
    c. Keratin
    d. Ketone

15. A desirable cholesterol level is _____milligrams/deciliter.
    a. less than 200
    b. 200–239
    c. 300–450
    d. 350–500

16. _____ measures the volume of the patient's red blood cells as a percentage of whole blood in relationship to the plasma.
    a. Hgb
    b. Hct
    c. FBS
    d. HDL

17. _____ is the iron-containing protein pigment of the red blood cells.
    a. FSB
    b. Hct
    c. Hgb
    d. LDL

18. The reference value range for a hematocrit for a female patient is _____ percent.
    a. 32–38
    b. 36–48
    c. 42–52
    d. 51–61

19. The normal values for PTT or APTT, when using whole blood, are _____ seconds.
    a. 24–34
    b. 38–56
    c. 72–94
    d. 93–127

20. The most common drug(s) detected in drug screens are all of the following except _____.
    a. alcohol
    b. crack cocaine
    c. marijuana
    d. acetaminophen

21. Before performing a modified Ivy bleeding time, determine whether the patient has consumed _____ or other salicylate-containing drugs in the past two weeks.
    a. aspirin
    b. bicarbonates
    c. vitamins
    d. alcohol

22. The phlebotomist performs a control "check" _____ to ensure that control specimens fall within established range values.
    a. prior to each test
    b. daily
    c. quarterly
    d. biannually

23. All of the following are considered point-of-care tests except _____.
    a. fecal occult blood test
    b. coagulation monitoring
    c. chemistry panels
    d. immune assay

24. _____ pertains to the condition in which the blood sugar is increased.
    a. Hyperthyroidism
    b. Hyperglycemia
    c. Hypoglycemia
    d. Hyperinsulinism

25. Increased cholesterol levels cause fats to deposit in the inner lining of the arteries, creating a condition known as _____.
    a. arteriosclerosis
    b. arthrosclerosis
    c. atherosclerosis
    d. arterisclerosis

26. Hemoglobin reference value ranges for a newborn are _____ grams/deciliter.
    a. 10.0–14.0
    b. 16.0–23.0
    c. 13.5–17.5
    d. 12.5–15.5

27. Which of the following medications may be taken by a patient scheduled for a glucose tolerance test (GTT)?
    a. Acetaminophen
    b. Diuretics
    c. Corticosteroids
    d. All of the above

28. A(n) _____ is performed by collecting a small volume of blood in a prewarmed special gray top evacuated tube.
    a. PT test
    b. ACT analysis
    c. toxicology profile
    d. CBC

29. Potassium plays a major role in all of the following except _____.
    a. osmotic pressure
    b. muscle function
    c. nerve conduction
    d. core body temperature

30. The normal range for arterial blood pH is _____.
    a. 7.53–7.63
    b. 7.43–7.53
    c. 7.35–7.45
    d. 7.45–7.53

31. A type of urine collection requiring a patient to void at specific time intervals is known as a _____ collection.
    a. 24-hour
    b. random
    c. timed
    d. double voided

32. A _____ collection method is used to ensure that the urinary opening is free of contaminants.
    a. random
    b. midstream
    c. timed
    d. 24-hour

33. Streptococcal infections can be diagnosed with the aid of a _____.
    a. semen specimen
    b. stool specimen
    c. throat culture
    d. urine specimen

34. The most concentrated urine specimen is a _____.
    a. first morning
    b. 24-hour collection
    c. midstream
    d. clean catch

35. A _____ specimen is collected when a patient is having trouble voiding.
    a. catheterized
    b. clean catch
    c. random
    d. 24-hour

36. The Schick test is used to test for _____.
    a. diphtheria
    b. coccidioidomycosis
    c. tuberculosis exposure
    d. scarlet fever

37. The syringe for an intradermal injection is held at a _____degree angle.
    a. 10- to 15-
    b. 15- to 20-
    c. 20- to 25-
    d. 25- to 30-

38. _____ is/are one element responsible the normal color of feces.
    a. Bilirubin
    b. Ketones
    c. Protein
    d. Urobilin

39. A nitrate test and a _____ test are both performed to screen for urinary tract infections.
    a. glucose
    b. leukocyte
    c. hemoglobin
    d. ketones

40. Which of the following types of specimens has a heightened concentration of analytes, with a heightened specific gravity?
    a. Random
    b. Fractional or double void
    c. First morning
    d. Midstream

41. _____ specimens are examined to help evaluate gastrointestinal disorders and conditions.
    a. Fecal
    b. Stomach acid
    c. Urine
    d. Throat

42. For the accurate testing of semen, the specimen should be collected in a _____.
    a. condom
    b. clean medicine bottle
    c. sterile urine container
    d. clean baby food jar

43. When instructing a patient about a fecal occult blood test, you must be sure to have the patient discontinue _____ for at least one week prior to the test.
    a. alcohol consumption
    b. aspirin
    c. smoking
    d. eating sugary foods

44. A skin test must be read for a reaction in _____ hours.
    a. 8–24
    b. 12–36
    c. 24–72
    d. 36–80

45. A strep A test is typically performed given the symptoms for which of the following conditions?
    a. appendicitis
    b. tonsillitis
    c. gastroenteritis
    d. all of the above

46. Freshly voided urine should have a distinctive _____ odor.
    a. ammonia
    b. aromatic
    c. fruity
    d. putrid

47. A pH of _____ is considered to be neutral for urine
    a. 5
    b. 7
    c. 8
    d. 9

48. A timed urine collection that requires a patient to drink approximately 200 milliliters of water and wait a required amount of time is called a _____.
    a. fractional or double void specimen
    b. 24-hour collection
    c. 2-hour collection
    d. midstream collection

49. The clean catch collection procedure requires a female patient to _____.
    a. open and use two prepackaged towelettes
    b. cleanse from back to front
    c. sit directly on the toilet
    d. void the first portion of urine into the toilet (midstream)

50. Which of the following is *not* considered a normal urine color?
    a. Straw
    b. Amber
    c. Pale green
    d. All of the above are considered normal

CRITICAL THINKING

1. Bill Jones arrives at your clinic for his preemployment drug screen; he is going to work for Homeland Security. You prepare your lavatory site according to NIDA guidelines; you have all the supplies you need except you're missing the blue dye for the toilet. Sarah was going to pick it up at lunch and hasn't returned with it yet. Mr. Jones looks like a nice honest man, so you take a chance and go ahead with the test. While Mr. Jones is in the lavatory, you begin the paperwork required for the collection. Upon his return, you ask for his picture identification and a signature for the consent form. Mr. Jones refuses to sign the consent form since his potential employer is the one requesting the drug screen. You explain that you must have it signed before you can continue processing the specimen. He refuses and leaves the clinic in a fury.
   - What procedural errors occurred?

2. Derek Johannes, a 55-year-old male, is a patient at the clinic where you work. During his appointment today he complained of increased lethargy. The physician orders a STAT hemoglobin to rule out anemia. You have a choice of a venipuncture or a capillary stick.
   - Which would you choose?
   - Explain your choice.
   - What should the reference value range be for Mr. Johannes?

3. Melanie was sent to the lab to have a GTT drawn. You ask her if she has eaten anything yet this morning. "Only water with my blood pressure pills," she replies. You think this will be okay; so you document it on Melanie's chart and you prepare her for the test. Your hospital's protocols require a 3-hour duration for GTT collections. Every half hour a blood specimen and a urine specimen will be collected. You draw baselines, give Melanie a commercially prepared glucose drink, and start timing. After 2 hours of testing, Melanie's glucose is 200 milligrams/deciliter. After 3 hours, it has dropped to 150 milligrams/deciliter.
   - What will these results tell the doctor?

MODULE **8**

Legal, Ethical, and Professional Communications, and Clerical Skills and Duties

I. LEGALITIES

A. The Patient Care Partnership
   1. The Patient Care Partnership, adopted in April 2003, is a document designed to protect the patient. Although not legally binding, it is accepted throughout the medical field as the standard for treating all patients.
   2. The Patient Care Partnership outlines what the patient can expect during a hospital stay.
      a. High-quality hospital care
      b. A clean and safe environment
      c. Involvement in the patient's care
         (1) Patient's right to discuss his or her medical condition
         (2) Patient's right to discuss his or her treatment plan
         (3) Patient's responsibility to give information to caregivers
         (4) Patient's responsibility to share health care goals and values
         (5) Patient's responsiblity to notify caregivers of who should make decisions when he or she cannot
      d. Protection of patient privacy
      e. Instruction and aid in preparation upon departure from hospital
      f. Help filing insurance claims and other billing matters
B. Two main divisions of law (civil and criminal) and preventive law
   1. Civil law—Is the law of private rights between persons or parties.
      a. Civil law actions comprise the majority of all health care cases.

   b. Types
      (1) Tort—Private wrong or injury, other than breach of contract, for which the court will provide a remedy; a civil wrong based on an act committed without just cause.
         (a) Intentional torts
            (i) Abandonment—Premature termination of the professional treatment relationship by the health care provider without adequate notice or the patient's consent
            (ii) Assault—Intentionally causing someone to fear that he or she is about to become the victim of battery
            (iii) Battery—Intentionally touching someone in a harmful or offensive manner without the person's consent
            (iv) Duty of care—Requirement that a person act toward others and the public with the watchfulness, attention, caution, and prudence that a reasonable person in the circumstances would use. If a person's actions do not meet this standard of care, then the acts are considered negligent, and any damages resulting may be claimed in a lawsuit for negligence.
            (v) False imprisonment—Intentionally and unjustifiably preventing someone from moving about

(vi) Fraud—Deliberate deception intended to produce unlawful gain

(vii) Intentional infliction of emotional distress—Willful infliction of emotions or actions, causing the patient to suffer duress

(viii) Invasion of privacy—Tort involving one or more of the following four categories: illegal appropriation of another's name for commercial use, intrusion into a person's privacy, placing a person in a false light, or disclosure of private facts

(ix) Libel—Written statement falsifying facts about someone that causes harm to the person's reputation

(x) Slander—Falsifying facts, which causes harm to a person's reputation (Slander is spoken; libel is written.)

(b) Negligence torts—Torts that occur when a duty of care is breached unintentionally, causing harm. Negligence is the failure to act with reasonable care when one should act, resulting in the harming of others.

(i) Negligence does not require intent.

(ii) Malpractice is a claim of improper treatment or negligence brought against a professional person and/or institution by means of a civil lawsuit.

(iii) Strict liability means that, in a few instances, a health care provider can be found guilty of a tort, even though it neither intentionally nor unintentionally committed a tort.

2. Criminal law—Concerned with violations of laws established by local, state, or federal government agencies; divided into two classifications: felonies and misdemeanors

a. Felony—Crime more serious than a misdemeanor, punishable by a sentence of more than one year in prison or death

b. Misdemeanor—Crime less serious than a felony, punishable by a fine or imprisonment of up to one year in jail

3. Preventive law—Avoidance of legal conflicts through education and planning

a. Informed consent—Agreement by the patient to a medical procedure or treatment after receiving adequate information about the procedure or treatment, including the benefits, alternatives, and consequences if the patient chooses not to have it

b. Burden of proof—Used in conjunction with the terms "malpractice" and "negligence," a legal term meaning that the client must show proof of a claimed accusation of malpractice or negligence, rather than the health care provider having to prove that none existed

c. Chain of custody—Procedure for ensuring that material obtained for diagnosis has been taken from the correct patient, is properly labeled, and has not been tampered with en route to the laboratory

C. Lawsuit prevention measures

1. Accurately and legibly document all information.

2. Acquire informed consent prior to specimen collection.

3. Document all incidents immediately.

4. Participate in continuing education.

5. Perform at the accepted standard of care.

6. Strictly adhere to all laboratory policies and procedures.

7. Use proper safety measures.

D. Proof of negligence

1. A standard of care must exist.

2. The standard of care must be breached.

3. An injury must be sustained.

4. It must be proved that the injury was caused by acts resulting from a breach of standard of care.

E. Ethics—Area of philosophical study that examines society's values, actions, and choices to determine right and wrong

1. Medical code of ethic—Constitutes the medical profession's rules of right and wrong

II. PROFESSIONAL COMMUNICATION SKILLS

A. The most important skill that a successful health care provider can possess is the ability to interact compassionately with patients.

B. Professionalism—Ability to perform work-related duties and responsibilities with a high degree of respect for the profession and for the patient

1. Ethics—Standards established to address the basic principles of right and wrong conduct.

Hospitals and laboratories have established codes of ethics.

    a. Do not intentionally harm anyone.

    b. Work within your scope of practice, using sound judgment, and act as any reasonable professional would act.

    c. Respect the rights of the patient (i.e., confidentiality, privacy, informed consent, and the right to refuse treatment).

  2. Integrity—Ability to do what is right even when no one is watching

C. Verbal and nonverbal communication—Skills that require two active participants: the person sending the message and the person receiving the message.

  1. If the message is not understood in the manner in which it was meant to be, we have failed to communicate.

  2. The messages can be sent verbally or nonverbally.

    a. Verbal communication—For effective verbal communication to take place, the sender of the message must be articulate. To be articulate is to distinctly and clearly enunciate words, phrases, and sentences.

    b. Nonverbal communication—It has been stated that approximately 80 percent of all communication is nonverbal. Nonverbal communication is multidimensional and involves body movement, gestures, facial expression, eye contact, touch, use of space, and appearance.

      (1) Appearance—Most facilities require a dress code because they know that the physical impression their employees give establishes how future interactions with other health care providers will go. Having a good appearance communicates to the patient that the phlebotomist is confident and capable.

        (a) Uniforms and/or lab coats must be clean and pressed and in good repair. Never wear anything that would distract or offend a patient.

        (b) Duty shoes are to be clean and in good repair.

        (c) Jewelry should be kept to a minimum. The use of perfume and cologne is discouraged.

        (d) Hair is neat and clean, with no extreme hairstyles or colors. It should be worn off the collar or pulled into a clip, ponytail, or braid.

        (e) Nails are always clean and well-groomed. Particular attention is always paid to personal hygiene. Shower or bathe daily.

        (f) Teeth are clean, breath is fresh.

        (g) The use of antiperspirant/ deodorant must be part of the phlebotomist's daily routine.

      (2) A sincere smile—The most lasting nonverbal communication from the phlebotomist is a warm smile. Smiling sincerely conveys to the patient that you care.

      (3) Eye contact—It tells the patient that the phlebotomist cares enough to recognize the patient as an individual, not just another case.

      (4) Gestures—Gestures should match the spoken word. People trust nonverbal communication messages over the spoken word, especially when the two conflict.

      (5) Observation of nonverbal communication from the patient—The patient also communicates nonverbally; the health care provider can use this feedback for clues as to how the patient is really feeling.

        (a) The study of body language is called kinesics.

      (6) Touch—Generally patients appreciate being touched in a thoughtful and caring manner by a health care professional. The phlebotomist must be sensitive to the patient's needs. It is impossible to perform a venipuncture without touching the patient. Establishing a favorable rapport in the beginning lessens a patient's apprehension about being touched with a needle. Communicating effectively comforts the patient. Verbally communicate to the patient what is to be expected and ask for permission before touching.

  3. Learning to be a good listener—As a phlebotomist you must be ready to actively listen. Listening is the result of understanding the words and taking action and/or responding appropriately.

    a. The average person can absorb approximately 500–600 words per minute. The average speaking rate is 120–150 words per minute.

    b. Not actively listening can cause valuable information to be missed and conveys to the patient a lack of interest and caring.

    c. With active listening, the health care provider can increase comprehension and retention of information.

d. To actively listen:
   (1) Give the patient undivided attention, acknowledge the message sent, and offer an appropriate response or take the appropriate action.
   (2) Stay focused on the patient. Do not allow distractions to interrupt.

4. Other considerations in health care communication—Patients commonly reach out for comfort and reassurance through conversation.
   a. The phlebotomist must respond to patients in a calm and respectful manner, using a communication style that includes trust, empowerment, and empathy.
   b. Empathy is an objective awareness of and insight into the feelings, emotions, and behaviors of another person.

5. Barriers to effective communication
   a. Medical terminology—Speak in terms that the patient understands, without talking down to the patient. Explain procedures thoroughly in lay terms.
   b. Hearing Impairment—A patient with a hearing impairment requires a different style of communication.
      (1) Enunciate terms distinctly and clearly.
      (2) Depending on the degree of the impairment, a sign language translator may be necessary.
      (3) If there is a concern about whether the patient understands a procedure, a patient advocate can be requested, or a family member or friend can be invited to be present.
   c. Non-English–speaking patients—Non-English–speaking patients and those for whom English is a second language have special concerns.
      (1) Often non-English–speaking patients understand basic directions through the use of hand signals or sign language.
      (2) Always treat the patient with respect and honor the dignity of the patient.
      (3) If you are learning the predominant, non-English language of the area, practice basic requests with a native speaker; the mispronunciation of terms may only further confuse patients.
   d. Level of consciousness—This and patient's state of health play an important role in communication. Often patients are heavily medicated or have altered levels of consciousness, posing a special communication challenge.

e. Comfort zone—The comfort zone, or an individual's "personal" space, must also be taken into consideration. Everyone has an area or space around the body that others should respect.
   (1) Comfort zones are also culturally based.

6. Telecommunications—The telephone is an essential communication tool and requires special communication consideration. The basic tenets of communication still apply. Enunciation of words, pitch, and voice quality become even more important than in face-to-face encounters.
   a. Professional telephone etiquette—Representation for the employer's business may be gained or lost through telephone manners. Telephone etiquette can be summed up in one phrase: *Be courteous*.
      (1) Answering the phone
         (a) Answer the phone within 3 rings.
         (b) Treat the person on the other end of the line as you would treat a person standing in front of you.
         (c) Be expressive; do not speak in a monotone. Be alert, attentive, and discreet.
         (d) Use good listening skills and avoid slang.
      (2) The conversation
         (a) Obtain the caller's name early in the conversation.
         (b) If you cannot help the caller, you must redirect the call.
      (3) Answering multiple phone lines
         (a) Answer all incoming calls in a timely manner by the third ring.
         (b) Do not wait until you have finished with the first call to answer a second. Put the first caller on hold, answer the second call, ask if you may put the caller on hold, and return to the first call.
         (c) If you suspect the first call may be lengthy, return to the additional caller and ask if you may take a message and return the call. Give the first caller an idea of how long it will be before the call is returned.
      (4) Putting a caller on hold—Sometimes the caller must be put on hold.
         (a) Ask the caller if you may put him or her on hold.
         (b) Wait for a response.

(c) Explain why you must put them on hold.

(d) Thank the caller for holding when you return.

(5) Taking a message—Sometimes the phlebotomist has to take a phone message. The following information is critical and must be recorded accurately:

(a) Whom the message is for

(b) The caller's name (spelled correctly)

(c) Company name (as applicable)

(d) Telephone number (including area code if it is a long distance call)

(e) The best time to return the call

(f) The time of the call

(g) The message (recorded exactly)

(h) Repeat all the information to the caller before hanging up.

(6) End of call

(a) Always end the call on a positive note. Repeat any actions that you and the caller agreed to during the conversation.

(b) Ask the caller if you can do anything else for him or her.

(c) Thank the caller for calling.

(d) Let the caller hang up first, so that the caller is not accidentally hung up on midsentence.

(e) Write down important information immediately after ending the call.

III. MANAGE TIME EFFECTIVELY

A. Invest in a daily planner that accommodates your particular needs.

B. Matrix your planner. Time management takes organization.

1. Fill in all the addresses and telephone numbers you use frequently or may need to access quickly.

2. Fill in commitments that do not change throughout the year, such as birthdays and anniversaries.

3. Then fill in your work schedule and regularly scheduled events. Also, if you have significant others, keep track of their events (e.g., hockey games, dance practice, dentist appointments).

4. Then schedule in tasks that must be accomplished on a routine basis, grocery shopping, laundry, etc.

IV. DOCUMENTATION

A. Laboratory requisition forms

1. Computer requisition forms—Typically preprinted, with self-adhesive labels attached

a. Advantages of computer generated forms

(1) Lists the specific test, the required specimen, and the specimen requirements.

(2) Prints the forms by means of the software program.

(3) Has the capability to sort tests by patient.

(4) Generates requisitions by draw times.

(5) Records test results.

(6) Prints multiple laboratory reports.

2. Manual requisition forms

a. There are a variety of manual requisition forms; they are typically not preprinted.

b. Manual forms are generally 3¼ to 7½ inches long and are easily attached to 8½ × 11-inch courier paper, the traditional size of patient's charts.

3. Bar codes

a. A barcode is a series of black and white bands of varying widths and lengths that are grouped together in specific sequences. The sequence represents patient information.

b. Both computer and manual requisition forms can contain bar codes.

4. Required information on requisition forms—Must be easy to handle, inexpensive, and produce legible copies; must include pertinent information

a. Patient's full name and address

b. Patient's identification number

c. Patient's date of birth (DOB)

d. Room number and bed (if applicable)

e. Physician's name requesting the test

f. Date of test

g. Diagnosis

h. Test requested

i. Test status (e.g., timed, fasting, priority)

j. Billing information (optional)

k. Special precautions (optional)

l. Physician's signature

5. Required information on specimen tube labels—Must be handwritten onto the specimen tube label *after* the collection of the specimen

a. Time of test

b. Patient's name and DOB

c. Initials of the phlebotomist who obtained the specimen

d. Accession number

6. Accession numbers—Alphanumerics assigned to each request for a laboratory specimen and used to identify all paperwork and supplies associated with a specific patient

7. Blood collection logbook—Serves as an excellent means of communication between the laboratory and the patient's other health care providers

   a. Manual log book—Can be used to:

      (1) Verify that a test was ordered.

      (2) Record when the specimen was collected.

      (3) Record any comments regarding the collection.

   b. Computerized logbooks—Increased accuracy

      (1) Laboratory software programs are able to perform automatic checks and balances.

      (2) Specimens are logged into the computer database when the specimen accession number is scanned.

      (3) The phlebotomist can access the most up-to-date information regarding the requested test, such as revised specimen collection requirements, delivery instructions, assay techniques, reference ranges, and fees.

8. Verbal laboratory requests—Given frequently in an outpatient setting and in emergency situations. Verbal requests must be:

   a. Documented on a laboratory requisition form prior to collection of the specimen.

   b. Executed quickly.

9. Transmission of laboratory requisition forms

   a. Manual requisition forms—Dispatched to the laboratory either by a pneumatic tube system, by courier, or by means of collections, or "sweeps," by the phlebotomist; must then be sorted and prioritized by date, time, and priority of collection

      (1) Pneumatic tube system—A unidirectional, continuously operating vacuum system that transfers specimens in Plexiglas carriers from the patient units to the laboratory

   b. Computer requisition forms—Either e-mailed or otherwise transmitted through the hospital's electronic communications system.

      (1) The physician orders tests for a patient from a computer.

      (2) The laboratory requisition form is printed at a computer terminal at the phlebotomist station in the laboratory.

B. Patient charting

   1. Manual lab reports are:

      a. Filed chronologically in the patient's paper chart.

      b. Shingled (attached to file with overlap of reports) with the most recent report on top.

      c. Typically color coded, with like test reports shingled on the same courier sheet.

   2. Computerized laboratory software programs—Computerized programs have automated the "filing" of the laboratory reports.

      a. The electronic (on-screen) patient file has a section labeled "laboratory tests."

      b. The test is ordered on the computer; the patient information and test request are either keyed or scanned.

      c. The lab request form is created and stored in the patient's electronic file.

      d. The completed test results are entered into the patient's electronic file.

      e. Lab results can be:

         (1) Printed and delivered.

         (2) Phoned and followed up by a hard copy of the report.

         (3) E-mailed or faxed to the physician.

C. Insurance billing/private pay

   1. Fee-for-service—Most traditional way to pay for health care

      a. A fee for a specific procedure or test is determined based on the usual or customary fee within the community (what other laboratories in the area are charging for the service).

      b. The laboratory charges the patient the set fee at the time the service is provided.

   2. Third-party payer—The health insurance provider that is paid for by the patient

      a. Third-party payers pay all or part of the cost of health care services on behalf of the patient.

      b. Each company sets its own requirements for eligibility.

      c. This type of payer is a private insurance company or from medical coverage through government agencies, such as Medicare, Medicaid, and Tricare.

         (1) Tricare is a managed health care program offered to spouses and dependents of military service personnel. Benefits and fees are implemented nationwide by the federal government.

d. The patient pays premiums typically each month for the coverage.

e. Since some policies pay only partially for services provided, the patient is required to make various types of additional payment at the time services are rendered.

   (1) Copayment—Predetermined amount paid regardless of the treatment

   (2) Deductible—Predetermined amount that the patient must pay directly for health care services prior to receiving insurance benefits

f. Explanation of benefits (EOB)—Form sent by the insurance carrier to the doctor that states the amount paid by the insurance company or that the patient has not met the deductible

3. Payment for services rendered—Once service is rendered to the patient, the laboratory has two options for receiving payment.

   a. The patient pays for the services at the time the service is rendered and then personally submits the claim to the insurance company.

   b. The laboratory bills the insurance company.

      (1) A claim form is filled out and signed by the patient at the time the service is rendered.

      (2) The laboratory can:

          (a) *Either* keep the originally signed claim form on file or submit it electronically via the computer.

          (b) *Or* type out the original claim form with the correct information and submit it to the insurance company.

      (3) The process then proceeds as if the patient submitted the claim.

   c. Diagnostic and procedure codes are used on claim forms to specifically classify the patient's diagnosis and treatment procedures.

      (1) The *International Classification of Diseases 9th Revision Clinical Modification* (ICD-9-CM) is the reference used to code diagnoses.

      (2) The *Current Procedural Terminology* (CPT) is the reference used to code procedures.

4. Health care revisions—The health care industry is continuously in revision in an attempt to contain costs, provide better health care to more people, and keep up with new technology.

   a. Diagnosis related groupings (DRGs) are a classification system categorizing patient procedures using like diagnoses and treatments.

   b. Health maintenance organizations (HMOs) are prepaid health plans.

      (1) In these group practices, members pay a fixed periodic payment in advance for all eligible services by participating providers who render these services.

      (2) Patients are required to obtain all their health care needs with the participating HMO providers. Unless preauthorized, services obtained from a nonparticipating provider are not reimbursed and must be paid for by the patient.

   c. Preferred provider organizations (PPOs) are health benefit programs in which enrollees receive the highest level of benefits when they obtain services from a physician, hospital, or other health care provider designated by the program as a "preferred provider."

      (1) Unlike HMO members, PPO members have the freedom to choose any physician or hospital for services.

      (2) However, when a patient selects a preferred provider they receive a higher level of benefits.

   d. Managed care evolved because the act of prepayment basically changed the relationships between the patient and the health care provider. (HMOs and PPOs were the precursors of managed care systems.)

      (1) Managed care places the financial risk on the health care provider rather than on the insurer.

      (2) The primary care physician's responsibility is to advise and coordinate the patient's health care needs and serve as a gatekeeper. The primary care physician must refer the patient to the appropriate specialist in order to receive the maximum benefits of the plan.

      (3) Provider networks are established—Contracts with local providers—To provide a complete network of services. The providers are paid by capitation.

5. Health insurance claim forms—The CMS-1500 is the standard form accepted by most insurance companies.

   a. CMS-1500 can be handwritten, typewritten, or processed using a computer.

   b. The form can be either mailed to the insurance company or sent electronically via the computer.

c. Diagnostic and procedure codes are used to specifically classify the patient's diagnosis and the procedures used to treat the patient.

D. Laboratory computer

1. Capabilities—The laboratory computer can perform many functions. Based on the specific software program the facility is using, the computer can be used to perform one or all of the following:
   a. Data entry
   b. Test requisitions
   c. Printing test request forms, labels, and accession numbers
   d. Printing schedules and collection lists
   e. Entering test results
   f. Maintenance of medical records
   g. Transfer of information

2. Common computer terms
   a. Backup—Duplicate of data files made to protect information
      (1) Records should be backed up daily. Some experts recommend twice daily.
   b. Batch—Accumulation of data to be processed
   c. Boot—To start up a computer
   d. Catalog—List of files on the storage media
   e. CD-ROM—Compact disk read-only memory; indicates the computer is capable of playing compact disks
   f. Characters per second—Term used to measure the speed of printer output
   g. Central processing unit (CPU)—Brain of the system
   h. Disk operating system (DOS)—Program that tells the computer how to use the disk drive
   i. Downtime—Period of lost work time during which a computer is not operating or is malfunctioning because of machine failure
   j. Initialize—To prepare a disk to receive data; usually referred to as "formatting" a disk
   k. Input—Data processed from peripheral equipment into the machine via the keyboard or disk for internal storage
   l. Interface—Hardware and software that enable individual computers and components to interact
   m. Log on—Signing on to a computer system by entering a username and a password
   n. Main memory—Internal memory of the computer

o. Menu—Display of available machine functions or other options for selection by the operator
p. Microprocessor—Single chip on which the computer computes
q. Modem—Peripheral device that enables a computer to communicate with other computers or terminals over normal telephone or cable lines
r. Peripheral—Anything you plug into a computer
s. Random access memory (RAM)—Temporary or programmable memory. You can put new information into RAM. When you turn off the computer, the data is deleted.
t. Software—Computer programs necessary to direct the hardware of a computer system to perform specific tasks
u. Terminal—Device used to communicate with a computer, usually a keyboard and monitor; depends on the main computer for its abilities
v. Write-protect—Process or code that prevents overwriting of data or programs on a disk

PRACTICE

1. _____ is (are) *not* a barrier to effective communication.
   a. English as a second language
   b. Hearing impairments
   c. Patient's level of consciousness
   d. Eye contact

2. What percentage of all communication is non-verbal?
   a. 20
   b. 50
   c. 80
   d. 75

3. Comfort zones are *not* typically based on _____.
   a. culture
   b. gender
   c. individual preference
   d. education

4. _____ is *not* a vital piece of information needed when taking a phone message.
   a. Caller's DOB
   b. Time of call
   c. Caller's phone number
   d. Caller's name

5. _____ should *not* be a daily part of a phlebotomist's routine.
   a. Use of perfumes or cologne
   b. Bathing
   c. Brushing teeth
   d. Use of deodorant

6. The average person speaks at approximately _____ words per minute.
   a. 50–100
   b. 120–150
   c. 140–200
   d. 500–600

7. The medical profession's rules of right and wrong are called _____.
   a. duty of care
   b. code of ethics
   c. laws
   d. conditions

8. _____ is a claim of improper treatment brought against a professional person and/or institution by means of a civil lawsuit.
   a. Duty of care
   b. Libel
   c. Malpractice
   d. Battery

9. _____ does *not* require intent.
   a. Fraud
   b. Libel
   c. Malpractice
   d. Negligence

10. _____ is the act of intentionally touching someone in a harmful or offensive manner without the person's consent.
   a. Assault
   b. Battery
   c. Intentional infliction of emotional duress
   d. Malpractice

11. _____ is a billing sent to an insurance carrier.
   a. Claim
   b. EOB
   c. Premium
   d. Ledger

12. Active listening requires all of the following *except* _____.
   a. undivided attention
   b. concentration
   c. skill
   d. physical contact

13. Personal _____ is the ability to do what is right when no one is watching.
   a. duty
   b. laws
   c. integrity
   d. morals

14. Manual requisition forms are generally 3¼ inches wide and _____ inches long.
   a. 2
   b. 5
   c. 7½
   d. 11

15. When completing insurance claim forms, you will find diagnosis codes in which of the following references?
   a. ICD-9-CM
   b. CPT
   c. HCPCs
   d. BBP

16. _____ is signing on to a computer system by entering a username and a password.
   a. Online
   b. Log-on
   c. Interface
   d. Hard copy

17. _____ is the area of philosophical study that examines society's values, actions, and choices to determine right and wrong.
   a. Ethics
   b. Fraud
   c. Morals
   d. Values

18. _____ torts occur when a duty of care is breached unintentionally, causing harm.
   a. Fraud
   b. Libel
   c. Malpractice
   d. Negligence

19. _____ is the responsibility of health care providers to protect others from harm.
   a. Due care
   b. A tort
   c. Respondeat superior
   d. Ethics

20. An agreement by the patient to a medical procedure or treatment after reasonable explanation is called _____.
   a. chain of custody
   b. burden of proof
   c. informed consent
   d. assumed consent

21. To prove negligence, which of the following conditions is *not* necessary?
   a. A standard of care must exist.
   b. The standard of care must not be breached.
   c. An injury must have occurred.
   d. The injury must be proven to be caused by the acts that result from the breach of care.

22. A _____ fee is a fee for a specific procedure or test based on what other laboratories in the area charge for the same service.
    a. negotiable
    b. premium-driven
    c. reasonable and fair
    d. usual and customary

23. An individual or organization covered for protection and loss under the specific terms of an insurance policy is called the _____.
    a. coinsured
    b. insured
    c. guarantor
    d. PPO

24. _____ is the standard form, accepted by most insurance companies, for submitting an insurance claim.
    a. HCFA-1000
    b. HCFA-200
    c. CMS-1000
    d. CMS-1500

25. _____ involves body movements, gestures, facial expression, eye contact, touch, use of space, and appearance.
    a. Articulation
    b. Verbal communication
    c. Kinesics
    d. Nonverbal communication

26. _____ is a private wrong or injury, other than a breach of contract.
    a. Malpractice
    b. Negligence
    c. Battery
    d. A tort

27. _____ is not a legally binding document. However, it is accepted throughout the medical health care industry as the standard to which all patients have the right to be treated.
    a. Patient Care Partnership
    b. Patient's Ledger of Rights
    c. Patient's Right for Quality Care
    d. Patient Informed Consent

28. According to the _____, a patient can expect high-quality hospital care, a clean and safe environment, involvement in care, protection of privacy, preparation for release, and help with billing and the filing of insurance claims.
    a. Patient's Right for Quality Care
    b. Patient's Ledger of Rights
    c. Patient Care Partnership
    d. Patient Informed Consent

29. "_____" is a legal term used in conjunction with the terms "malpractice" and "negligence."
    a. Chain of custody
    b. Burden of proof
    c. Informed consent
    d. Duty of care

30. The most important skill that a successful health care provider can possess is _____.
    a. integrity
    b. compassion
    c. professionalism
    d. communication

31. To enunciate words, phrases, and sentences distinctly and clearly is to _____.
    a. communicate
    b. verbalize
    c. vocalize
    d. articulate

32. An objective awareness of and insight into the feelings, emotions, and behaviors of another person is known as _____.
    a. sympathy
    b. empathy
    c. compassion
    d. commiseration

33. _____ are a classification system categorizing patient procedures using like diagnoses and treatments.
    a. DRGs
    b. PPOs
    c. HMOs
    d. CDLs

34. Which of the following functions is a laboratory computer *not* typically capable of?
    a. Data entry
    b. Transferring Information
    c. Decoding lab tests
    d. Maintenance of medical records

35. _____ is a managed health care program offered to spouses and dependents of military personnel.
    a. Champus
    b. Tricare
    c. Medicare
    d. Medicaid

36. Which one of the following is *not* part of the basic guidelines for a phlebotomist to prevent a lawsuit?
    a. Use of safety measures
    b. Clean professional background
    c. Continuing education
    d. Accurately documenting all information

37. _____ actions comprise the majority of all health care cases.
    a. Government law
    b. Civil law
    c. Federal law
    d. Tort

38. _____ is the failure to act with reasonable care, resulting in the harming of others.
    a. Malpractice
    b. Assault
    c. Negligence
    d. Battery

39. A(n) _____ explains to health care providers that the insurance is not responsible to pay the provider the full amount billed.
    a. EOB
    b. deductible
    c. preexisting condition
    d. copayment

40. Lawsuits brought against phlebotomists commonly involve _____.
    a. causing an infection
    b. injury to a vein
    c. breech of confidentiality
    d. All of the above

41. A patient has the responsibility and the right to all of the following *except* _____.
    a. discussing treatment plans
    b. discussing medical conditions
    c. submitting a medical history
    d. diagnosing and ordering lab tests

42. A type of health care program that authorizes services from preselected providers is _____.
    a. Medicare
    b. HMO
    c. PPO
    d. Medicaid

43. To make informed decisions with the attending doctor, the patient needs to understand _____.
    a. the financial consequences of using in-network providers
    b. the financial consequences of using covered services
    c. the financial consequences of using out-of-network providers
    d. both a and b

44. Caregivers need to be informed of _____.
    a. past allergic reactions
    b. spiritual beliefs
    c. health coverage
    d. all of the above

45. The spoken act of falsifying facts that causes harm to a person's reputation is _____.
    a. libel
    b. slander
    c. fraud
    d. duty of care

46. In 1990, the federal government issued the _____, which was enacted to protect health care workers and patients from injuries caused by health care devices.
    a. Safe Medical Devices Act
    b. Medical Devices Protection Act
    c. Health Care Safe Device Act
    d. Health Care Protection Act

47. The responsibility not to infringe on another's rights by either intentionally or carelessly causing him or her harm is called _____.
    a. libel
    b. slander
    c. invasion of privacy
    d. duty of care

48. A mode or rule for comparison of measurement that is established by custom or authority is called _____.
    a. professionalism
    b. a standard
    c. ethics
    d. integrity

49. When verbally communicating with a patient, always speak _____ to ensure that the patient understands.
    a. in modern slang
    b. in medical terms
    c. with lengthy explanations
    d. none of the above

50. The telephone should be answered before a maximum of _____ rings.
    a. two
    b. three
    c. four
    d. five

CRITICAL THINKING

1. Karen works for ABC Laboratory as the phlebotomist. Her main responsibility is to collect and process specimens. She is an excellent employee and is thorough and diligent in all of her responsibilities. Karen is always willing to cover extra shifts, and Dr. Korn relies on her to keep the lab running smoothly. Karen has just finished working 10 days

straight, covering for vacations. Today, however, Karen is having one of "those" days. She has missed two very easy venipuncture draws and a butterfly draw. Dr. Korn is very angry with Karen for taking so long to collect the specimens and wasting supplies. He demanded Karen meet with him in his office, and he spent 10 minutes berating her. He began yelling and swearing. He told Karen she was worthless and incompetent. By the time he was done Karen was in tears. Dr. Korn told her to stop crying immediately and get back to work, and she had better not miss any more draws the remainder of the day or she would not be employed tomorrow.

- Did Dr. Korn break any civil or criminal laws?
- If so, explain which and why.

2. As part of an annual physical, Mr. Leonard wants to have an HIV blood test drawn. Cheryl is the clinic's phlebotomist and is going to draw the specimen. The clinic follows HIPAA protocol, and Cheryl is required to have Mr. Leonard sign a consent form, required by HIPPA, in order to bill the insurance company. Mr. Leonard does not wish his insurance company to be billed, and he elects to sign the form requesting this and pay for the test out of his pocket. A month later Mr. Leonard is calling to complain that he received an EOB stating his HIV test isn't covered by his insurance as part of his physical.

- What do you think happened?
- Why do you think Mr. Leonard is so upset?

3. Jim is a patient at the downtown health clinic. He likes the staff that works there; everyone is always happy, smiling, and laughing with one other. They make him feel like one of the family. Everyone greets him by name. There have been several times when he was upset and frightened about a procedure, and one of the health care practitioners held his hand or gave him a gentle pat on the arm. No one ever seems in too much of a hurry not to take the time to listen, and everyone seems to have a heartfelt concern for his health. Jim wouldn't think of going anywhere else for health care.

- What do you think makes Jim feel this way about the health clinic?

MODULE 9

Regulatory Agencies, Safety Standards, and Infection Control

I. REGULATORY AGENCIES

A. Occupational Safety and Health Administration (OSHA)—Is a division of the U.S. Department of Labor responsible for enforcing OSHA standards.

1. Several areas of these standards directly affect the health care industry.
   a. Blood-borne pathogens
   b. Personal protective equipment
   c. Formaldehyde (standard)
   d. Eye wash protection
   e. Respirator (standard)
   f. Maintenance of injury and illness log
   g. Electrical systems
   h. Biohazardous waste

B. Clinical Laboratory Improvement Amendments (CLIA)—The CLIA law stipulates that all clinical laboratories use the same standards, regardless of their location, type, or size. CLIA also establishes levels of laboratory testing certification based on the complexity of the test.

1. CLIA-waived tests are simple to perform, require a minimum of quality control, and have an insignificant risk of harm to the patient.
   a. Urinalysis by reagent strip
   b. Microscopic urine sediment
   c. Urine pregnancy tests
   d. Occult blood/guaiac tests
   e. Microscopic examination
   f. Screen slide card agglutination test
   g. Ovulation tests
   h. Whole blood clotting time
   i. Glucose reagent strip screening
   j. Spun microhematocrit
   k. Erythrocyte sedimentation rate

2. Level 1—Moderate-complexity tests:
   a. Are more complicated to perform than waived tests.

b. Require an understanding of methodology, quality control, reagent stability, and instrument calibration.

2. Level 2—High-complexity tests:
   a. Include sophisticated testing methodology.
   b. Often require independent judgment for interpretation.

C. The Clinical Laboratory Standards Institute (CLSI) has set guidelines and standards for phlebotomy curriculum. Most certification agencies base their certification standards on these guidelines.

D. The Centers for Disease Control and Prevention (CDC).

1. The CDC, along with OSHA, the Joint Commission on Accreditation of Healthcare Organizations (JCAHO), and the CDC's Healthcare Infection Control and Prevention Advisory Committee (HICPAC), assists hospitals, clinics, and laboratories to:
   a. Maintain up-to-date isolation practices.
   b. Establish guidelines and enforce regulations governing infection control.

2. The CDC published a detailed manual entitled *Isolation Techniques for Use in Hospitals* to assist general hospitals with isolation precautions. Category-specific isolation is as follows:
   a. Strict isolation
      (1) Complete isolation is required for all patients with highly contagious diseases, which may be spread through direct contact and/or by air.
      (2) Strict isolation requires anyone entering the patient's room to wear:
         (a) Gloves.
         (b) Mask.
         (c) Gown.

(3) All items taken into room must be left in the room or disposed of properly in biohazardous waste containers.

b. Contact isolation

(1) Contact isolation was designed for highly transmittable diseases spread primarily by direct contact, not warranting strict isolation.

(2) If soiling is likely, contact isolation protocols require the wearing of:

(a) Gloves.

(b) Mask.

(c) Gown.

c. Respiratory isolation

(1) Respiratory isolation is required for patients with infections that can be spread from short distances through the air by means of droplet transmission.

(2) Masks must be worn by anyone coming in close contact with these patients.

(3) All supplies should be disposed of inside the patient's room.

d. AFB (acid-fast-bacilli) isolation

(1) AFB isolation is required for patients with infectious tuberculosis.

(2) OSHA implemented a new policy, requiring the use of a high-efficiency particulate air (HEPA) respirator as a minimum level of respiratory protection for all health care workers who care for AFB patients.

(3) Gowns and gloves are also required as part of the barrier precautions.

(4) All supplies must be disposed of inside the patient's room.

e. Drainage/secretion isolation

(1) Drainage/secretion isolation is required for patients:

(a) With skin infections.

(b) With open wounds.

(c) With burns.

(d) Sometimes when recovering from surgery.

(2) Patient are restricted to their rooms.

(3) Anyone entering the room is required to wear gowns and gloves.

(4) If soiling is likely, protocols require the wearing of:

(a) Gloves.

(b) Mask.

(c) Gown.

f. Enteric precautions

(1) Enteric isolation procedures are used with patients with intestinal infections that may be transmitted by ingestion.

(2) Anyone entering the room must wear:

(a) Gloves.

(b) Mask.

(c) Gown.

(3) The patient's bathroom facilities should not be used by anyone other than the patient.

(4) All contaminated materials must be disposed of in the patient's room.

II. QUALITY ASSURANCE AND CONTROL

A. The Joint Commission on Accreditation of Healthcare Organizations (JCAHO)—The leading national accreditation body for hospitals

B. Terminology

1. Quality assurance (QA)—A group of activities and programs designed to guarantee the highest level of quality patient care

2. Total quality management (TQM)—Based on improving services and client care, directed at customer satisfaction

3. Quality control (QC)—Component of quality assurance, built on procedural steps to obtain accurate and reliable test results

4. Risk management—Used in conjunction with QA/QC, designed to minimize the exposure to risk of loss or injury, for both the health care provider and the patient; policies and procedures developed to protect employees, employer, and clients

III. SAFETY STANDARDS

A. Laboratory hazards

1. Biological, or biohazards, are any materials that are dangerous to health. Most commonly in the medical laboratory they are items contaminated by blood or body fluids containing blood.

2. Sharps—Take precautions to prevent injuries caused by needles, glass slides, and other sharp instruments during procedures, when cleaning used instruments, when disposing of used needles, and when handling sharp instruments.

3. Chemical hazards

a. Examples:

(1) Preservatives for a 24-hour urine collection

(2) Cleaning solutions

(3) Laboratory chemicals

b. Mixing the wrong chemicals can be very hazardous and create toxic gases.

    (1) Example:

        (a) Bleach and ammonia

c. A material safety data sheets (MSDS) is required by OSHA from chemical manufacturers for every hazardous chemical they manufacture or import.

    (1) The MSDS provides detailed information regarding special conditions, safe handling, and properties of the chemical and antidotes where applicable.

    (2) The MSDS must be kept in a laboratory logbook or binder, and every lab employee must know where it is kept and how it is organized.

d. Hazardous chemical containers must be labeled to clearly identify the hazard.

e. Chemical spills require special cleanup kits containing neutralizer materials, which are used depending on the type of spill.

    (1) Disposal of chemicals is regulated by the Environmental Protection Agency (EPA).

f. Safety shower and eye wash stations

    (1) Employees of the lab must be instructed in the locations and use of these stations at the time of employment.

    (2) Eyes or affected body parts must be flushed for a minimum of 15 minutes, followed by an ER visit for evaluation.

    (3) Some chemicals are activated by water and should not be flushed.

4. Electrical hazards—The phlebotomist is at risk of electrical hazards whenever using electrical equipment, such as a centrifuge. If an accident occurs:

a. The first thing you should do is shut off the source of electricity immediately.

b. If this is impossible, move the electrical hazard away from the injured person. Use a substance that does not conduct electricity to do so, such as something made of glass or wood, like a glass beaker or a broom handle.

c. Call for medical assistance.

d. Start cardiopulmonary resuscitation (CPR), if necessary, and keep the victim warm.

5. Radioactive hazards

a. Radiation hazard signs must be posted in areas where exposure is possible.

b. Precautions include wearing lead aprons and lead lined gloves.

c. Phlebotomists who are or may be pregnant should refrain from collecting specimens from patients who may present a radioactive hazard and should avoid areas labeled with radioactive hazard signs.

6. Fire or explosion hazards

a. Every policy and procedure manual should contain a section on fire safety.

b. Every employee should be aware of the procedures to follow in case of fire, be able to locate a fire extinguisher, and know how to use it.

c. There are four classifications of fire and fire extinguishers:

    (1) Class A—Ordinary combustibles, such as wood, paper, or clothing

        (a) Class A fires require extinguishers of water or water-based solutions.

    (2) Class B—Flammable liquids and vapors, such as paint, oil, grease, or gasoline

        (a) Class B fires require extinguishers that can block the source of oxygen, such as foam, dry chemical, or carbon dioxide materials.

    (3) Class C—Electrical equipment fires

        (a) Class C fires require extinguishers of nonconductible agents, such as dry chemical, carbon dioxide, or halon.

    (4) Class D—Combustible or reactive metals, such as sodium, potassium, magnesium, uranium, powdered aluminum, and lithium

        (a) Class D fires require extinguishers of dry powder agents or sand. These are the most difficult fires to control and often lead to explosions.

    (5) Class ABC (multipurpose)—Use dry chemical reagents to smother the fire; can be used on Class A, B, or C fires. This eliminates some of the confusion of finding the right extinguisher when it's needed. Multipurpose extinguishers are the kind most often found in health care facilities.

B. Laboratory safety

1. Employers are mandated by OSHA to provide a safe working environment for their employees, the goal of every health care facility.

2. Guidelines are implemented to minimize the risks of these hazards, and precautions are taken to prevent accidents.

3. List of general laboratory safety rules

a. *Never* eat, drink, chew gum, or smoke in the laboratory.

b. *Never* put anything in your mouth, such as pens, pencils, or fingers, while working in the laboratory.

c. *Never* store food or beverages in the laboratory refrigerator used to store reagents or specimens.

d. *Never* apply cosmetics, handle contact lenses, or rub your eyes in the laboratory.

e. *Never* wear excessive jewelry, such as long chains, large or dangling earrings, or loose bracelets.

f. *Always* wear your hair back away from your face if it is shoulder length or longer.

g. *Always* wear uniforms or work clothes that are neither formfitting nor floppy. Work clothes should *always* be neat and clean.

h. *Always* wear a buttoned lab coat when working in the laboratory.

i. *Never* wear a lab coat to lunch, on breaks, or when leaving the lab to go home.

j. *Never* wear any of the PPE items outside their designated areas.

k. *Always* wear closed-toe, leather or nonporous, nonskid sole shoes. Sandals, slippers, or high heels are inappropriate.

l. *Never* pipettes specimens or reagents by mouth.

m. *Always* wear a face shield when performing specimen collections or processing specimens that might generate splashes or aerosol of body fluids.

n. *Always* wear gloves for phlebotomy procedures and specimen processing.

4. General guidelines for safety outside the laboratory
   a. Perform all activities using standard precautions.
   b. *Never* recap contaminated needles.
   c. Properly dispose of all contaminated material in the appropriate biohazardous waste container.
   d. Properly dispose of all sharps in the appropriate puncture-resistant container.
   e. Replace bed rails of the patient's bed after performing a specimen collection.
   f. Report infiltrated IVs or any other concerns about a patient's IV.
   g. Report unresponsive patients to the nurse.
   h. Report unusual odors to the nurse.
   i. Report any spills or items dropped on the floor to the nurse or to housekeeping.
   j. Avoid running or yelling.

k. Know what procedure to follow if a patient has fainted or is unconscious.

l. Know basic lifesaver cardiopulmonary resuscitation.

IV. THE INFECTION CYCLE

A. Microbes—The thousands of microorganisms we live with everyday
   1. Microbes are classified as bacteria, virus, fungi, or protozoa.
   2. The majority of these microbes are nonpathogenic. However, some microbes are pathogenic.
      a. Pathogen—Organism or substance capable of causing a disease, condition, or infection
      b. Nonpathogenic—Microbe that is nondisease producing
   3. Environmental conditions required for pathogen growth
      a. Nutrients
      b. Water
      c. Oxygen or the lack of it
      d. Proper pH
      e. Proper temperature of 37.5 degrees Celsius (98.6 degrees Fahrenheit)
      f. Darkness

B. Chain of infection
   1. Reservoir host—Breeding ground for transmission of pathogens to others; any person, animal, arthropod, plant, soil, or substance in which an infectious agent normally lives, reproduces, and depends on for survival, that allows transmission to a susceptible host
   2. Means of exit—Route by which pathogens leave the reservoir host
   3. Susceptible host—Person capable of being infected by the pathogen
   4. Means of transmission—Method of transmission from one host to another
      a. Direct contact—Direct physical transfer of pathogens from a reservoir host to a susceptible host
      b. Indirect contact—Exposing a susceptible host to a pathogen by means of an inanimate object
      c. Droplet transmission—When droplets containing microorganisms generated from the infected person are propelled a short distance through the air and deposited on the host's conjunctivae, nasal mucosa, or mouth
      d. Airborne transmission—Dissemination of either airborne droplet nuclei or dust particles containing the infectious agent

(1) Microorganisms carried in this manner can be dispersed widely by air currents and may become inhaled by a susceptible host within the same room or over a longer distance from the source patient, depending on environmental factors.

e. Vehicle transmission—Infection by means of a microorganism being transmitted by contaminated items such as food, water, medications, devices, and equipment

f. Vector-borne—When vectors, such as mosquitoes, flies, rats, and other vermin, transmit microorganisms

(1) This route of transmission is of less significance in hospitals in the United States than in other regions of the world.

C. Breaking the chain of infection—Either by reducing the susceptibility of the host or by eliminating the means of transmission

1. Means of reducing susceptibility
   a. Proper nutrition
   b. Sleep
   c. Stress reduction
   d. Immunizations
2. Means of eliminating transmission
   a. Hand washing
   b. Wearing personal protective equipment (gloves, gowns, masks)
   c. Proper disposal of contaminated waste
   d. Insect and rodent control
   e. Decontamination of equipment, instruments, and other surfaces.
   f. Isolation procedures

V. UNIVERSAL PRECAUTIONS VERSUS STANDARD PRECAUTIONS

A. Universal precautions

1. In 1985, due to the HIV epidemic, isolation practices were dramatically altered. The revised procedures became known as Universal Precautions.
2. Universal precautions, as defined by the CDC, are designed to prevent the transmission of human immunodeficiency virus (HIV), hepatitis B virus (HBV), and other blood-borne pathogens when personnel are providing first aid or health care.
   a. Human immunodeficiency virus (HIV)—Retrovirus that causes acquired immunodeficiency syndrome (AIDS)
   b. Hepatitis B (HBV)—Blood-borne pathogen that causes a severe acute infection and may

progress to chronic infection and permanent liver damage; caused by the hepatitis B virus, an enveloped, double-stranded DNA virus

c. Blood-borne pathogen—Any infectious microorganism present in the blood and/or other body fluids and tissues; commonly applied to the hepatitis B virus and the human immunodeficiency virus

B. Standard precautions

1. These were designed to reduce the risk of transmission of microorganisms from both recognized and unrecognized sources of infection.
2. Standard precautions apply to the following:
   a. Blood
   b. All body fluids, secretions and excretions (except sweat), regardless of whether they contain visible blood
   c. Nonintact skin
   d. Mucous membranes

VI. PERSONAL PROTECTIVE EQUIPMENT (PPE)

A. Gloves—Worn for two important reasons:

1. Gloves are worn to provide a protective barrier and to prevent gross contamination of the hands when touching blood, body fluids, secretions, excretions, mucous membranes, and nonintact skin.
2. Gloves are worn also to reduce the likelihood of microorganisms present on the hands of personnel being transmitted to patients during invasive or other patient care procedures that involve touching a patient's mucous membranes and nonintact skin.

B. Masks, respiratory protection, protective eye wear (goggles), face shields—Mandated by the OSHA blood-borne pathogens final rule

1. A surgical mask is generally worn to provide protection from the spread of infectious large-particle droplets.
2. Large-particle droplets, which are transmitted by infected patients who are coughing or sneezing in close contact, generally travel only short distances (up to 3 feet).

C. Protective apparel (gowns, aprons, laboratory coats)—Worn to prevent contamination of clothing and to protect the skin of personnel from blood and body fluid exposures

1. Gowns may be:
   a. Disposable and discarded in a biohazardous container.
   b. Nondisposable and laundered on the premises.

2. Laboratory coats—Worn to prevent contamination of clothing during lab procedures.
   a. Laboratories must provide the phlebotomists with a laboratory coat.
   b. The coat remains at the laboratory and is:
     (1) *Either* laundered on the premises
     (2) *Or* disposable.

VII. HANDWASHING

A. Handwashing is the first line of defense in the fight against the spread of infection.
B. It must be performed:
  1. Before and after *every* patient contact.
  2. Between different procedures on the same patient.
  3. Whenever hands are visibly contaminated.
  4. Before and after using the lavatory.
  5. Before leaving the lab.
  6. Before and after breaks and lunch.
  7. Before and after wearing and removing gloves.

VIII. MEDICAL/SURGICAL ASEPSIS

A. Two types of asepsis:
  1. Medical asepsis is the destruction of microorganisms after having left the body to prevent transmission of microorganisms to another person.
   a. To maintain medical asepsis, hands and wrists are washed for a minimum of 2 minutes with antimicrobial/antibacterial soap.
  2. Surgical asepsis is the process of destroying microorganisms before they enter the body.
   a. This process maintains sterility when entering a normally sterile part of the body.

IX. BLOOD-BORNE PATHOGENS—OSHA REGULATIONS

A. Risk
  1. All health care professionals are at risk of occupational exposure to blood-borne pathogens, including hepatitis B (HBV), hepatitis C (HCV), and human immunodeficiency virus (HIV).
  2. The chance of preventing disease if exposure occurs is greatly improved by:
   a. Understanding the precautions taken to reduce the risk of exposure.
   b. Knowing the protocols to follow upon exposure.
B. Common reasons for exposure
  1. Contaminated needle sticks, cuts from other sharp contaminated items such as glass slides, or pipettes

2. Direct contact with an infected patient's blood or body fluids
C. Prevention of occupational exposure
  1. Most contaminated needle sticks and other punctures or lacerations can be prevented by using safety techniques.
   a. Examples:
     (1) Not recapping needles by hand
     (2) Disposing of used needles in the appropriate sharps containers
     (3) Using medical devices with safety features designed to prevent injuries
  2. Using the appropriate barrier precautions, such as gloves, face shields, protective eyewear, or gowns, can prevent exposure to the eyes, nose, mouth, and hands.
D. Personal exposure control plan
  1. To be in compliance with OSHA standards, employers must have a written exposure control plan. Therefore, every medical facility has its own exposure control plan documented in their policies and procedures manual.
  2. The written plan must include:
   a. A list of all job classifications in which occupational exposure may occur.
   b. A standard precautions statement.
   c. Identification of engineering controls, such as accessible handwashing facilities, sharps containers, self-sheathing needles, autoclaves, and biohazardous waste symbols.
   d. Identification of work practice controls, such as:
     (1) Prohibiting the recapping of needles by hand.
     (2) Requiring handwashing after glove removal.
     (3) No eating, drinking, or smoking in the laboratory.
   e. Requirements of personal protective equipment.
   f. Housekeeping standards, such as decontamination of surfaces and blood spill cleanup.
  3. Hepatitis B vaccinations
   a. Requirements
     (1) All health care professionals who have a reasonable risk of being exposed to blood or body fluids should receive the hepatitis B vaccine.
     (2) Vaccinations must be offered free of charge to employees within 10 days of assignment to duties of occupational exposure risk.

(3) The ideal time to be vaccinated is during the training period.

b. The hepatitis B vaccine is a series of three vaccinations. After the first dose is given:

   (1) The second dose follows at 1 month.

   (2) The third dose is given 5 months later.

c. After completion of the vaccination series, the health care professional should be tested to make sure the vaccination has provided immunity to HBV.

   (1) Approximately 87 percent of those who take the series develop immunity after the second dose.

   (2) Ninety-six percent develop immunity after the third dose.

d. The employee has the right to decline the vaccine series.

e. If the vaccination is declined, a signed and dated statement of refusal must be retained in the employee's personnel file.

4. Warning labels and signs must be affixed to appropriate biohazardous waste containers.

a. Labels must be fluorescent orange or orange-red.

b. They must be printed with the words "Biohazardous Waste" on the label.

5. Training in dealing with blood-borne pathogens must be provided to all employees at risk for occupational exposure free of charge.

6. Record keeping—Employers who hire employees at risk for occupational exposure must maintain confidential medical records as well as records documenting all training sessions.

E. Postexposure action plan

1. Basic guidelines have been approved by OSHA and recommended by the CDC for the postexposure action plan that is maintained at every facility.

2. Immediately following an exposure:

a. Wash needle sticks, punctures, or lacerations with soap and water.

b. Flush splashes to the nose, mouth, or skin with water.

c. Irrigate eyes with clean water, saline, or sterile irrigants.

3. Not recommended

a. No scientific evidence shows that using antiseptics or squeezing the wound reduces the risk of transmission of blood-borne pathogens.

b. Using a caustic agent such as bleach is not recommended.

4. After taking immediate steps following exposure, you should:

a. Report the exposure to the appropriate personnel. Prompt reporting is imperative because in some cases postexposure treatment is recommended and should be started as soon as possible.

b. Seek treatment, if applicable.

   (1) Hepatitis B immune globulin (HBIG) is effective in preventing HBV infection after an exposure.

   (2) There is not a vaccine for hepatitis C and no treatment after an exposure that prevents infection. Immune globulin is not recommended. For this reason alone following recommended infection control practices is essential.

   (3) There is no vaccine for HIV.

      (a) However, results from a small number of studies suggest that the use of zidovudine after certain occupational exposures may reduce the chance of HIV transmission.

      (b) Postexposure treatment is not recommended for all occupational exposures to HIV. Many types of exposures do not lead to an HIV infection, and the medications may have serious side effects.

      (c) In 1996, the CDC recommended the preventative treatment of AZT and other drugs in combination after a possible occupational exposure to HIV. It is believed that the action of AZT prevents the virus from entering the cell. However, to be most effective, chemoprophylaxis must begin immediately within a 1- to 2-hour window after exposure.

c. Follow-up treatment

   (1) HBV

      (a) The CDC does not recommend follow-up treatment because postexposure treatment is highly effective in preventing HBV.

      (b) However, any symptoms suggesting hepatitis, such as yellow eyes or skin, loss of appetite, nausea, vomiting, fever, stomach or joint pain, extreme tiredness, should be reported to your health care provider.

   (2) HCV

      (a) You should have an antibody test for the hepatitis C virus and a liver enzyme test as soon as possible after the exposure. This creates a baseline and at 4 to 6 months another test should be performed.

    (b) Report any symptoms suggesting hepatitis to your health care provider.

   (3) HIV

    (a) You should be tested for the HIV antibody as soon as possible after exposure for a baseline and periodically for at least 6 months after exposure.

    (b) The recommended sequence of testing is at 6 weeks, 12 weeks, and then again at 6 months.

  d. Precautions taken during the follow-up period

   (1) HBV—If you are exposed to HBV and you are treated postexposure, it is unlikely you will become infected; therefore, no treatment is recommended.

   (2) HCV—The risk of becoming infected and passing the infection on to others is very low, and no precautions are recommended.

   (3) HIV—During the first 6–12 weeks of postexposure, you should follow the recommendations for preventing the transmission of HIV. These include not donating blood, semen, or organs and not having sexual intercourse.

    (a) If you do choose to have sexual intercourse, using a condom consistently and correctly may reduce the risk of HIV transmission.

    (b) HIV may be transmitted through breast milk.

PRACTICE

1. A microbe that is nondisease producing is called a _____ organism.
   a. pathogenic
   b. nonpathogenic
   c. causative
   d. palliative

2. _____ is a retrovirus that causes AIDS.
   a. HBV
   b. HIV
   c. BBP
   d. DNA

3. After a contaminated exposure, a phlebotomist should be tested for the HIV antibody as soon as possible for a baseline and then periodically for at least _____.
   a. 3 weeks
   b. 6 weeks
   c. 3 months
   d. 6 months

4. _____ isolation is required for patients with infectious tuberculosis.
   a. Strict
   b. Contact
   c. AFB
   d. Drainage

5. _____ isolation procedures are used for patients with intestinal infections that may be transmitted by ingestion.
   a. Strict
   b. Contact
   c. Drainage/secretion
   d. Enteric

6. _____ is a blood-borne pathogen that causes a severe acute infection and may progress to a chronic infection and permanent liver damage.
   a. HIV
   b. HBV
   c. Fomite
   d. BBP

7. "_____" is the correct term used to describe any infectious microorganism present in blood and/or other body fluids and tissues.
   a. HIV
   b. Blood-borne pathogen
   c. Fomites
   d. Germ

8. When transmitted by infected patients by means of coughing or sneezing at close range, large-particle droplets generally travel only short distances, up to _____ feet.
   a. 2
   b. 3
   c. 5
   d. 6

9. _____ hazards are any materials that are dangerous to health and are contaminated with blood or body fluids containing blood.
   a. Biological
   b. Chemical
   c. Electrical
   d. Radioactive

10. _____ is the act of exposing a susceptible host to a pathogen by means of an inanimate object.
    a. Direct contact
    b. Droplet transmission
    c. Indirect contact
    d. Airborne transmission

11. _____ is/are *not* required by OSHA to be worn when you are handling body fluids.
    a. Protective face gear
    b. Disposable lab coat
    c. Disposable gloves
    d. Disposable hair cover

12. _____ is/are the first line of defense in the fight against the spread of infection.
    a. Gloves
    b. Hand washing
    c. Lab coats
    d. A face shield

13. Which of the following requires cleanup kits containing absorbent and neutralizer materials?
    a. Biological spills
    b. Chemical spills
    c. Electrical hazards
    d. Radioactive hazards

14. The disposal of chemicals is regulated by _____.
    a. DEA
    b. EPA
    c. OSHA
    d. CDC

15. The EPA recommends that a _____ bleach solution be used to decontaminate surfaces at the end of each shift.
    a. 1:10
    b. 10:1
    c. 10:10
    d. 10:100

16. A Class _____ fire extinguisher is used to contain electrical equipment fires.
    a. A
    b. B
    c. C
    d. D

17. _____ provides detailed information for each hazardous chemical manufactured or imported.
    a. A laboratory operating manual
    b. A material safety data sheet
    c. A laboratory chemical composition sheet
    d. OSHA

18. Disposable _____ should not be disposed of in a biohazards waste container.
    a. gloves
    b. gowns
    c. instruments
    d. lab coats

19. To maintain medical asepsis, hands and wrists should be washed for a minimum of _____ minutes with antimicrobial or antibacterial soap.
    a. 1
    b. 2
    c. 3
    d. 4

20. If an electrical accident occurs, the first thing you must do is _____.
    a. call the electric company
    b. move the patient from the area of the electrical source
    c. start CPR
    d. shut off the source of electricity

21. _____ is/are a group of activities and programs designed to guarantee the highest level of quality patient care.
    a. Standards of care
    b. Due process
    c. Quality assurance
    d. Quality control

22. _____ is a program, used in conjunction with QA/QC, designed to minimize the risk of loss or injury for both the health care provider and the patient.
    a. JCAHO
    b. NCCLS
    c. Risk management
    d. Total quality management

23. All of the following are standards regulated by OSHA *except* _____.
    a. biohazardous waste
    b. personal protection equipment
    c. blood-borne pathogens
    d. outpatient scheduling

24. According to CLIA, _____ require an understanding of methodology, quality control, reagent stability, and instrument calibration.
    a. moderate-complexity tests
    b. high-complexity tests
    c. waived tests
    d. low-complexity tests

25. _____ is the leading national accreditation body for hospitals.
    a. JACHO
    b. CLSI
    c. NACCLS
    d. HIPAA

26. A _____ is considered the breeding ground for the transmission of pathogens to others.
    a. susceptible host
    b. reservoir host
    c. carrier
    d. fomite

27. A _____ organism is capable of causing disease.
    a. nonpathogenic
    b. pathogenic
    c. curative
    d. corroborative

28. All of the following assist hospitals, clinics, and laboratories to maintain up-to-date isolation practices except _____.
    a. JCAHO
    b. HIPAA
    c. CDC
    d. OSHA

29. Contact isolation was designed for highly transmittable diseases that are spread primarily by direct contact and that do not warrant strict isolation, such as _____.
    a. pneumonia
    b. measles
    c. meningococcal meningitis
    d. chickenpox

30. In 1970, the _____ published a detailed manual entitled *Isolation Techniques for Use in Hospitals*.
    a. OSHA
    b. CLIA
    c. CDC
    d. NCCLS

CRITICAL THINKING

1. Jennie is the phlebotomist for the county's STD clinic. Yesterday morning Jennie noticed an elderly gentleman sitting in the crowded waiting area. He was coughing uncontrollably into a dirty handkerchief and was as pale as a sheet. Jennie had not seen the man at the clinic before and was very concerned he might collapse. Jennie decided she would go talk with him and take him a cup of water. After speaking with the man for a few minutes, Jennie found out that Mr. Franklin lived alone in a small trailer on the outskirts of town. The trailer had no running water and no electricity. Jennie also found out that Mr. Franklin had had the cough for the past 2 years, but it had been getting worse the past three weeks. Jennie left the water and went to find a doctor. Dr. Mills was on duty. After Jennie related what Mr. Franklin had told her, Dr. Mills asked Jennie to find an empty exam room and escort Mr. Franklin to it. After examining Mr. Franklin, Dr Mills ordered a chest X-ray to rule out pneumonia. The chest X-ray revealed Mr. Franklin has active tuberculosis.
   • What is the mechanism of exposure of tuberculosis? Explain.
   • What are the appropriate protocols for isolating Mr. Franklin? Explain.

2. Phyllis is a phlebotomist at Geneva General and is on duty this weekend when a call comes in for a stat draw on the peds unit. She gathers her lab tray and runs to the unit. The order is for a CBC, PT/INR on a 2-year-old little boy. Phyllis looks for a vein, assembles a butterfly collection kit, and sets up with pediatric evacuated tubes. The boy seems cooperative, but Phyllis has a nurse holding her young patient on her lap in a semirestraint. However, both of the boy's arms are free. Phyllis dons her PPEs and is ready to begin. Phyllis ties the tourniquet, cleans the site, leans over, and inserts the needle. Just as she inserts the needle, the boy reaches out and grabs Phyllis's loop earring and pulls hard. Phyllis has the needle in the patient, it is a stat draw, and she probably won't get a second chance at the draw, but the boy will not let go of her earring—And it really hurts!
   • What should Phyllis do?
   • Has Phyllis violated any laboratory safety rules or OSHA regulations?

3. Dena has been hired at a local lab in her small hometown. The lab allows Dena to perform not only blood draws, but UAs, pregnancy tests, ECGs, CBC, lipid panels, and strep tests. She hopes to be busy with all the new challenges. She is very excited to be home and working in her field. On the first day, the lab manager takes her under her wing, teaches her how to calibrate and run the CBC machine, and shows her the latest and greatest cholesterol, glucose, and protime machines. Dena has had a great first day and is meeting some friends after work to celebrate. Dena talks nonstop about all of the things the lab manager showed her and her new responsibilities. One of Dena's friends is an MLT and quizzes Dena by asking her what level the laboratory is, based on CLIA regulations. Dena didn't know the answer.
   • Do you?
   • Explain your response.

Appendix A

Answers to Practice Questions

MODULE 4: MEDICAL TERMINOLOGY AND ANATOMY AND PHYSIOLOGY

1. *ANS:* D

   Word roots are the basis from which all medical terms are derived. A prefix is added at the beginning of a word root to change the meaning of the word. A suffix is added to the end of a word root or combining vowel to add to or change its meaning.

   ### References

   Kalanick, K. *Phlebotomy Technician Specialist.* Clifton Park, N.Y.: Thomson Delmar Learning, 2004, p. 34.

2. *ANS:* B

   A combining vowel is an extension of the word root and may be used to modify the spelling of a term, generally by using the letters "o" or "i."

   ### References

   Kalanick, K. *Phlebotomy Technician Specialist.* Clifton Park, N.Y.: Thomson Delmar Learning, 2004, p. 35.

3. *ANS:* D

   "ABG" is the correct way to abbreviate the medical term arterial blood gases; all of the others are incorrect.

   ### References

   Kalanick, K. *Phlebotomy Technician Specialist.* Clifton Park, N.Y.: Thomson Delmar Learning, 2004, p. 46.

4. *ANS:* B

   "Thromb/o" refers to a clot, "ven/o" refers to a vein, "corpuscul/o" means little body, and "abrupt/o" refers to broken away from.

   ### References

   Kalanick, K. *Phlebotomy Technician Specialist.* Clifton Park, N.Y.: Thomson Delmar Learning, 2004, p. 38.

5. *ANS:* A

   The medical abbreviation for hemoglobin is "hgb"; all of the others are incorrect.

References

Kalanick, K. *Phlebotomy Technician Specialist.* Clifton Park, N.Y.: Thomson Delmar Learning, 2004, p. 47.

6. *ANS:* B

   The midsagittal plane is a lengthwise plane running from front to back, dividing the body or any of its parts into equal right and left halves. The sagittal plane is a longitudinal imaginary line dividing the entire body into equal right and left parts. The frontal plane divides the body into anterior and posterior portions. The transverse plane divides the body into a top and bottom portion.

   ### References

   Kalanick, K. *Phlebotomy Technician Specialist.* Clifton Park, N.Y.: Thomson Delmar Learning, 2004, p. 65.

   Hoeltke, L. *The Complete Textbook of Phlebotomy,* 3rd ed. Clifton Park, N.Y.: Thomson Delmar Learning, 2006, p. 81.

7. *ANS:* A

   A ventricle is a cavity of a bodily part or organ. For example, a chamber of the heart receives blood from the corresponding atrium; from it, blood is forced into the arteries and a system of communicating cavities in the brain that are continuous with the central canal of the spinal cord. The atria are the upper chambers of the heart and are not referenced as a chamber of the brain. The Purkinje fibers and the bundle of His are both associated with the electrical conduction system of the heart, and neither one is considered a cavity or chamber.

   ### References

   Kalanick, K. *Phlebotomy Technician Specialist.* Clifton Park, N.Y.: Thomson Delmar Learning, 2004, p. 123.

   Hoeltke, L. *The Complete Textbook of Phlebotomy,* 3rd ed. Clifton Park, N.Y.: Thomson Delmar Learning, 2006, p. 113.

   Merriam-Webster's Medical Desk Dictionary, rev. ed. Clifton Park, N.Y.: Thomson Delmar Learning, 2006.

8. *ANS:* B

The bicuspid valve, also called the mitral valve, is a valve in the heart that guards the opening between the left atrium and the left ventricle, preventing the blood in the ventricle from returning to the atrium. It consists of two triangular flaps attached at the base of the ventricular walls; it is called "bicuspid" because of the two triangular flaps. The tricuspid valve is a three-part valve located between the right atrium and right ventricle. The pulmonary semilunar valve is the half-moon–shaped valve between the right ventricle and the pulmonary artery. The aortic semilunar valve is the valve between the left ventricle and the ascending aorta and is made up of three half-moon–shaped cups.

References

Kalanick, K. *Phlebotomy Technician Specialist.* Clifton Park, N.Y.: Thomson Delmar Learning, 2004, p. 124.

Hoeltke, L. *The Complete Textbook of Phlebotomy,* 3rd ed. Clifton Park, N.Y.: Thomson Delmar Learning, 2006, p. 113.

Merriam-Webster's Medical Desk Dictionary, rev. ed. Clifton Park, N.Y.: Thomson Delmar Learning, 2006.

9. *ANS:* B

The myocardium is the middle cardiac muscular layer of the heart wall and makes up the major portion of the heart. The pericardium is the closed membranous sac surrounding the heart. The endocardium is the membrane lining the interior of the heart. The epicardium is the visceral part of the pericardium.

References

Kalanick, K. *Phlebotomy Technician Specialist.* Clifton Park, N.Y.: Thomson Delmar Learning, 2004, p. 125.

Hoeltke, L. *The Complete Textbook of Phlebotomy,* 3rd ed. Clifton Park, N.Y.: Thomson Delmar Learning, 2006, p. 116.

Merriam-Webster's Medical Desk Dictionary, rev. ed. Clifton Park, N.Y.: Thomson Delmar Learning, 2006.

10. *ANS:* A

Tunica adventitia is the outer layer of a tubular organ or structure, especially a blood vessel. It is composed of collagenous and elastic fibers, and is not covered with peritoneum. The tunica media is the middle layer in the wall of a blood vessel, and the tunica intima is the inside lining of a blood vessel. The lumen is a passageway or opening to a tubular structure such as a blood vessel or a phlebotomy or hypodermic needle.

References

Kalanick, K. *Phlebotomy Technician Specialist.* Clifton Park, N.Y.: Thomson Delmar Learning, 2004, p. 131.

Hoeltke, L. *The Complete Textbook of Phlebotomy,* 3rd ed. Clifton Park, N.Y.: Thomson Delmar Learning, 2006, p. 108.

Merriam-Webster's Medical Desk Dictionary, rev. ed. Clifton Park, N.Y.: Thomson Delmar Learning, 2006.

11. *ANS:* D

Phlebitis is inflammation of the lining of a vein, accompanied by clotting of the blood in the vein. Symptoms include edema of the affected area, pain, and redness along the length of the vein. An aneurysm occurs when a weakened artery bulges or balloons out. A CVA is a cerebrovascular accident, or stroke. Hemorrhoids are varicose veins in the walls of the lower rectum and tissues around the anus.

References

Kalanick, K. *Phlebotomy Technician Specialist.* Clifton Park, N.Y.: Thomson Delmar Learning, 2004, p. 135.

12. *ANS:* C

The average adult has 4.5 to 5.0 million RBCs per cubic millimeter of blood. The other answers are incorrect.

References

Kalanick, K. *Phlebotomy Technician Specialist.* Clifton Park, N.Y.: Thomson Delmar Learning, 2004, p. 138.

13. *ANS:* A

Hemostasis is the stoppage or sluggishness of blood flow, the arrest of bleeding or of circulation. Homeostasis is the state of dynamic equilibrium of the internal environment of the body. Hemopoiesis is the production and development of blood cells. Hemolysis is the lysis of red blood cells with liberation of hemoglobin.

References

Kalanick, K. *Phlebotomy Technician Specialist.* Clifton Park, N.Y.: Thomson Delmar Learning, 2004, p. 141.

Merriam-Webster's Medical Desk Dictionary, rev. ed. Clifton Park, N.Y.: Thomson Delmar Learning, 2006.

14. *ANS:* C

An individual belonging to the AB blood group can accept blood from all blood types. Type AB blood lacks antibodies in its plasma, so it cannot agglutinate the red blood cells of any donor. Therefore, type AB blood is the considered the universal recipient. Type O is considered the universal donor but can receive blood only from a type O donor. Types A and B are antigen specific.

References

Kalanick, K. *Phlebotomy Technician Specialist*. Clifton Park, N.Y.: Thomson Delmar Learning, 2004, p. 143.

15. *ANS:* C

Leukopenia is a condition in which the number of white blood cells circulating in the blood is abnormally low; it is most commonly due to a decreased production of new cells in conjunction with various infectious diseases, as a reaction to various drugs or other chemicals, or in response to irradiation. Anemia is a condition in which the blood is deficient in red blood cells. Leukocytosis is an increase in the number of white blood cells in the circulating blood that occurs normally (after a meal) or abnormally (as in some infections). Polycythemia is a condition marked by an abnormal increase in the number of circulating red blood cells.

References

Kalanick, K. *Phlebotomy Technician Specialist*. Clifton Park, N.Y.: Thomson Delmar Learning, 2004, p. 144.

Merriam-Webster's Medical Desk Dictionary, rev. ed. Clifton Park, N.Y.: Thomson Delmar Learning, 2006.

16. *ANS:* C

Leukemia is an acute or chronic disease of unknown cause in humans and other warm-blooded animals that involves the blood-forming organs It is characterized by an abnormal increase in the number of white blood cells in the tissues of the body, with or without a corresponding increase of those in the circulating blood, and is classified according to the type of white blood cell most prominently involved. Anemia is a condition in which the blood is deficient in red blood cells. Hemophilia is a hereditary blood disease marked by greatly prolonged blood coagulation time. Polycythemia is a condition marked by an abnormal increase in the number of circulating red blood cells.

References

Kalanick, K. *Phlebotomy Technician Specialist*. Clifton Park, N.Y.: Thomson Delmar Learning, 2004, p. 144.

Merriam-Webster's Medical Desk Dictionary, rev. ed. Clifton Park, N.Y.: Thomson Delmar Learning, 2006.

17. *ANS:* A

The outer membrane of the human red blood cell may also contain a D antigen, better known as the Rh factor, in addition to the AB antigens. The Rh/D antigen was first discovered in Rhesus monkeys; hence the term "Rh" was given to the D antigen. All of the other responses are distracters.

References

Kalanick, K. *Phlebotomy Technician Specialist*. Clifton Park, N.Y.: Thomson Delmar Learning, 2004, p. 143.

18. *ANS:* D

Veins carry deoxygenated blood toward the heart. The one exception is the pulmonary vein, which carries oxygenated blood from the lungs back to the heart. Arterioles carry oxygenated blood from the arteries to the capillaries. Arteries carry oxygenated blood. Capillaries carry a mixture of venous and arterial blood and are the site of oxygen/carbon dioxide and nutrient/waste material exchange.

References

Kalanick, K. *Phlebotomy Technician Specialist*. Clifton Park, N.Y.: Thomson Delmar Learning, 2004, p. 130.

Hoeltke, L. *The Complete Textbook of Phlebotomy*, 3rd ed. Clifton Park, N.Y.: Thomson Delmar Learning, 2006, p. 113.

19. *ANS:* C

Serum is blood that has been removed from the body and allowed to clot 30–60 minutes before centrifuging. Chemistry and immunological tests are performed on serum. Electrolytes are found in plasma and consist of calcium, sodium, potassium, and magnesium. Plasma is the liquid portion of whole blood that has not been allowed to clot. Whole blood consists of plasma and formed elements (WBCs, RBCs, platelets).

References

Kalanick, K. *Phlebotomy Technician Specialist*. Clifton Park, N.Y.: Thomson Delmar Learning, 2004, p. 137.

20. *ANS:* D

Portal circulation is a division of systemic venous circulation. Coronary circulation takes oxygenated blood directly to the cells of the heart muscle. Fetal circulation is the circulation that takes place in a fetus. Caudal circulation is a nonsense distracter.

References

Kalanick, K. *Phlebotomy Technician Specialist*. Clifton Park, N.Y.: Thomson Delmar Learning, 2004, p. 129.

21. *ANS:* C

The median cubital vein is usually large and well anchored. This makes it the first choice for venipuncture and it is typically less painful. The cephalic vein is the second choice; it is also well anchored but is often more difficult to palpate. The basilic vein is usually easy to palpate, but it is not well anchored, which causes it to roll and bruise more easily. Radial is a distracter response.

References

Kalanick, K. *Phlebotomy Technician Specialist*. Clifton Park, N.Y.: Thomson Delmar Learning, 2004, p. 133.

Hoeltke, L. *The Complete Textbook of Phlebotomy*, 3rd ed. Clifton Park, N.Y.: Thomson Delmar Learning, 2006, p. 119.

22. *ANS:* A

The upper two chambers are called the atria, the receiving chambers of the heart. "Atrium" is singular and refers to only one of the upper two chambers. The ventricles are the lower two chambers of the heart. The pericardium is the outer covering of the heart and is not a chamber.

References

Kalanick, K. *Phlebotomy Technician Specialist*. Clifton Park, N.Y.: Thomson Delmar Learning, 2004, p. 123.

Hoeltke, L. *The Complete Textbook of Phlebotomy*, 3rd ed. Clifton Park, N.Y.: Thomson Delmar Learning, 2006, p. 113.

23. *ANS:* A

The medical prefix "infra-" means inferior to. The prefix "a-" or "an-" means without. Either "en-" or "endo-" means within, and "fore-" means in front of.

References

Kalanick, K. *Phlebotomy Technician Specialist*. Clifton Park, N.Y.: Thomson Delmar Learning, 2004, p. 40.

24. *ANS:* B

Hemolysis occurs when red blood cells rupture. Hemopoiesis is the production and development of blood cells. Hemostasis is the stoppage or sluggishness of blood flow, the arrest of bleeding or of circulation. Hemocytosis is a distracter.

References

Kalanick, K. *Phlebotomy Technician Specialist*. Clifton Park, N.Y.: Thomson Delmar Learning, 2004, p. 138.

Hoeltke, L. *The Complete Textbook of Phlebotomy*, 3rd ed. Clifton Park, N.Y.: Thomson Delmar Learning, 2006, p. 209.

25. *ANS:* B

The medical suffix "-ectasis" means stretching, dilation, and enlargement. The suffix "-iasis" means a condition, pathologic state, or abnormal condition; "-exis" means condition; "-esis" means state or abnormal condition.

References

Kalanick, K. *Phlebotomy Technician Specialist*. Clifton Park, N.Y.: Thomson Delmar Learning, 2004, p. 42.

26. *ANS:* D

Eosinophils are granulocytes. Their numbers increase in allergic reactions and parasitic infestations, and their primary function is in the defense of invading organisms. Neutrophils have a many-lobed nucleus and phagocytize bacteria. Basophils are essential to nonspecific immune response to inflammation. Monocytes are large mononuclear leukocytes with deeply indented nuclei and slate gray cytoplasm.

References

Kalanick, K. *Phlebotomy Technician Specialist*. Clifton Park, N.Y.: Thomson Delmar Learning, 2004, p. 140.

27. *ANS:* B

A universal donor is an individual with type O blood, which has no A or B antigens and can be donated to all blood types.

References

Kalanick, K. *Phlebotomy Technician Specialist*. Clifton Park, N.Y.: Thomson Delmar Learning, 2004, p. 143.

28. *ANS:* D

Type B blood accounts for 12 percent of the U.S. population. Type AB accounts for 3 percent, type O accounts for 44 percent, and type A accounts for 41 percent.

References

Kalanick, K. *Phlebotomy Technician Specialist*. Clifton Park, N.Y.: Thomson Delmar Learning, 2004, p. 142.

29. *ANS:* C

In the prevention of erythroblastosis fetalis, a special injection of immune globulin, Rho-GAM, can be given to an RH− mother within 72 hours after delivery of a viable or nonviable fetus or a miscarriage. All other answers are incorrect and are distracters.

References

Kalanick, K. *Phlebotomy Technician Specialist*. Clifton Park, N.Y.: Thomson Delmar Learning, 2004, pp. 143–144.

30. *ANS:* C

Plasma, which makes up about 55 percent of the total blood volume, is the straw-colored liquid portion of blood minus the cellular elements. It is approximately 92 percent water. All other answers are incorrect and are distracters.

References

Kalanick, K. *Phlebotomy Technician Specialist*. Clifton Park, N.Y.: Thomson Delmar Learning, 2004, p. 136.

Hoeltke, L. *The Complete Textbook of Phlebotomy*, 3rd ed. Clifton Park, N.Y.: Thomson Delmar Learning, 2006, p. 101.

MODULE 5: HEALTH CARE SYSTEMS

1. *ANS:* A

   An anesthesiologist is an individual with a medical degree who is board-certified and state-licensed to administer anesthetics. An oncologist is an individual who works specifically with cancer patients or patients with tumors. A neurologist is a physician skilled in the diagnosis and treatment of diseases of the nervous system. A surgeon is an individual qualified to treat those diseases that are amenable to or require surgery.

   ## References

   Kalanick, K. *Phlebotomy Technician Specialist*. Clifton Park, N.Y.: Thomson Delmar Learning, 2004, p. 13.

   Hoeltke, L. *The Complete Textbook of Phlebotomy*, 3rd ed. Clifton Park, N.Y.: Thomson Delmar Learning, 2006, pp. 6–8.

2. *ANS:* C

   Surgery is the branch of medicine dealing with manual and operative procedures for the correction of deformities and defects, repairs or injuries, and diagnosis and cure of certain diseases. Internal medicine is the department that treats diseases of the internal organs. The intensive care unit is the department within the hospital for patients who require continuous monitoring by specially trained personnel. The emergency room specializes in emergency care of the acutely ill and injured.

   ## References

   Kalanick, K. *Phlebotomy Technician Specialist*. Clifton Park, N.Y.: Thomson Delmar Learning, 2004, p. 12.

   Hoeltke, L. *The Complete Textbook of Phlebotomy*, 3rd ed. Clifton Park, N.Y.: Thomson Delmar Learning, 2006, pp. 6–8.

3. *ANS:* A

   A registered nurse (RN) has graduated from an accredited nursing program, passed the state examination for licensure, and is registered and licensed to practice by state authority. A licensed practical nurse (LPN) has graduated from an accredited school of practical nursing, passed the state examination for licensure, and is licensed to practice by a state authority. A nurse practitioner—Advanced practice registered nurse (NP or APRN) is a registered nurse with a minimum of a master's degree in nursing and advanced education in a particular health care specialty from family practice to midwifery in collaboration with a physician. A certified nursing assistant is an unlicensed nursing staff member who assists with basic patient care. Nursing assistants usually must complete a training course.

   ## References

   Kalanick, K. *Phlebotomy Technician Specialist*. Clifton Park, N.Y.: Thomson Delmar Learning, 2004, p. 13.

   Hoeltke, L. *The Complete Textbook of Phlebotomy*, 3rd ed. Clifton Park, N.Y.: Thomson Delmar Learning, 2006, pp. 6–8.

4. *ANS:* B

   Oncology is the diagnosis and treatment of malignant tumors and blood disorders. Internal medicine is the department that treats diseases of the internal organs. Radiology is the department concerned with the diagnosis, treatment, and prevention of disease through the use of X-rays, radioactive isotopes, ionizing radiations, ultrasonography, and magnetic resonance imaging. Neurology specializes in the diagnosis and treatment of diseases of the nervous system.

   ## References

   Kalanick, K. *Phlebotomy Technician Specialist*. Clifton Park, N.Y.: Thomson Delmar Learning, 2004, p. 12.

   Hoeltke, L. *The Complete Textbook of Phlebotomy*, 3rd ed. Clifton Park, N.Y.: Thomson Delmar Learning, 2006, pp. 6–8.

5. *ANS:* C

   The phlebotomist's primary function is the collection of blood samples from patients using venipuncture or microcollection techniques. Medical laboratory technicians (MLTs) or clinical laboratory technicians (CLTs) have graduated from a two-year associate degree program and have completed the required credit hours of hands-on clinical training as part of their degree. The medical technologist (MT) or clinical laboratory scientist (CLS) has a four-year bachelor's degree in medical technology. MTs are authorized to perform any and all clinical laboratory tests. A pharmacist is a specialist in formulating and dispensing medications and is licensed by individual states to practice pharmacy. Training consists of two years of postgraduate study in pharmacology.

   ## References

   Kalanick, K. *Phlebotomy Technician Specialist*. Clifton Park, N.Y.: Thomson Delmar Learning, 2004, p. 10.

   Hoeltke, L. *The Complete Textbook of Phlebotomy*, 3rd ed. Clifton Park, N.Y.: Thomson Delmar Learning, 2006, pp. 16–20.

6. *ANS:* B

A pathologist is a physician who practices, evaluates, or supervises diagnostic tests, using materials removed from living or dead patients. A medical technologist (MT) or clinical laboratory scientist (CLS) has a four-year bachelor's degree in medical technology. MTs are authorized to perform any and all clinical laboratory tests. Medical laboratory technicians or clinical laboratory technicians have graduated from a two-year associate degree program and have completed the required credit hours of hands-on clinical training as part of their degree. The phlebotomist's primary function is the collection of blood samples from patients using venipuncture or microcollection techniques.

References

Kalanick, K. (2004) *Phlebotomy Technician Specialist.* Clifton Park, N.Y.: Thomson Delmar Learning. p. 14.

Hoeltke, L. *The Complete Textbook of Phlebotomy*, 3rd ed. Clifton Park, N.Y.: Thomson Delmar Learning, 2006, pp. 16–20.

7. *ANS:* C

The medical technologist (MT) or clinical laboratory scientist (CLS) has a four-year bachelor's degree in medical technology. MTs are authorized to perform any and all clinical laboratory tests. A clinical laboratory clerical staff person is a clerical staff employee who is generally required to have a high school diploma and some prior clinical training. The medical laboratory technicians and clinical laboratory technicians have graduated from a two-year associate degree program and have completed the required credit hours of hands-on clinical training as part of their degree. The phlebotomist's primary function is the collection of blood samples from patients using venipuncture or microcollection techniques.

References

Kalanick, K. *Phlebotomy Technician Specialist.* Clifton Park, N.Y.: Thomson Delmar Learning, 2004, p. 14.

Hoeltke, L. *The Complete Textbook of Phlebotomy*, 3rd ed. Clifton Park, N.Y.: Thomson Delmar Learning, 2006, pp. 16–20.

8. *ANS:* C

A physician's assistant (PA) is a health care professional who provides patient services ranging from physical examination to surgical procedures and works under the supervision of a physician. A medical assistant (MA) is a multiskilled allied health care practitioner who is competent in a wide variety of clinical and laboratory procedures, as well as many administrative roles. A licensed practical nurse (LPN) has graduated from an accredited school of practical nursing, passed the state examination for licensure, and is licensed to practice by a state authority. A registered nurse (RN) has graduated from an accredited nursing program, passed the state exam for licensure, and is registered and licensed to practice by state authority.

References

Kalanick, K. *Phlebotomy Technician Specialist.* Clifton Park, N.Y.: Thomson Delmar Learning, 2004, p. 12

Hoeltke, L. *The Complete Textbook of Phlebotomy*, 3rd ed. Clifton Park, N.Y.: Thomson Delmar Learning, 2006, pp. 6–8.

9. *ANS:* A

Cardiology is a subspecialty of internal medicine dealing with the blood vessels and the heart. Neurology specializes in the diagnosis and treatment of diseases of the nervous system. Physiology is a branch of biology that deals with the functions and activities of life or of living matter and with the physical and chemical phenomena involved. Oncology is the diagnosis and treatment of malignant tumors and blood disorders.

References

Kalanick, K. *Phlebotomy Technician Specialist.* Clifton Park, N.Y.: Thomson Delmar Learning, 2004, p. 11.

Hoeltke, L. *The Complete Textbook of Phlebotomy*, 3rd ed. Clifton Park, N.Y.: Thomson Delmar Learning, 2006, pp. 6–8.

10. *ANS:* B

The laboratory manager is responsible for the overseeing of all the business operations of the laboratory, such as developing and maintaining the clinical laboratory budget, hiring laboratory personnel, setting goals and objectives, and providing continuing education. The laboratory director/pathologist is a PhD or physician who practices, evaluates, or supervises diagnostic tests, using materials removed from living or dead patients. Medical laboratory technicians (MLTs) or clinical laboratory technicians (CLTs) have graduated from a two-year associate degree program and have completed the required credit hours of hands-on clinical training as part of their degree. The phlebotomist's primary function is the collection of blood samples from patients using venipuncture or microcollection techniques.

References

Kalanick, K. *Phlebotomy Technician Specialist.* Clifton Park, N.Y.: Thomson Delmar Learning, 2004, p. 14.

Hoeltke, L. *The Complete Textbook of Phlebotomy*, 3rd ed. Clifton Park, N.Y.: Thomson Delmar Learning, 2006, pp. 16–20.

11. *ANS:* A

APRN is an advanced practice registered nurse or nurse practitioner is a registered nurse with a minimum of a master's degree in nursing and advanced education in a particular type of care. LPN is a licensed practical nurse. PT is the abbreviation for physical therapist and an RT is a respiratory technician.

References

Kalanick, K. *Phlebotomy Technician Specialist.* Clifton Park, N.Y.: Thomson Delmar Learning, 2004, p. 13.

Hoeltke, L. *The Complete Textbook of Phlebotomy,* 3rd ed. Clifton Park, N.Y.: Thomson Delmar Learning, 2006, pp. 6–8.

12. *ANS:* C

Gynecology is the department concerned with women's health issues. Oncology provides the diagnosis and treatment of malignant tumors and blood disorders. Internal medicine is the department that treats diseases of the internal organs. Neurology specializes in the diagnosis and treatment of diseases of the nervous system.

References

Kalanick, K. *Phlebotomy Technician Specialist.* Clifton Park, N.Y.: Thomson Delmar Learning, 2004, pp. 11–12.

Hoeltke, L. *The Complete Textbook of Phlebotomy,* 3rd ed. Clifton Park, N.Y.: Thomson Delmar Learning, 2006, pp. 6–8.

13. *ANS:* C

A physician is a person who has been educated, trained, and state-licensed to practice the art and science of medicine. A registered nurse has graduated from an accredited nursing program, passed the state exam for licensure, and is registered and licensed to practice by state authority. The phlebotomist's primary function is the collection of blood samples from patients using venipuncture or microcollection techniques. The medical laboratory technicians or clinical laboratory technicians have graduated from a two-year associate degree program and have completed the required credit hours of hands-on clinical training as part of their degree.

References

Kalanick, K. *Phlebotomy Technician Specialist.* Clifton Park, N.Y.: Thomson Delmar Learning, 2004, p. 12.

Hoeltke, L. *The Complete Textbook of Phlebotomy,* 3rd ed. Clifton Park, N.Y.: Thomson Delmar Learning, 2006, pp. 6–8.

14. *ANS:* A

A clinical laboratory clerical staff person is a clerical staff employee who is generally required to have a high school diploma and some prior clinical training. The medical laboratory technicians or clinical laboratory technicians have graduated from a two-year associate degree program and have completed the required credit hours of hands-on clinical training as part of their degree. The medical technologist (MT) or clinical laboratory scientist (CLS) has a four-year bachelor's degree in medical technology. MTs are authorized to perform any and all clinical laboratory tests. The laboratory manager is responsible for the overseeing of all the business operations of the laboratory, such as developing and maintaining the clinical laboratory budget, hiring laboratory personnel, setting goals and objectives, and providing continuing education.

References

Kalanick, K. *Phlebotomy Technician Specialist.* Clifton Park, N.Y.: Thomson Delmar Learning, 2004, p. 15.

Hoeltke, L. *The Complete Textbook of Phlebotomy,* 3rd ed. Clifton Park, N.Y.: Thomson Delmar Learning, 2006, pp. 16–20.

15. *ANS:* A

Occupational therapists help people with physical or mental disabilities, using the activities of everyday living to achieve maximum functioning and independence at home and in the workplace. A physical therapist is a medical practitioner with either a bachelor's or master's degree in physical therapy. A physical therapist treats patients to restore physical strength and endurance, coordination, and range of motion through exercises, heat or cold therapy, and massage. A respiratory therapist is a licensed allied health professional trained to provide respiratory care. A respiratory therapist works under the direction of a physician, educating patients, treating and assessing patient response to therapy, and managing and monitoring patients with deficiencies and abnormalities of cardiopulmonary function. A physician's assistant works under the supervision of a physician and provides patient services ranging from physical examinations to surgical procedures.

References

Kalanick, K. *Phlebotomy Technician Specialist.* Clifton Park, N.Y.: Thomson Delmar Learning, 2004, p. 14.

Hoeltke, L. *The Complete Textbook of Phlebotomy,* 3rd ed. Clifton Park, N.Y.: Thomson Delmar Learning, 2006, pp. 6–8.

16. *ANS:* C

Medical laboratory technicians or clinical laboratory technicians have graduated from a two-year associate degree program and have completed the required credit hours of hands-on clinical training as part of their degree. The laboratory manager is responsible for the overseeing of all the business operations of the laboratory, such as developing and maintaining the clinical laboratory budget, hiring laboratory personnel, setting goals and objectives, and providing continuing education. The medical technologist (MT) or clinical laboratory scientist (CLS) has a four-year bachelor's degree in medical technology. MTs are authorized to perform any and all clinical laboratory tests. A pharmacist is a specialist in formulating and dispensing medications.

References

Kalanick, K. *Phlebotomy Technician Specialist*. Clifton Park, N.Y.: Thomson Delmar Learning, 2004, p. 15.

Hoeltke, L. *The Complete Textbook of Phlebotomy*, 3rd ed. Clifton Park, N.Y.: Thomson Delmar Learning, 2006, pp. 16–20.

17. *ANS:* D

CPR and AED certifications, ability to obtain blood samples, and electrocardiography are some of the skills required of entry-level phlebotomists.

References

Kalanick, K. *Phlebotomy Technician Specialist*. Clifton Park, N.Y.: Thomson Delmar Learning, 2004, p. 11.

Hoeltke, L. *The Complete Textbook of Phlebotomy*, 3rd ed. Clifton Park, N.Y.: Thomson Delmar Learning, 2006, pp. 16–20.

18. *ANS:* C

A certified nursing assistant is an unlicensed nursing staff member who assists with basic patient care, such as giving baths, checking vital signs, bed making, and positioning.

References

Kalanick, K. *Phlebotomy Technician Specialist*. Clifton Park, N.Y.: Thomson Delmar Learning, 2004, p. 13.

Hoeltke, L. *The Complete Textbook of Phlebotomy*, 3rd ed. Clifton Park, N.Y.: Thomson Delmar Learning, 2006, pp. 6–8.

19. *ANS:* C

A respiratory therapist works under the direction of a physician, educating patients, treating and assessing patient response to therapy, and managing and monitoring patients with deficiencies and abnormalities of cardiopulmonary function. A physical therapist is a medical practitioner with either a bachelor's or master's degree in physical therapy. A physical therapist treats patients to restore physical strength and endurance, coordination, and range of motion through exercises, heat or cold therapy, and massage. A cardiologist is a physician who specializes in the study of the heart, its action, and its diseases. An

oncologist provides the diagnosis and treatment of malignant tumors and blood disorders.

References

Kalanick, K. *Phlebotomy Technician Specialist*. Clifton Park, N.Y.: Thomson Delmar Learning, 2004, p. 12.

Hoeltke, L. *The Complete Textbook of Phlebotomy*, 3rd ed. Clifton Park, N.Y.: Thomson Delmar Learning, 2006, pp. 6–8.

20. *ANS:* D

Pathology is the study of the nature and cause of disease through clinical laboratory test results. Radiology is the department concerned with the diagnosis, treatment, and prevention of disease through the use of X-rays, radioactive isotopes, ionizing radiations, ultrasonography, and magnetic resonance imaging. Oncology is the diagnosis and treatment of malignant tumors and blood disorders. Gynecology is the department concerned with women's health issues.

References

Kalanick, K. *Phlebotomy Technician Specialist*. Clifton Park, N.Y.: Thomson Delmar Learning, 2004, p. 12.

Hoeltke, L. *The Complete Textbook of Phlebotomy*, 3rd ed. Clifton Park, N.Y.: Thomson Delmar Learning, 2006, pp. 6–8.

MODULE 6: SPECIMEN COLLECTION

1. *ANS:* A

A lancet puncture of deeper than 2.4 millimeters administered to an infant or newborn can penetrate the calcaneous bone which can cause complication, such as sepsis and osteomyelitis. Osteoblastomas, anemia, and hemorrhaging would not occur from a puncture of 2.4 millimeters on an infant.

References

Kalanick, K. *Phlebotomy Technician Specialist*. Clifton Park, N.Y.: Thomson Delmar Learning, 2004, p. 331.

Hoeltke, L. *The Complete Textbook of Phlebotomy*, 3rd ed. Clifton Park, N.Y.: Thomson Delmar Learning, 2006, p. 235.

2. *ANS:* D

Too small a needle will not cause a hematoma.

A hematoma may occur if any or all of the following occur:

- Inadequate pressure is applied to the venipuncture site for an inadequate amount of time.
- Excessive probing is used to locate a vein.
- The needle is only partially in the vein, thereby allowing blood to seep into the tissue.

- The needle penetrates all the way through the vein, thereby allowing blood to seep into the tissue.
- The tourniquet is not removed before the needle is withdrawn.
- Too large a needle is used for the vein size.

References

Kalanick, K. *Phlebotomy Technician Specialist*. Clifton Park, N.Y.: Thomson Delmar Learning, 2004, pp. 431–432.

Hoeltke, L. *The Complete Textbook of Phlebotomy*, 3rd ed. Clifton Park, N.Y.: Thomson Delmar Learning, 2006, p. 207.

3. *ANS:* C

Patients allergic to isopropyl alcohol can have their skin cleaned with povidone iodine. All remaining answers are distracters.

References

Kalanick, K. *Phlebotomy Technician Specialist*. Clifton Park, N.Y.: Thomson Delmar Learning, 2004, p. 426.

Hoeltke, L. *The Complete Textbook of Phlebotomy*, 3rd ed. Clifton Park, N.Y.: Thomson Delmar Learning, 2006, p. 207.

4. *ANS:* B

A hematoma is an accumulation of blood at the venipuncture site. It is caused by leaking into the tissues around the site and identified by swelling and discoloration. All remaining answers are nonsense distracters.

References

Kalanick, K. *Phlebotomy Technician Specialist*. Clifton Park, N.Y.: Thomson Delmar Learning, 2004, p. 430.

Hoeltke, L. *The Complete Textbook of Phlebotomy*, 3rd ed. Clifton Park, N.Y.: Thomson Delmar Learning, 2006, p. 207.

5. *ANS:* C

Instruct patients to remove the bandage 5 to 10 minutes after the draw. All remaining answers are distracters.

References

Kalanick, K. *Phlebotomy Technician Specialist*. Clifton Park, N.Y.: Thomson Delmar Learning, 2004, p. 329.

6. *ANS:* B

Sodium citrate is the additive in the light blue top evacuated tube. A royal blue top tube contains EDTA (ethylenediaminetetraacetic acid) and sodium heparin. A green-black top tube contains a gel barrier. The light gray top tube is a distracter.

References

Kalanick, K. *Phlebotomy Technician Specialist*. Clifton Park, N.Y.: Thomson Delmar Learning, 2004, p. 341.

Hoeltke, L. (2006) *The Complete Textbook of Phlebotomy,* 3rd ed. Clifton Park, N.Y.: Thomson Delmar Learning, p. 191.

7. *ANS:* D

A yellow top evacuated tube is drawn for the collection of blood cultures. A red top evacuated tube is drawn for serology, routine chemistries, blood banking, and therapeutic drug levels. A light blue evacuated tube is drawn for coagulation studies, such as prothrombin time (PT) or activated partial thromboplastin time. A brown top evacuated tube is drawn for lead determinations.

References

Kalanick, K. *Phlebotomy Technician Specialist*. Clifton Park, N.Y.: Thomson Delmar Learning, 2004, p. 341.

Hoeltke, L. *The Complete Textbook of Phlebotomy*, 3rd ed. Clifton Park, N.Y.: Thomson Delmar Learning, 2006, p. 191.

8. *ANS:* A

A red top evacuated tube must not be inverted. Tube inversion must occur for proper mixing in a lavender, yellow, or black top evacuated tube.

References

Kalanick, K. *Phlebotomy Technician Specialist*. Clifton Park, N.Y.: Thomson Delmar Learning, 2004, p. 341.

Hoeltke, L. *The Complete Textbook of Phlebotomy*, 3rd ed. Clifton Park, N.Y.: Thomson Delmar Learning, 2006, p. 191.

9. *ANS:* A

Paper tape and a 2 × 2-inch gauze pad are used in place of adhesive bandages. All remaining answers are distracters.

References

Kalanick, K. *Phlebotomy Technician Specialist*. Clifton Park, N.Y.: Thomson Delmar Learning, 2004, p. 426.

Hoeltke, L. *The Complete Textbook of Phlebotomy*, 3rd ed. Clifton Park, N.Y.: Thomson Delmar Learning, 2006, p. 72.

10. *ANS:* D

All fingertips may be used, with the exception of the 5th digit.

References

Kalanick, K. *Phlebotomy Technician Specialist*. Clifton Park, N.Y.: Thomson Delmar Learning, 2004, p. 356.

Hoeltke, L. *The Complete Textbook of Phlebotomy*, 3rd ed. Clifton Park, N.Y.: Thomson Delmar Learning, 2006, 236.

11. *ANS:* D

If an elderly patient tells you his or her veins are fragile, you should use a pediatric evacuated tube set, use a butterfly infusion set, or use a syringe and a small-gauge needle.

References

Kalanick, K. *Phlebotomy Technician Specialist*. Clifton Park, N.Y.: Thomson Delmar Learning, 2004, p. 335.

Hoeltke, L. *The Complete Textbook of Phlebotomy*, 3rd ed. Clifton Park, N.Y.: Thomson Delmar Learning, 2006, p. 360.

12. *ANS:* C

The patient in anaphylactic shock presents with acute respiratory distress, hypotension, edema, hives, tachycardia, pale cool skin, convulsions, and cyanosis. All remaining answers are distracters.

References

Kalanick, K. *Phlebotomy Technician Specialist*. Clifton Park, N.Y.: Thomson Delmar Learning, 2004, p. 427.

13. *ANS:* B

Hemophilia is a hereditary blood disease marked by greatly prolonged blood coagulation time, failure of the blood to clot and abnormal bleeding. Anaphylactic shock is an immediate allergic reaction characterized by acute respiratory distress, hypotension, edema, and rash. Erythroblastosis occurs when there is an abnormal presence of erythroblasts in the blood. CHF is congestive heart failure.

References

Kalanick, K. *Phlebotomy Technician Specialist*. Clifton Park, N.Y.: Thomson Delmar Learning, 2004, p. 427.

14. *ANS:* B

If an artery is accidentally punctured, the phlebotomist should apply pressure for a minimum of 5 minutes. All remaining answers are distracters.

References

Kalanick, K. *Phlebotomy Technician Specialist*. Clifton Park, N.Y.: Thomson Delmar Learning, 2004, p. 426.

Hoeltke, L. *The Complete Textbook of Phlebotomy*, 3rd ed. Clifton Park, N.Y.: Thomson Delmar Learning, 2006, p. 349.

15. *ANS:* C

Alcohol pads, or alcohol wipes, containing 70 percent isopropyl alcohol solution, are used prior to the puncture to disinfect the patient's skin at the site of needle insertion. All remaining answers are distracters.

References

Kalanick, K. *Phlebotomy Technician Specialist*. Clifton Park, N.Y.: Thomson Delmar Learning, 2004, p. 329.

Hoeltke, L. *The Complete Textbook of Phlebotomy*, 3rd ed. Clifton Park, N.Y.: Thomson Delmar Learning, 2006, 194.

16. *ANS:* A

Tourniquets should not be left in place for longer than 1 to 2 minutes because blood may become more concentrated and adversely affects test results. All remaining answers are distracters.

References

Kalanick, K. *Phlebotomy Technician Specialist*. Clifton Park, N.Y.: Thomson Delmar Learning, 2004, p. 339.

Hoeltke, L. *The Complete Textbook of Phlebotomy*, 3rd ed. Clifton Park, N.Y.: Thomson Delmar Learning, 2006, p. 149.

17. *ANS:* B

Try not to select a vein that feels hard or cordlike, because these veins may be sclerosed and are more difficult to penetrate with the needle. All remaining answers are distracters.

References

Kalanick, K. *Phlebotomy Technician Specialist*. Clifton Park, N.Y.: Thomson Delmar Learning, 2004, p. 383.

Hoeltke, L. *The Complete Textbook of Phlebotomy*, 3rd ed. Clifton Park, N.Y.: Thomson Delmar Learning, 2006, p. 179.

18. *ANS:* B

If an antecubital site is not suitable on either arm, check the wrist and back of each hand for a vein. If a suitable site cannot be located, warm the arm or hand by wrapping a warm, moist towel around the site, leaving it in place for 3 to 5 minutes. All remaining answers are distracters.

References

Kalanick, K. *Phlebotomy Technician Specialist*. Clifton Park, N.Y.: Thomson Delmar Learning, 2004, p. 384.

Hoeltke, L. *The Complete Textbook of Phlebotomy*, 3rd ed. Clifton Park, N.Y.: Thomson Delmar Learning, 2006, p. 179.

19. *ANS:* A

The point of the needle that has been cut on a slant for ease of entry is called the bevel. All other answers are distracters.

References

Kalanick, K. *Phlebotomy Technician Specialist*. Clifton Park, N.Y.: Thomson Delmar Learning, 2004, p. 387.

Hoeltke, L. *The Complete Textbook of Phlebotomy*, 3rd ed. Clifton Park, N.Y.: Thomson Delmar Learning, 2006, p. 129.

20. *ANS:* C

The butterfly needle is typically 23 gauge and 5/8 inch in length. All remaining answers are distracters.

References

Kalanick, K. *Phlebotomy Technician Specialist*. Clifton Park, N.Y.: Thomson Delmar Learning, 2004, p. 397.

Hoeltke, L. *The Complete Textbook of Phlebotomy*, 3rd ed. Clifton Park, N.Y.: Thomson Delmar Learning, 2006, p. 141.

21. *ANS:* D

All of the answers cause hemolysis. If the gauge of the needle is too small for the pressure of the evacuated tube, as the blood is forced through the needle, the cells lyze. The same is true of using a larger evacuated tube with a butterfly infusion set. The force behind the vacuum of the tube causes the cells to lyze as they are drawn through the needle attached to the butterfly infusion set. Forcing blood that has been drawn into a syringe into an evacuated tube also causes hemolysis; the blood should be allowed to flow from the syringe into the evacuated tube from the pressure of the vacuum of the tube rather than manually pushing the plunger of the syringe.

References

Kalanick, K. *Phlebotomy Technician Specialist*. Clifton Park, N.Y.: Thomson Delmar Learning, 2004, p. 398.

Hoeltke, L. *The Complete Textbook of Phlebotomy*, 3rd ed. Clifton Park, N.Y.: Thomson Delmar Learning, 2006, p. 209.

22. *ANS:* B

When you are using a butterfly infusion set, the needle should be inserted into the vein at a 10- to 15-degree angle. All remaining answers are distracters.

References

Kalanick, K. *Phlebotomy Technician Specialist*. Clifton Park, N.Y.: Thomson Delmar Learning, 2004, p. 399.

Hoeltke, L. *The Complete Textbook of Phlebotomy*, 3rd ed. Clifton Park, N.Y.: Thomson Delmar Learning, 2006, p. 200.

23. *ANS:* A

Sclerosed or occluded veins are often the result of inflammation and disease, or they occur in patients who have had repeated punctures to veins. All remaining answers are distracters.

References

Kalanick, K. *Phlebotomy Technician Specialist*. Clifton Park, N.Y.: Thomson Delmar Learning, 2004, p. 383.

Hoeltke, L. *The Complete Textbook of Phlebotomy*, 3rd ed. Clifton Park, N.Y.: Thomson Delmar Learning, 2006, p. 179.

24. *ANS:* B

The phlebotomist may draw at least 2 inches below the IV site once permission has been given by the patient's physician. All remaining answers are distracters.

References

Kalanick, K. *Phlebotomy Technician Specialist*. Clifton Park, N.Y.: Thomson Delmar Learning, 2004, p. 405.

Hoeltke, L. *The Complete Textbook of Phlebotomy*, 3rd ed. Clifton Park, N.Y.: Thomson Delmar Learning, 2006, p. 211.

25. *ANS:* B

Ask the nurse to turn off the IV for a minimum of 2 minutes prior to the draw. All remaining answers are distracters.

References

Kalanick, K. *Phlebotomy Technician Specialist*. Clifton Park, N.Y.: Thomson Delmar Learning, 2004, p. 405.

Hoeltke, L. *The Complete Textbook of Phlebotomy*, 3rd ed. Clifton Park, N.Y.: Thomson Delmar Learning, 2006, p. 211.

26. *ANS:* C

Immediately after removing the tube from the needle and tube adapter, gently invert the tube 5 to 8 times before setting it down. All remaining answers are distracters.

References

Kalanick, K. *Phlebotomy Technician Specialist*. Clifton Park, N.Y.: Thomson Delmar Learning, 2004, p. 388.

27. *ANS:* C

Red top tubes are drawn for blood banking and must not be inverted. Lavender, red, and gray tubes must be inverted for proper mixing to occur.

References

Kalanick, K. *Phlebotomy Technician Specialist*. Clifton Park, N.Y.: Thomson Delmar Learning, 2004, p. 341.

Hoeltke, L. *The Complete Textbook of Phlebotomy*, 3rd ed. Clifton Park, N.Y.: Thomson Delmar Learning, 2006, p. 191.

28. *ANS:* B

Lancets are small, sterile, single-use instruments used to puncture the capillaries of the skin. Microhematocrit tubes are disposable glass pipettes designed to hold 50 to 75 microliters of blood. Hypodermic needles are syringes with a needle attached.

References

Kalanick, K. *Phlebotomy Technician Specialist*. Clifton Park, N.Y.: Thomson Delmar Learning, 2004, p. 331.

Hoeltke, L. *The Complete Textbook of Phlebotomy*, 3rd ed. Clifton Park, N.Y.: Thomson Delmar Learning, 2006, p. 236.

29. *ANS:* C

A syringe should be used when drawing blood from fragile veins. Lancets are used to puncture the capillaries of the skin. Microhematocrit tubes are designed to hold 50 to 75 microliters of blood. An evacuated tube fills immediately because of the premeasured amount of vacuum in the tube and could damage fragile veins.

References

Kalanick, K. *Phlebotomy Technician Specialist*. Clifton Park, N.Y.: Thomson Delmar Learning, 2004, p. 333.

30. *ANS:* B

Use a 15- to 30-degree angle of insertion. All remaining answers are distracters.

References

Kalanick, K. *Phlebotomy Technician Specialist*. Clifton Park, N.Y.: Thomson Delmar Learning, 2004, p. 395.

Hoeltke, L. *The Complete Textbook of Phlebotomy*, 3rd ed. Clifton Park, N.Y.: Thomson Delmar Learning, 2006, p. 188.

31. *ANS:* C

Using the syringe method, the phlebotomist can control the amount of pressure by pulling the plunger of the syringe back slowly. All remaining answers are distracters.

References

Kalanick, K. *Phlebotomy Technician Specialist*. Clifton Park, N.Y.: Thomson Delmar Learning, 2004, p. 393.

Hoeltke, L. *The Complete Textbook of Phlebotomy*, 3rd ed. Clifton Park, N.Y.: Thomson Delmar Learning, 2006, p. 183.

32. *ANS:* C

Positioning the patient is important when performing a venipuncture. Position the patient in either a sitting or lying down position prior to the blood draw. Never allow the patient to be standing.

References

Kalanick, K. *Phlebotomy Technician Specialist*. Clifton Park, N.Y.: Thomson Delmar Learning, 2004, p. 379.

Hoeltke, L. *The Complete Textbook of Phlebotomy*, 3rd ed. Clifton Park, N.Y.: Thomson Delmar Learning, 2006, p. 178.

33. *ANS:* A

Most frequently, venipuncture is performed in the antecubital area of the arm where the median cubital, cephalic, and basilic veins are located close to the surface. All remaining answers are distracters.

References

Kalanick, K. *Phlebotomy Technician Specialist*. Clifton Park, N.Y.: Thomson Delmar Learning, 2004, p. 380.

Hoeltke, L. *The Complete Textbook of Phlebotomy*, 3rd ed. Clifton Park, N.Y.: Thomson Delmar Learning, 2006, p. 179.

34. *ANS:* A

Use the tip of the index finger to palpate their vein. All remaining answers are distracters.

References

Kalanick, K. *Phlebotomy Technician Specialist*. Clifton Park, N.Y.: Thomson Delmar Learning, 2004, p. 383.

Hoeltke, L. *The Complete Textbook of Phlebotomy*, 3rd ed. Clifton Park, N.Y.: Thomson Delmar Learning, 2006, p. 181.

35. *ANS:* C

Apply direct pressure to the site for 3 to 5 minutes. All remaining answers are distracters.

References

Kalanick, K. *Phlebotomy Technician Specialist*. Clifton Park, N.Y.: Thomson Delmar Learning, 2004, p. 383

Hoeltke, L. *The Complete Textbook of Phlebotomy*, 3rd ed. Clifton Park, N.Y.: Thomson Delmar Learning, 2006, p. 188.

36. *ANS:* B

Microhematocrit tubes are commonly referred to as capillary tubes because they fill with capillary action. All remaining answers are distracters.

References

Kalanick, K. *Phlebotomy Technician Specialist*. Clifton Park, N.Y.: Thomson Delmar Learning, 2004, p. 332.

Hoeltke, L. *The Complete Textbook of Phlebotomy*, 3rd ed. Clifton Park, N.Y.: Thomson Delmar Learning, 2006, p. 151.

37. *ANS:* A

Ammonium-heparin–coated tubes have a red band at one end; plain tubes have a blue band. Green and yellow are distracters.

References

Kalanick, K. *Phlebotomy Technician Specialist*. Clifton Park, N.Y.: Thomson Delmar Learning, 2004, p. 332.

Hoeltke, L. *The Complete Textbook of Phlebotomy*, 3rd ed. Clifton Park, N.Y.: Thomson Delmar Learning, 2006, p. 191.

38. *ANS:* A

Microcollection containers are small plastic containers or tubes often referred to as "bullets" because of their size and shape. All remaining answers are distracters.

References

Kalanick, K. *Phlebotomy Technician Specialist*. Clifton Park, N.Y.: Thomson Delmar Learning, 2004, p. 333.

Hoeltke, L. *The Complete Textbook of Phlebotomy*, 3rd ed. Clifton Park, N.Y.: Thomson Delmar Learning, 2006, p. 151.

39. *ANS:* C

The 10-cc syringe is most commonly used for routine venipuncture. All remaining answers are distracters.

References

Kalanick, K. *Phlebotomy Technician Specialist*. Clifton Park, N.Y.: Thomson Delmar Learning, 2004, p. 334.

Hoeltke, L. *The Complete Textbook of Phlebotomy*, 3rd ed. Clifton Park, N.Y.: Thomson Delmar Learning, 2006, p. 129.

40. *ANS:* B

Complete blood counts should be drawn in a lavender top evacuated tube. Coagulation studies should be drawn on a light blue evacuated tube. Sedimentation rate testing is drawn on a black evacuated tube. Toxicology profiles are drawn on a royal blue evacuated tube.

References

Kalanick, K. *Phlebotomy Technician Specialist*. Clifton Park, N.Y.: Thomson Delmar Learning, 2004, p. 341.

Hoeltke, L. *The Complete Textbook of Phlebotomy*, 3rd ed. Clifton Park, N.Y.: Thomson Delmar Learning, 2006, p. 191.

41. *ANS:* A

Arterial blood gases provide the physician with vital information about the respiratory status and acid-base balance. The hematocrit measures the volume of the patient's red blood cells as a percentage of whole blood in relationship to the plasma. Hemoglobin aids in the transportation of oxygen to all the cells of the body and the return of carbon dioxide to the lungs as a waste product to be expelled. Glucose testing allows the patient and physician to monitor glucose levels in the blood.

References

Kalanick, K. *Phlebotomy Technician Specialist*. Clifton Park, N.Y.: Thomson Delmar Learning, 2004, p. 345.

Hoeltke, L. *The Complete Textbook of Phlebotomy*, 3rd ed. Clifton Park, N.Y.: Thomson Delmar Learning, 2006, p. 220.

42. *ANS:* B

The puncture should be made perpendicular to the fingerprint, causing a drop to form. Punctures made horizontal to or going with the fingerprint cause blood to run down the finger instead of forming a drop. The remaining answer is a distracter.

References

Kalanick, K. *Phlebotomy Technician Specialist*. Clifton Park, N.Y.: Thomson Delmar Learning, 2004, p. 356.

Hoeltke, L. *The Complete Textbook of Phlebotomy*, 3rd ed. Clifton Park, N.Y.: Thomson Delmar Learning, 2006, p. 236.

43. *ANS:* A

When you are performing a bleeding time, a small incision is made in the patient's forearm, and the blood is blotted at 30-second intervals. All remaining answers are distracters.

References

Kalanick, K. *Phlebotomy Technician Specialist*. Clifton Park, N.Y.: Thomson Delmar Learning, 2004, pp. 495–496.

Hoeltke, L. *The Complete Textbook of Phlebotomy*, 3rd ed. Clifton Park, N.Y.: Thomson Delmar Learning, 2006, p. 281.

44. *ANS:* C

Fainting, or syncope, is a common complication of blood collection. Syncope is a transient loss of consciousness resulting from an inadequate flow of blood to the brain. A hematoma is a swelling or mass of blood (usually clotted), confined to an organ, tissue, or space and caused by a break in a blood vessel. Shock, or anaphylactic shock, is an immediate allergic reaction characterized by acute respiratory distress, hypotension, edema, and rash. A seizure is a sudden attack of pain, a disease, or certain symptoms—An epileptic attack or convulsion.

References

Kalanick, K. *Phlebotomy Technician Specialist*. Clifton Park, N.Y.: Thomson Delmar Learning, 2004, p. 428.

Hoeltke, L. *The Complete Textbook of Phlebotomy*, 3rd ed. Clifton Park, N.Y.: Thomson Delmar Learning, 2006, p. 349.

45. *ANS:* D

Several million Americans fear needles so intensely that being stuck with one for an injection or a blood test can trigger fainting, convulsions, and, in 23 reported cases, death.

References

Kalanick, K. *Phlebotomy Technician Specialist*. Clifton Park, N.Y.: Thomson Delmar Learning, 2004, p. 428.

Hoeltke, L. *The Complete Textbook of Phlebotomy*, 3rd ed. Clifton Park, N.Y.: Thomson Delmar Learning, 2006, p. 349.

46. *ANS:* D

The patient should be instructed on the appropriate method to use the ice pack at home: Apply it for 20 minutes; then remove it for 20 minutes. All remaining answers are distracters.

References

Kalanick, K. *Phlebotomy Technician Specialist*. Clifton Park, N.Y.: Thomson Delmar Learning, 2004, p. 430.

Hoeltke, L. *The Complete Textbook of Phlebotomy*, 3rd ed. Clifton Park, N.Y.: Thomson Delmar Learning, 2006, p. 357.

47. *ANS:* C

"Hitting" a nerve is painful and can cause permanent damage. All remaining answers are distracters.

References

Kalanick, K. *Phlebotomy Technician Specialist*. Clifton Park, N.Y.: Thomson Delmar Learning, 2004, p. 432.

Hoeltke, L. *The Complete Textbook of Phlebotomy*, 3rd ed. Clifton Park, N.Y.: Thomson Delmar Learning, 2006, p. 205.

48. *ANS:* D

Combative, drug-overdosed, and very ill patients can cause a phlebotomist to resort to restraining them to collect a specimen.

References

Kalanick, K. *Phlebotomy Technician Specialist*. Clifton Park, N.Y.: Thomson Delmar Learning, 2004, p. 432.

Hoeltke, L. *The Complete Textbook of Phlebotomy*, 3rd ed. Clifton Park, N.Y.: Thomson Delmar Learning, 2006, p. 245.

49. *ANS:* C

As a matter of routine and as a prevention to allergic reaction by the patient, the phlebotomist should routinely ask the patient if they are allergic to antiseptics, adhesives, and latex. The remaining answers are distracters.

References

Kalanick, K. *Phlebotomy Technician Specialist*. Clifton Park, N.Y.: Thomson Delmar Learning, 2004, p. 426.

Hoeltke, L. *The Complete Textbook of Phlebotomy*, 3rd ed. Clifton Park, N.Y.: Thomson Delmar Learning, 2006, p. 200.

50. *ANS:* A

Ointments prescribed by a physician, applied topically, will cause a rash to subside and soothe the itching. "Sublingually" is under the tongue. "Subcutaneously" is under the skin. The remaining answer is a distracter.

References

Kalanick, K. *Phlebotomy Technician Specialist*. Clifton Park, N.Y.: Thomson Delmar Learning, 2004, p. 427.

51. *ANS:* B

Royal blue top evacuated tube is used for toxicology profiles. A black top evacuated tube is used for hematology-Westergren sedimentation rate. A lavender top evacuated tube is used for complete blood counts. A red top tube is used for serology, routine chemistries, blood banking, and therapeutic drug levels.

References

Kalanick, K. *Phlebotomy Technician Specialist*. Clifton Park, N.Y.: Thomson Delmar Learning, 2004, p. 341.

Hoeltke, L. *The Complete Textbook of Phlebotomy*, 3rd ed. Clifton Park, N.Y.: Thomson Delmar Learning, 2006, p. 191.

52. *ANS:* D

A puncture of a vein for any reason is called venipuncture. ABG means arterial blood gas, referring to any of the gases present in blood and, clinically, to the determination of levels in the blood of oxygen and carbon dioxide. A capillary stick is the procedure by which the skin is punctured with a lance. A glucose test is only one type of test and does not encompass all other punctures of a vein.

References

Kalanick, K. *Phlebotomy Technician Specialist*. Clifton Park, N.Y.: Thomson Delmar Learning, 2004, p. 376.

Hoeltke, L. *The Complete Textbook of Phlebotomy*, 3rd ed. Clifton Park, N.Y.: Thomson Delmar Learning, 2006, p. 159.

53. *ANS:* B

Making a fist helps to make the vein more prominent. Do not, however, request the patient to open and close the fist vigorously, because doing so can contribute to hemoconcentration, which can cause test results to be inaccurate. All remaining answers are distracters.

References

Kalanick, K. *Phlebotomy Technician Specialist*. Clifton Park, N.Y.: Thomson Delmar Learning, 2004, p. 383.

Hoeltke, L. *The Complete Textbook of Phlebotomy*, 3rd ed. Clifton Park, N.Y.: Thomson Delmar Learning, 2006, p. 181.

54. *ANS:* B

If an antecubital vein cannot be located on either arm, check the wrists and hands. If a suitable site cannot be located the feet and ankle veins may be drawn with permission from the patient's physician. All remaining answers are distracters.

References

Kalanick, K. *Phlebotomy Technician Specialist.* Clifton Park, N.Y.: Thomson Delmar Learning, 2004, p. 384.

Hoeltke, L. *The Complete Textbook of Phlebotomy*, 3rd ed. Clifton Park, N.Y.: Thomson Delmar Learning, 2006, p. 179.

55. *ANS:* B

Lavender top tubes drawn for hematology studies are never centrifuged. All remaining answers are distracters.

References

Kalanick, K. *Phlebotomy Technician Specialist.* Clifton Park, N.Y.: Thomson Delmar Learning, 2004, p. 407.

Hoeltke, L. *The Complete Textbook of Phlebotomy*, 3rd ed. Clifton Park, N.Y.: Thomson Delmar Learning, 2006, p. 191.

56. *ANS:* A

Cleanse the venipuncture site in a circular motion from the center to the periphery. All remaining answers are distracters.

References

Kalanick, K. *Phlebotomy Technician Specialist.* Clifton Park, N.Y.: Thomson Delmar Learning, 2004, p. 385.

Hoeltke, L. *The Complete Textbook of Phlebotomy*, 3rd ed. Clifton Park, N.Y.: Thomson Delmar Learning, 2006, p. 181.

57. *ANS:* C

Light blue top evacuated tube must be a full draw or rejection occurs. Black and brown top evacuated tubes must be no less than three-quarters of a tube. However, a full draw is preferred. A red-gray topped evacuated tube does not have a minimum volume per tube.

References

Kalanick, K. *Phlebotomy Technician Specialist.* Clifton Park, N.Y.: Thomson Delmar Learning, 2004, p. 341.

Hoeltke, L. *The Complete Textbook of Phlebotomy*, 3rd ed. Clifton Park, N.Y.: Thomson Delmar Learning, 2006, p. 191.

58. *ANS:* D

If the evacuated tube is not filling with blood, the phlebotomist should make sure the tube is properly seated into the needle, the tube hasn't lost its vacuum, or the needle is not in the correct position to the vein.

References

Kalanick, K. *Phlebotomy Technician Specialist.* Clifton Park, N.Y.: Thomson Delmar Learning, 2004, p. 402.

59. *ANS:* B

If the client/patient is an inpatient at the hospital, verify the information in the patient's identification bracelet against the laboratory orders and the information supplied by the patient. All remaining answers are distracters.

References

Kalanick, K. *Phlebotomy Technician Specialist.* Clifton Park, N.Y.: Thomson Delmar Learning, 2004, p. 355.

Hoeltke, L. *The Complete Textbook of Phlebotomy*, 3rd ed. Clifton Park, N.Y.: Thomson Delmar Learning, 2006, p. 170.

60. *ANS:* B

Once the equipment and supplies have been assembled, the next step is to identify the client/patient. First, introduce yourself. All remaining answers are distracters.

References

Kalanick, K. *Phlebotomy Technician Specialist.* Clifton Park, N.Y.: Thomson Delmar Learning, 2004, p. 355.

Hoeltke, L. *The Complete Textbook of Phlebotomy*, 3rd ed. Clifton Park, N.Y.: Thomson Delmar Learning, 2006, p. 170.

61. *ANS:* D

Capillary punctures can be performed on fingertips, heels, toes, or earlobes. Wrists are not to be used for a capillary puncture.

References

Kalanick, K. *Phlebotomy Technician Specialist.* Clifton Park, N.Y.: Thomson Delmar Learning, 2004, p. 356.

Hoeltke, L. *The Complete Textbook of Phlebotomy*, 3rd ed. Clifton Park, N.Y.: Thomson Delmar Learning, 2006, p. 236.

62. *ANS:* A

VADs (vascular access devices) are inserted to administer fluids and medications, monitoring pressures, and drawing blood. They are not inserted to monitor a patient's acid-base balance.

References

Kalanick, K. *Phlebotomy Technician Specialist.* Clifton Park, N.Y.: Thomson Delmar Learning, 2004, p. 468.

Hoeltke, L. *The Complete Textbook of Phlebotomy*, 3rd ed. Clifton Park, N.Y.: Thomson Delmar Learning, 2006, p. 212.

63. *ANS:* C

The risk of infection increases with a puncture of the femoral artery, because of the pubic hair. All remaining answers are distracters.

References

Kalanick, K. *Phlebotomy Technician Specialist.* Clifton Park, N.Y.: Thomson Delmar Learning, 2004, p. 445.

Hoeltke, L. *The Complete Textbook of Phlebotomy,* 3rd ed. Clifton Park, N.Y.: Thomson Delmar Learning, 2006, p. 179.

64. *ANS:* D

Evacuated tubes should not be used for collection of ABGs because the tubes alter the partial pressure of the gas in the blood example. All remaining answers are distracters.

References

Kalanick, K. *Phlebotomy Technician Specialist.* Clifton Park, N.Y.: Thomson Delmar Learning, 2004, p. 446.

Hoeltke, L. *The Complete Textbook of Phlebotomy,* 3rd ed. Clifton Park, N.Y.: Thomson Delmar Learning, 2006, p. 215.

65. *ANS:* C

The patient must have been resting comfortably for a minimum of 30 minutes with no exercise, treatments, or respiratory changes. All remaining answers are distracters.

References

Kalanick, K. *Phlebotomy Technician Specialist.* Clifton Park, N.Y.: Thomson Delmar Learning, 2004, p. 447.

Hoeltke, L. *The Complete Textbook of Phlebotomy,* 3rd ed. Clifton Park, N.Y.: Thomson Delmar Learning, 2006, p. 182.

66. *ANS:* C

Wrap the bilirubin specimen in aluminum foil to protect it from light. All the remaining answers are distracters.

References

Kalanick, K. *Phlebotomy Technician Specialist.* Clifton Park, N.Y.: Thomson Delmar Learning, 2004, p. 391.

Hoeltke, L. *The Complete Textbook of Phlebotomy,* 3rd ed. Clifton Park, N.Y.: Thomson Delmar Learning, 2006, p. 316.

67. *ANS:* C

Tourniquets are designed to temporarily reduce the flow of venous blood in the arm. All remaining answers are distracters.

References

Kalanick, K. *Phlebotomy Technician Specialist.* Clifton Park, N.Y.: Thomson Delmar Learning, 2004, p. 339.

Hoeltke, L. *The Complete Textbook of Phlebotomy,* 3rd ed. Clifton Park, N.Y.: Thomson Delmar Learning, 2006, p. 149.

68. *ANS:* A

Face gear is an example of a personal protective equipment (PPE). All remaining answers are distracters.

References

Kalanick, K. *Phlebotomy Technician Specialist.* Clifton Park, N.Y.: Thomson Delmar Learning, 2004, p. 175.

Hoeltke, L. *The Complete Textbook of Phlebotomy,* 3rd ed. Clifton Park, N.Y.: Thomson Delmar Learning, 2006, p. 57.

69. *ANS:* B

Bandages should not be used on a patient under the age of 2, because of the danger of aspiration and suffocation by a loose bandage. All remaining answers are distracters.

References

Kalanick, K. *Phlebotomy Technician Specialist.* Clifton Park, N.Y.: Thomson Delmar Learning, 2004, p. 329.

Hoeltke, L. *The Complete Textbook of Phlebotomy,* 3rd ed. Clifton Park, N.Y.: Thomson Delmar Learning, 2006, p. 257.

70. *ANS:* D

According to guidelines recommended by the National Committee for Clinical Laboratory Standards (NCCLS), the depth of the puncture should not exceed 2.4 millimeters in depth. All remaining answers are distracters.

References

Kalanick, K. *Phlebotomy Technician Specialist.* Clifton Park, N.Y.: Thomson Delmar Learning, 2004, p. 357.

Hoeltke, L. *The Complete Textbook of Phlebotomy,* 3rd ed. Clifton Park, N.Y.: Thomson Delmar Learning, 2006, p. 236.

71. *ANS:* B

When performing a capillary puncture, position the patient seated or lying down with the palmar side of the hand facing up. Dorsal is relating to the back side. Ventral is relating to the front side of the body. And plantar is relating to the bottom of the foot.

References

Kalanick, K. *Phlebotomy Technician Specialist.* Clifton Park, N.Y.: Thomson Delmar Learning, 2004, p. 359.

Hoeltke, L. *The Complete Textbook of Phlebotomy,* 3rd ed. Clifton Park, N.Y.: Thomson Delmar Learning, 2006, p. 236.

72. *ANS:* A

Perform a capillary puncture using a quick darting motion. The remaining answers are distracters.

References

Kalanick, K. *Phlebotomy Technician Specialist.* Clifton Park, N.Y.: Thomson Delmar Learning, 2004, p. 360.

Hoeltke, L. *The Complete Textbook of Phlebotomy*, 3rd ed. Clifton Park, N.Y.: Thomson Delmar Learning, 2006, p. 236.

73. *ANS:* D

The first tube in the correct order of evacuated tube filling from a syringe draw is a sterile specimen, which is drawn in a yellow sterile evacuated tube. All remaining answers are distracters.

References

Kalanick, K. *Phlebotomy Technician Specialist.* Clifton Park, N.Y.: Thomson Delmar Learning, 2004, p. 397.

Hoeltke, L. *The Complete Textbook of Phlebotomy*, 3rd ed. Clifton Park, N.Y.: Thomson Delmar Learning, 2006, p. 191.

74. *ANS:* B

When an artery has been effectively entered, a flash of blood appears in the hub of the needle. All remaining answers are distracters.

References

Kalanick, K. *Phlebotomy Technician Specialist.* Clifton Park, N.Y.: Thomson Delmar Learning, 2004, p. 450.

Hoeltke, L. *The Complete Textbook of Phlebotomy*, 3rd ed. Clifton Park, N.Y.: Thomson Delmar Learning, 2006, p. 215.

75. *ANS:* A

The most critical factor in collecting blood culture specimens is antisepsis of the patient's skin. The site must be as clean as possible to avoid contamination of the specimen with surface microorganisms, which will produce a false-positive blood culture. The remaining answers are distracters.

References

Kalanick, K. *Phlebotomy Technician Specialist.* Clifton Park, N.Y.: Thomson Delmar Learning, 2004, p. 453.

Hoeltke, L. *The Complete Textbook of Phlebotomy*, 3rd ed. Clifton Park, N.Y.: Thomson Delmar Learning, 2006, p. 231.

76. *ANS:* A

One of the most common blood-banking tests performed is a type and crossmatch. Hematocrit, ESR, and a CBC are not blood-banking tests.

References

Kalanick, K. *Phlebotomy Technician Specialist.* Clifton Park, N.Y.: Thomson Delmar Learning, 2004, p. 464.

Hoeltke, L. *The Complete Textbook of Phlebotomy*, 3rd ed. Clifton Park, N.Y.: Thomson Delmar Learning, 2006, p. 11.

77. *ANS:* B

An external AV (arteriovenous) shunt is a temporary connection between a vein and artery used for dialysis and for drawing blood. A peripherally inserted central catheter (PICC) is inserted into the peripheral venous system and is then threaded into the central venous system. A PICC tends to collapse on aspiration; drawing blood from a PICC is not recommended. An arterial line is most commonly located in the radial artery and is used to provide continuous monitoring of a patient's blood pressure. It can also be used for the collection of arterial blood gases. A central venous catheter (CVC) is a catheter inserted into the superior vena cava to permit intermittent or continuous monitoring of central venous pressure and to facilitate collecting blood samples for chemical analysis.

References

Kalanick, K. *Phlebotomy Technician Specialist.* Clifton Park, N.Y.: Thomson Delmar Learning, 2004, p. 470.

Hoeltke, L. *The Complete Textbook of Phlebotomy*, 3rd ed. Clifton Park, N.Y.: Thomson Delmar Learning, 2006, p. 211.

78. *ANS:* A

Transferring blood from a syringe to an evacuated tube poses a greater risk to the phlebotomist for accidental needle sticks than collection from an evacuated tube. All remaining answers are distracters.

References

Kalanick, K. *Phlebotomy Technician Specialist.* Clifton Park, N.Y.: Thomson Delmar Learning, 2004, p. 335.

Hoeltke, L. *The Complete Textbook of Phlebotomy*, 3rd ed. Clifton Park, N.Y.: Thomson Delmar Learning, 2006, p. 188.

79. ANS: B

Hands must be washed thoroughly for a minimum of 3 minutes. All remaining answers are distracters.

References

Kalanick, K. *Phlebotomy Technician Specialist.* Clifton Park, N.Y.: Thomson Delmar Learning, 2004, p. 362.

Hoeltke, L. *The Complete Textbook of Phlebotomy*, 3rd ed. Clifton Park, N.Y.: Thomson Delmar Learning, 2006, p. 55.

80. *ANS:* D

When you are performing a finger stick, the activity to be done first should be assemble and prepare equipment and supplies. After washing the hands and donning gloves, identify the patient, then explain the procedure. Dispose of the lancet immediately after the puncture.

References

Kalanick, K. *Phlebotomy Technician Specialist*. Clifton Park, N.Y.: Thomson Delmar Learning, 2004, p. 359.

Hoeltke, L. *The Complete Textbook of Phlebotomy*, 3rd ed. Clifton Park, N.Y.: Thomson Delmar Learning, 2006, p. 236.

81. *ANS:* A

Alcohol wipes should not be used for draws when testing blood alcohol. All remaining answers are distracters.

References

Kalanick, K. *Phlebotomy Technician Specialist*. Clifton Park, N.Y.: Thomson Delmar Learning, 2004, p. 411.

Hoeltke, L. *The Complete Textbook of Phlebotomy*, 3rd ed. Clifton Park, N.Y.: Thomson Delmar Learning, 2006, p. 271.

82. *ANS:* B

A reflectively contracted artery during an ABG can be caused by an arteriospasm. All remaining answers are nonsense distracters.

References

Kalanick, K. *Phlebotomy Technician Specialist*. Clifton Park, N.Y.: Thomson Delmar Learning, 2004, p. 447.

Hoeltke, L. *The Complete Textbook of Phlebotomy*, 3rd ed. Clifton Park, N.Y.: Thomson Delmar Learning, 2006, p. 215.

83. *ANS:* B

Goggles protect the phlebotomist from aerosol exposure. All remaining answers are distracters.

References

Kalanick, K. *Phlebotomy Technician Specialist*. Clifton Park, N.Y.: Thomson Delmar Learning, 2004, p. 328.
Hoeltke, L. *The Complete Textbook of Phlebotomy*, 3rd ed. Clifton Park, N.Y.: Thomson Delmar Learning, 2006, p. 51.

84. *ANS:* D

The risk of using a small-gauge needle is long draw time, hard-to-draw large quantities, and hemolysis. Vasoconstriction is a decrease in the caliber of blood vessels.

References

Kalanick, K. *Phlebotomy Technician Specialist*. Clifton Park, N.Y.: Thomson Delmar Learning, 2004, p. 335.

85. *ANS:* C

Collateral circulation means that blood is supplied to the area by more than one artery. Coronary circulation takes oxygenated blood directly to the cells of the heart muscle. Both arterial circulation and venous circulation are distracters.

References

Kalanick, K. *Phlebotomy Technician Specialist*. Clifton Park, N.Y.: Thomson Delmar Learning, 2004, p. 443.

86. *ANS:* B

A donor unit is a specific amount of blood, approximately 1 pint, supplied by a volunteer as part of a blood bank procedure. All remaining answers are distracters.

References

Kalanick, K. *Phlebotomy Technician Specialist*. Clifton Park, N.Y.: Thomson Delmar Learning, 2004, p. 466.

87. *ANS:* C

A PICC is a catheter inserted into the peripheral venous system and then threaded into the central venous system. An arterial line is a hemodynamic monitoring system consisting of a catheter in an artery connected to pressure tubing, a transducer, and an electronic monitor. It is used to measure systemic blood pressure and to provide ease of access for the drawing of blood for the study of gases present. A central venous catheter (CVC) is a catheter inserted into the superior vena cava to permit intermittent or continuous monitoring of central venous pressure and to facilitate collecting blood samples for chemical analysis. A vascular access device (VAD), also called an indwelling catheter, consists mainly of tubing inserted into a main artery or vein. This main vein or artery is customarily the subclavian, which is located in the chest below the clavicle. VADs are usually inserted for administering fluids and medications, monitoring pressures, and drawing blood.

References

Kalanick, K. *Phlebotomy Technician Specialist*. Clifton Park, N.Y.: Thomson Delmar Learning, 2004, p. 469.

Hoeltke, L. *The Complete Textbook of Phlebotomy*, 3rd ed. Clifton Park, N.Y.: Thomson Delmar Learning, 2006, p. 211.

88. *ANS:* B

Coagulation studies cannot be drawn from a heparin lock. All remaining answers are distracters.

References

Kalanick, K. *Phlebotomy Technician Specialist*. Clifton Park, N.Y.: Thomson Delmar Learning, 2004, p. 469.

Hoeltke, L. *The Complete Textbook of Phlebotomy*, 3rd ed. Clifton Park, N.Y.: Thomson Delmar Learning, 2006, p. 142.

89. *ANS:* A

Withdrawal of large quantities of blood over a long period of time can cause a pediatric patient to become anemic. All remaining answers are distracters.

References

Kalanick, K. *Phlebotomy Technician Specialist*. Clifton Park, N.Y.: Thomson Delmar Learning, 2004, p. 439.

Hoeltke, L. *The Complete Textbook of Phlebotomy*, 3rd ed. Clifton Park, N.Y.: Thomson Delmar Learning, 2006, p. 262.

90. *ANS:* C

Removal of over 10 percent of an infant's blood can cause cardiac arrest. All remaining answers are distracters.

References

Kalanick, K. *Phlebotomy Technician Specialist*. Clifton Park, N.Y.: Thomson Delmar Learning, 2004, p. 439.

Hoeltke, L. *The Complete Textbook of Phlebotomy*, 3rd ed. Clifton Park, N.Y.: Thomson Delmar Learning, 2006, p. 207.

91. *ANS:* B

PPE consists of items required by OSHA, such as the gloves that a phlebotomist is required to wear when in contact with body fluids. All remaining answers are nonsense distracters.

References

Kalanick, K. *Phlebotomy Technician Specialist*. Clifton Park, N.Y.: Thomson Delmar Learning, 2004, p. 328.

Hoeltke, L. *The Complete Textbook of Phlebotomy*, 3rd ed. Clifton Park, N.Y.: Thomson Delmar Learning, 2006, p. 62.

92. *ANS:* B

Hypodermic needles are typically single-sample needles, used when performing syringe draws. All remaining answers are distracters.

References

Kalanick, K. *Phlebotomy Technician Specialist*. Clifton Park, N.Y.: Thomson Delmar Learning, 2004, p. 337.

Hoeltke, L. *The Complete Textbook of Phlebotomy*, 3rd ed. Clifton Park, N.Y.: Thomson Delmar Learning, 2006, p. 129.

93. *ANS:* B

The most common multisample needle length used is 1–1½ inches. All remaining answers are distracters.

References

Kalanick, K. *Phlebotomy Technician Specialist*. Clifton Park, N.Y.: Thomson Delmar Learning, 2004, p. 336.

Hoeltke, L. *The Complete Textbook of Phlebotomy*, 3rd ed. Clifton Park, N.Y.: Thomson Delmar Learning, 2006, p. 129.

94. *ANS:* C

The most common gauge multisample needle used by a phlebotomist is 20–21. All remaining answers are distracters.

References

Kalanick, K. *Phlebotomy Technician Specialist*. Clifton Park, N.Y.: Thomson Delmar Learning, 2004, p. 336.

Hoeltke, L. *The Complete Textbook of Phlebotomy*, 3rd ed. Clifton Park, N.Y.: Thomson Delmar Learning, 2006, p. 129.

95. *ANS:* B

When lead determinations are being made, the brown top tube is drawn. Trace elements, nutrient studies, and toxicology profiles are drawn on a royal blue top evacuated tube. With a green-gray evacuated tube, chemistry polymer gel separates plasma from cells when properly centrifuged. Blue is a distracter.

References

Kalanick, K. *Phlebotomy Technician Specialist*. Clifton Park, N.Y.: Thomson Delmar Learning, 2004, p. 341.

Hoeltke, L. *The Complete Textbook of Phlebotomy*, 3rd ed. Clifton Park, N.Y.: Thomson Delmar Learning, 2006, p. 191.

96. *ANS:* C

A multisample needle is most commonly used with the evacuated tube system because it has two sharp ends, one beveled and the other covered with a rubber sheath. All remaining answers are distracters.

References

Kalanick, K. *Phlebotomy Technician Specialist*. Clifton Park, N.Y.: Thomson Delmar Learning, 2004, p. 336.

Hoeltke, L. *The Complete Textbook of Phlebotomy*, 3rd ed. Clifton Park, N.Y.: Thomson Delmar Learning, 2006, p. 129.

97. *ANS:* C

Interstitial fluid is fluid between the tissues, surrounding a cell. Arterial blood is blood in the arteries. Capillary blood is a mixture of venous and arterial blood. Venous blood is blood in the veins.

References

Kalanick, K. *Phlebotomy Technician Specialist*. Clifton Park, N.Y.: Thomson Delmar Learning, 2004, p. 354.

Hoeltke, L. *The Complete Textbook of Phlebotomy*, 3rd ed. Clifton Park, N.Y.: Thomson Delmar Learning, 2006, p. 231.

98. *ANS:* C

Capillary blood flow can be greatly increased when the site is warm. All remaining answers are distracters.

References

Kalanick, K. *Phlebotomy Technician Specialist*. Clifton Park, N.Y.: Thomson Delmar Learning, 2004, p. 359.

Hoeltke, L. *The Complete Textbook of Phlebotomy*, 3rd ed. Clifton Park, N.Y.: Thomson Delmar Learning, 2006, p. 231.

99. *ANS:* D

Firm pressure, milking, and massaging can be applied to ensure a steady flow of blood.

References

Kalanick, K. *Phlebotomy Technician Specialist*. Clifton Park, N.Y.: Thomson Delmar Learning, 2004, p. 360.

Hoeltke, L. *The Complete Textbook of Phlebotomy*, 3rd ed. Clifton Park, N.Y.: Thomson Delmar Learning, 2006, p. 232.

100. *ANS:* B

In order to collect blood specimens safely, accurately, and in the most cost-effective manner, the phlebotomist must have the correct "tools of the trade." These are gloves, goggles, antiseptics, gauze pads, bandages, and sharps containers. A utility tray is not considered a tool of the trade.

References

Kalanick, K. *Phlebotomy Technician Specialist*. Clifton Park, N.Y.: Thomson Delmar Learning, 2004, pp. 328–330.

Hoeltke, L. *The Complete Textbook of Phlebotomy*, 3rd ed. Clifton Park, N.Y.: Thomson Delmar Learning, 2006, p. 160.

101. *ANS:* C

A butterfly infusion set contains a 1/2 to 3/4-inch stainless steel needle connected to a 5- to 12-inch length of tubing. All remaining answers are distracters.

References

Kalanick, K. *Phlebotomy Technician Specialist*. Clifton Park, N.Y.: Thomson Delmar Learning, 2004, p. 334.

Hoeltke, L. *The Complete Textbook of Phlebotomy*, 3rd ed. Clifton Park, N.Y.: Thomson Delmar Learning, 2006, p. 141.

102. *ANS:* C

A clay sealer tray is used to plug the open end of microhematocrit tubes and to hold filled tubes until the specimens are ready to be centrifuged. All remaining answers are distracters.

References

Kalanick, K. *Phlebotomy Technician Specialist*. Clifton Park, N.Y.: Thomson Delmar Learning, 2004, p. 332.

Hoeltke, L. *The Complete Textbook of Phlebotomy*, 3rd ed. Clifton Park, N.Y.: Thomson Delmar Learning, 2006, p. 151.

103. *ANS:* D

OSHA alert: Never recap needles. Never bend, cut, or unscrew a needle from the tube adapter or syringe prior to disposal.

References

Kalanick, K. *Phlebotomy Technician Specialist*. Clifton Park, N.Y.: Thomson Delmar Learning, 2004, p. 330.

Hoeltke, L. *The Complete Textbook of Phlebotomy*, 3rd ed. Clifton Park, N.Y.: Thomson Delmar Learning, 2006, p. 62.

104. *ANS:* B

Lancets are primarily used on infants, children, and the elderly, or when microcollection techniques are required. All remaining answers are distracters.

References

Kalanick, K. *Phlebotomy Technician Specialist*. Clifton Park, N.Y.: Thomson Delmar Learning, 2004, p. 331.

Hoeltke, L. *The Complete Textbook of Phlebotomy*, 3rd ed. Clifton Park, N.Y.: Thomson Delmar Learning, 2006, p. 151.

105. *ANS:* B

The green-gray evacuated tube has the special requirement of tube inversion for proper mixing to occur. A royal blue evacuated tube does not have a special requirement of inversion. A red-gray evacuated tube has a special requirement of a clot activator and polymer gel.

References

Kalanick, K. *Phlebotomy Technician Specialist*. Clifton Park, N.Y.: Thomson Delmar Learning, 2004, p. 342.

Hoeltke, L. *The Complete Textbook of Phlebotomy*, 3rd ed. Clifton Park, N.Y.: Thomson Delmar Learning, 2006, p. 191.

106. *ANS:* A

A well stocked blood drawing tray includes glass slides, povidone-iodine swabs, and microhematocrit tubes. A hemostat is not commonly found in a well stocked blood drawing tray.

References

Kalanick, K. *Phlebotomy Technician Specialist*. Clifton Park, N.Y.: Thomson Delmar Learning, 2004, pp. 343–344.

Hoeltke, L. *The Complete Textbook of Phlebotomy*, 3rd ed. Clifton Park, N.Y.: Thomson Delmar Learning, 2006, p. 60.

107. *ANS:* A

Puncturing the bone during a heel stick on an infant may not only be painful, but can cause osteomyelitis and/or osteochondritis. All remaining answers are nonsense distracters.

References

Kalanick, K. *Phlebotomy Technician Specialist*. Clifton Park, N.Y.: Thomson Delmar Learning, 2004, pp. 357.

Hoeltke, L. *The Complete Textbook of Phlebotomy*, 3rd ed. Clifton Park, N.Y.: Thomson Delmar Learning, 2006, p. 236.

108. *ANS:* D

The infant's leg should be held securely with the nondominant hand and arm, while the dominant hand uses a pediatric lancet to perform a capillary heel stick. All remaining answers are distracters.

References

Kalanick, K. *Phlebotomy Technician Specialist*. Clifton Park, N.Y.: Thomson Delmar Learning, 2004, p. 358.

Hoeltke, L. *The Complete Textbook of Phlebotomy*, 3rd ed. Clifton Park, N.Y.: Thomson Delmar Learning, 2006, p. 236.

109. *ANS:* B

The standard for measuring the diameter of the lumen of a needle is called needle gauge. A lumen is a passageway or opening to a tubular structure, such as a hypodermic needle. A bevel is the point of a needle that has been cut on a slant for ease of entry. Dialogue and lunar are distracters.

References

Kalanick, K. *Phlebotomy Technician Specialist*. Clifton Park, N.Y.: Thomson Delmar Learning, 2004, p. 335.

Hoeltke, L. *The Complete Textbook of Phlebotomy*, 3rd ed. Clifton Park, N.Y.: Thomson Delmar Learning, 2006, p. 129.

110. *ANS:* D

In the area of phlebotomy, medical supply manufacturers have produced innovative new products to accommodate the new OSHA regulations. All remaining answers are distracters.

References

Kalanick, K. *Phlebotomy Technician Specialist*. Clifton Park, N.Y.: Thomson Delmar Learning, 2004, p. 337.

Hoeltke, L. *The Complete Textbook of Phlebotomy*, 3rd ed. Clifton Park, N.Y.: Thomson Delmar Learning, 2006, p. 62.

111. *ANS:* B

Wrap the tourniquet around the patient's arm approximately 3 to 4 inches above the venipuncture site. All remaining answers are distracters.

References

Kalanick, K. *Phlebotomy Technician Specialist*. Clifton Park, N.Y.: Thomson Delmar Learning, 2004, p. 381.

Hoeltke, L. *The Complete Textbook of Phlebotomy*, 3rd ed. Clifton Park, N.Y.: Thomson Delmar Learning, 2006, p. 183.

112. *ANS:* A

The loose ends of a tourniquet should be running up the patient's arm and away from the venipuncture site. All remaining answers are distracters.

References

Kalanick, K. *Phlebotomy Technician Specialist*. Clifton Park, N.Y.: Thomson Delmar Learning, 2004, p. 382.

Hoeltke, L. *The Complete Textbook of Phlebotomy*, 3rd ed. Clifton Park, N.Y.: Thomson Delmar Learning, 2006, p. 183.

113. *ANS:* C

Outpatients should remain sitting for 15 minutes before attempting a venipuncture for certain procedures. All remaining answers are distracters.

References

Kalanick, K. *Phlebotomy Technician Specialist*. Clifton Park, N.Y.: Thomson Delmar Learning, 2004, p. 405.

Hoeltke, L. *The Complete Textbook of Phlebotomy*, 3rd ed. Clifton Park, N.Y.: Thomson Delmar Learning, 2006, p. 182.

114. *ANS:* C

If the patient tells you he or she feels faint or starts to faint during the procedure, take the following steps: remove the tourniquet and withdraw the needle as quickly as possible, divert the patient's attention, ask the patient to lower his or her head between the knees, ask the patient to breathe slowly and deeply, physically support the patient to prevent further injury, loosen any tight clothing, apply a cold compress, use an ammonia inhalant, if necessary, alert the nurse and/or physician, and monitor the patient's vital signs until normal.

References

Kalanick, K. *Phlebotomy Technician Specialist*. Clifton Park, N.Y.: Thomson Delmar Learning, 2004, pp. 429–430.

Hoeltke, L. *The Complete Textbook of Phlebotomy*, 3rd ed. Clifton Park, N.Y.: Thomson Delmar Learning, 2006, p. 206.

115. *ANS:* B

Once the patient has stopped seizing, he should stay in the area for at least 15 minutes. He should be instructed not to operate a vehicle for at least 30 minutes. All remaining answers are distracters.

References

Kalanick, K. *Phlebotomy Technician Specialist*. Clifton Park, N.Y.: Thomson Delmar Learning, 2004, p. 430.

Hoeltke, L. *The Complete Textbook of Phlebotomy*, 3rd ed. Clifton Park, N.Y.: Thomson Delmar Learning, 2006, p. 206.

116. *ANS:* A

A hematoma occurs when an improperly placed needle results in blood escaping from a vein. All remaining answers are nonsense distracters.

References

Kalanick, K. *Phlebotomy Technician Specialist*. Clifton Park, N.Y.: Thomson Delmar Learning, 2004, p. 431.

Hoeltke, L. *The Complete Textbook of Phlebotomy*, 3rd ed. Clifton Park, N.Y.: Thomson Delmar Learning, 2006, p. 207.

117. *ANS:* D

Given that children's blood vessels are smaller and thus more difficult to visualize and palpate, the process of collecting blood is not the only concern or consideration of the phlebotomist. To auscultate is to examine by auscultation, that is, to listen for sounds within the body.

References

Kalanick, K. *Phlebotomy Technician Specialist*. Clifton Park, N.Y.: Thomson Delmar Learning, 2004, p. 438.

Hoeltke, L. *The Complete Textbook of Phlebotomy*, 3rd ed. Clifton Park, N.Y.: Thomson Delmar Learning, 2006, p. 254.

118. *ANS:* C

Personnel who are required to perform ABGs must be specially trained and, as a rule, are certified by their health care institution as having met the qualifications to perform this advanced procedure. NCCLS has determined the criteria for meeting these qualifications. All remaining answers are distracters.

References

Kalanick, K. *Phlebotomy Technician Specialist*. Clifton Park, N.Y.: Thomson Delmar Learning, 2004, pp. 442–443.

Hoeltke, L. *The Complete Textbook of Phlebotomy*, 3rd ed. Clifton Park, N.Y.: Thomson Delmar Learning, 2006, p. 215.

119. *ANS:* A

Blood smears that are improperly prepared will have an uneven distribution of cells, which will give inaccurate test results. All remaining answers are distracters.

References

Kalanick, K. *Phlebotomy Technician Specialist*. Clifton Park, N.Y.: Thomson Delmar Learning, 2004, p. 364.

Hoeltke, L. *The Complete Textbook of Phlebotomy*, 3rd ed. Clifton Park, N.Y.: Thomson Delmar Learning, 2006, p. 271.

120. *ANS:* A

Syringes come in a variety of sizes: 3 cc, 5 cc, 10 cc, 20 cc, and 60 cc. 0.5 cc is a distracter.

References

Kalanick, K. *Phlebotomy Technician Specialist*. Clifton Park, N.Y.: Thomson Delmar Learning, 2004, p. 334.

Hoeltke, L. *The Complete Textbook of Phlebotomy*, 3rd ed. Clifton Park, N.Y.: Thomson Delmar Learning, 2006, p. 129.

121. *ANS:* D

Two basic types of needles are used when performing venipuncture: multisample needles and single-sample or hypodermic needles. An 18-gauge IV catheter needle is not typically used when performing a venipuncture.

References

Kalanick, K. *Phlebotomy Technician Specialist*. Clifton Park, N.Y.: Thomson Delmar Learning, 2004, p. 336.

Hoeltke, L. *The Complete Textbook of Phlebotomy*, 3rd ed. Clifton Park, N.Y.: Thomson Delmar Learning, 2006, p. 129.

122. *ANS:* B

The phlebotomist may use up to a 1½-inch blood collection needle when using the Saf-T Clik needle adaptor. All remaining answers are distracters.

References

Kalanick, K. *Phlebotomy Technician Specialist*. Clifton Park, N.Y.: Thomson Delmar Learning, 2004, p. 338.

Hoeltke, L. *The Complete Textbook of Phlebotomy*, 3rd ed. Clifton Park, N.Y.: Thomson Delmar Learning, 2006, p. 129.

123. *ANS:* A

A tourniquet is used to distend veins to facilitate venipuncture of intravenous injections. All remaining answers are distracters.

References

Kalanick, K. *Phlebotomy Technician Specialist.* Clifton Park, N.Y.: Thomson Delmar Learning, 2004, p. 339.

Hoeltke, L. *The Complete Textbook of Phlebotomy,* 3rd ed. Clifton Park, N.Y.: Thomson Delmar Learning, 2006, p. 183.

124. *ANS:* A

The Penrose drain tubing is 18 to 20 inches in length and 1/2 to 1 inch wide. All remaining answers are distracters.

References

Kalanick, K. *Phlebotomy Technician Specialist.* Clifton Park, N.Y.: Thomson Delmar Learning, 2004, p. 339.

Hoeltke, L. *The Complete Textbook of Phlebotomy,* 3rd ed. Clifton Park, N.Y.: Thomson Delmar Learning, 2006, p. 149.

125. *ANS:* B

Light blue and yellow sterile tubes or bottles have a full draw requirement. Lavender top tubes prefer a full draw but no less than three-quarters of the tube.

References

Kalanick, K. *Phlebotomy Technician Specialist.* Clifton Park, N.Y.: Thomson Delmar Learning, 2004, p. 341.

Hoeltke, L. *The Complete Textbook of Phlebotomy,* 3rd ed. Clifton Park, N.Y.: Thomson Delmar Learning, 2006, p. 191.

126. *ANS:* B

Some phlebotomists prefer nitrile gloves because they are durable, hard to tear, and comfortable to wear. Nitrile gloves, however, are expensive and not reusable.

References

Kalanick, K. *Phlebotomy Technician Specialist.* Clifton Park, N.Y.: Thomson Delmar Learning, 2004, p. 328.

Hoeltke, L. *The Complete Textbook of Phlebotomy,* 3rd ed. Clifton Park, N.Y.: Thomson Delmar Learning, 2006, p. 58.

127. *ANS:* D

Evacuated tubes are made of either glass of plastic and are available in a range of sizes from 2 to 15 milliliters. All remaining answers are distracters.

References

Kalanick, K. *Phlebotomy Technician Specialist.* Clifton Park, N.Y.: Thomson Delmar Learning, 2004, p. 340.

Hoeltke, L. *The Complete Textbook of Phlebotomy,* 3rd ed. Clifton Park, N.Y.: Thomson Delmar Learning, 2006, p. 136.

128. *ANS:* C

The equipment and supplies needed to perform a successful arterial puncture are as follows: adhesive bandage, alcohol pad, 2×2-inch gauze squares, lidocaine 0.5–1 percent to numb the site, 10- to 22-gauge needle, 25- to 26-gauge needle, plastic bag or cup with crushed ice and water, povidone-iodine swabs, syringe (prefilled heparinized), syringe for lidocaine administration, and waterproof ink pen. A lancet is used for a capillary puncture.

References

Kalanick, K. *Phlebotomy Technician Specialist.* Clifton Park, N.Y.: Thomson Delmar Learning, 2004, p. 346.

Hoeltke, L. *The Complete Textbook of Phlebotomy,* 3rd ed. Clifton Park, N.Y.: Thomson Delmar Learning, 2006, p. 215.

129. *ANS:* C

EDTA is an additive found in the lavender and royal blue evacuated tubes. A light blue evacuated tube contains the additive sodium citrate. Lithium heparin and polymer gel are the additives in a green-gray evacuated tube. A gray evacuated tube contains the additives potassium oxalate/sodium fluoride, sodium fluoride, lithium iodoacetate, and lithium iodoacetate/lithium heparin.

References

Kalanick, K. *Phlebotomy Technician Specialist.* Clifton Park, N.Y.: Thomson Delmar Learning, 2004, p. 341.

Hoeltke, L. *The Complete Textbook of Phlebotomy,* 3rd ed. Clifton Park, N.Y.: Thomson Delmar Learning, 2006, p. 191.

130. *ANS:* B

It is more appropriate to perform a capillary puncture than a venipuncture, when:
- Only a small amount of blood is required to perform a test.
- Collecting specimens on children and infants.
- A substantial vein cannot be located.
- A patient is not cooperative or is overly apprehensive about having a venipuncture.
- The client has severe burns or scar tissue over venipuncture sites.
- The patient has very fragile or superficial veins.

References

Kalanick, K. *Phlebotomy Technician Specialist.* Clifton Park, N.Y.: Thomson Delmar Learning, 2004, p. 354.

Hoeltke, L. *The Complete Textbook of Phlebotomy*, 3rd ed. Clifton Park, N.Y.: Thomson Delmar Learning, 2006, p. 230.

131. *ANS:* A

When handling routine specimens after the blood draw, additive tubes must be gently inverted 8 to 10 times. All remaining answers are distracters.

References

Kalanick, K. *Phlebotomy Technician Specialist*. Clifton Park, N.Y.: Thomson Delmar Learning, 2004, p. 406.

Hoeltke, L. *The Complete Textbook of Phlebotomy*, 3rd ed. Clifton Park, N.Y.: Thomson Delmar Learning, 2006, p. 307.

132. *ANS:* B

When using the centrifuge, it is important that the machine be balanced by placing equal tubes and volumes of specimens opposite each other. If there are not an equal number of blood-filled evacuated glass tubes available for testing, an empty evacuated glass tube is filled with water and is used in place of a blood specimen to balance the centrifuge. All remaining answers are distracters.

References

Kalanick, K. *Phlebotomy Technician Specialist*. Clifton Park, N.Y.: Thomson Delmar Learning, 2004, p. 408.

Hoeltke, L. *The Complete Textbook of Phlebotomy*, 3rd ed. Clifton Park, N.Y.: Thomson Delmar Learning, 2006, p. 109.

133. *ANS:* C

When you are operating a centrifuge, the tubes must remain stoppered to prevent blood from splashing out of the tube, the specimen from evaporating, the pH of the specimen from changing, or the blood from forming aerosol. The tubes do not need to remain stoppered to prevent formation of condensation.

References

Kalanick, K. *Phlebotomy Technician Specialist*. Clifton Park, N.Y.: Thomson Delmar Learning, 2004, p. 408.

Hoeltke, L. *The Complete Textbook of Phlebotomy*, 3rd ed. Clifton Park, N.Y.: Thomson Delmar Learning, 2006, p. 109.

134. *ANS:* B

To obtain a serum specimen, a red-gray top evacuated tube must be used. All remaining answers are distracters.

References

Kalanick, K. *Phlebotomy Technician Specialist*. Clifton Park, N.Y.: Thomson Delmar Learning, 2004, p. 342.

Hoeltke, L. *The Complete Textbook of Phlebotomy*, 3rd ed. Clifton Park, N.Y.: Thomson Delmar Learning, 2006, p. 191.

135. *ANS:* C

Interstitial fluid is released into the blood during the process of a capillary puncture. Interstitial fluid contaminates the blood sample. All remaining answers are nonsense distracters.

References

Kalanick, K. *Phlebotomy Technician Specialist*. Clifton Park, N.Y.: Thomson Delmar Learning, 2004, p. 354.

Hoeltke, L. *The Complete Textbook of Phlebotomy*, 3rd ed. Clifton Park, NY.: Thomson Delmar Learning, 2006, p. 232.

136. *ANS:* D

Glucose levels are higher in capillary blood specimens; potassium, calcium, and total proteins are lower. All remaining answers are distracters.

References

Kalanick, K. *Phlebotomy Technician Specialist*. Clifton Park, N.Y.: Thomson Delmar Learning, 2004, p. 354.

137. *ANS:* B

Osteomyelitis is an inflammation of the bone (especially the bone marrow) caused by a pathogenic organism. All remaining answers are nonsense distracters.

References

Kalanick, K. *Phlebotomy Technician Specialist*. Clifton Park, N.Y.: Thomson Delmar Learning, 2004, p. 357.

138. *ANS:* A

The equipment and supplies needed for a finger stick include: lancet, latex gloves, alcohol prep pads, 2 × 2-inch gauze pads, microcollection container, required point-of-care testing equipment, biohazardous waste container, bandage, and pen. A multisample needle is not needed for a finger stick.

References

Kalanick, K. *Phlebotomy Technician Specialist*. Clifton Park, N.Y.: Thomson Delmar Learning, 2004, p. 359.

Hoeltke, L. *The Complete Textbook of Phlebotomy*, 3rd ed. Clifton Park, N.Y.: Thomson Delmar Learning, 2006, p. 151.

139. *ANS:* A

The blood smear is performed immediately after wiping away the 1st drop of blood of a capillary puncture. All remaining answers are distracters.

References

Kalanick, K. *Phlebotomy Technician Specialist.* Clifton Park, N.Y.: Thomson Delmar Learning, 2004, p. 364.

Hoeltke, L. *The Complete Textbook of Phlebotomy*, 3rd ed. Clifton Park, N.Y.: Thomson Delmar Learning, 2006, p. 270.

140. *ANS:* B

"Antecubital" means in front of the elbow, or at the end of the elbow. All remaining answers are distracters.

References

Kalanick, K. *Phlebotomy Technician Specialist.* Clifton Park, N.Y.: Thomson Delmar Learning, 2004, p. 380.

141. *ANS:* C

When collecting a specimen for blood alcohol levels, the typical 70 percent isopropyl alcohol wipes are not used in skin preparation, because they may affect the results of the alcohol content determination. Iodine preparations also contain alcohol and likewise are not used. A nonalcohol-containing alternative, such as green soap and water, are used instead.

References

Kalanick, K. *Phlebotomy Technician Specialist.* Clifton Park, N.Y.: Thomson Delmar Learning, 2004, p. 499.

Hoeltke, L. *The Complete Textbook of Phlebotomy*, 3rd ed. Clifton Park, N.Y.: Thomson Delmar Learning, 2006, p. 271.

142. *ANS:* C

During the centrifuge process, specimens are spun down for 5 minutes. All remaining answers are distracters.

References

Kalanick, K. *Phlebotomy Technician Specialist.* Clifton Park, N.Y.: Thomson Delmar Learning, 2004, p. 482.

Hoeltke, L. *The Complete Textbook of Phlebotomy*, 3rd ed. Clifton Park, N.Y.: Thomson Delmar Learning, 2006, p. 109.

143. *ANS:* B

A 23-gauge butterfly infusion set with a 2- to 3-milliliter evacuated tube provides the best results on an infant. All remaining answers are distracters.

References

Kalanick, K. *Phlebotomy Technician Specialist.* Clifton Park, N.Y.: Thomson Delmar Learning, 2004, p. 441.

Hoeltke, L. *The Complete Textbook of Phlebotomy*, 3rd ed. Clifton Park, N.Y.: Thomson Delmar Learning, 2006, p. 141.

144. *ANS:* C

A concern for a phlebotomist is the number of times a day blood may be drawn from a patient. Although the maximum number may vary from facility to facility, the average is typically three times a day. All remaining answers are distracters.

References

Kalanick, K. *Phlebotomy Technician Specialist.* Clifton Park, N.Y.: Thomson Delmar Learning, 2004, p. 404.

145. *ANS:* D

Cytogenics testing is drawn in a green tube. Glucose determinations are drawn in a gray tube.

Hematology-Westergren sedimentation rate is drawn on a black evacuated tube. Tests requiring blood serum are drawn in a green-black evacuated tube.

References

Kalanick, K. *Phlebotomy Technician Specialist.* Clifton Park, N.Y.: Thomson Delmar Learning, 2004, p. 341.

Hoeltke, L. *The Complete Textbook of Phlebotomy*, 3rd ed. Clifton Park, N.Y.: Thomson Delmar Learning, 2006, p. 12.

146. *ANS:* A

Arterial blood is used for blood gases because its composition is the same throughout the body. All remaining answers are distracters.

References

Kalanick, K. *Phlebotomy Technician Specialist.* Clifton Park, N.Y.: Thomson Delmar Learning, 2004, p. 345.

Hoeltke, L. *The Complete Textbook of Phlebotomy*, 3rd ed. Clifton Park, N.Y.: Thomson Delmar Learning, 2006, p. 215.

147. *ANS:* A

The National Committee for Clinical Laboratory Standards (NCCLS) guidelines state which areas may be punctured and how deep the puncture may be. All remaining answers are distracters.

References

Kalanick, K. *Phlebotomy Technician Specialist.* Clifton Park, N.Y.: Thomson Delmar Learning, 2004, p. 357.

148. *ANS:* A

While having blood drawn, patients must not be permitted to eat, drink, or have anything in their mouths, such as candy, thermometers, or lozenges. All remaining answers are distracters.

References

Kalanick, K. *Phlebotomy Technician Specialist.* Clifton Park, N.Y.: Thomson Delmar Learning, 2004, p. 380.

Hoeltke, L. *The Complete Textbook of Phlebotomy*, 3rd ed. Clifton Park, N.Y.: Thomson Delmar Learning, 2006, p. 182.

149. *ANS:* A

Pulling the skin taut with your thumb secures the vein and helps to keep it from rolling. It also eases the insertion of the needle into the patient's skin. All remaining answers are distracters.

References

Kalanick, K. *Phlebotomy Technician Specialist*. Clifton Park, N.Y.: Thomson Delmar Learning, 2004, pp. 368–387.

Hoeltke, L. *The Complete Textbook of Phlebotomy*, 3rd ed. Clifton Park, N.Y.: Thomson Delmar Learning, 2006, p. 187.

150. *ANS:* A

It is recommended that pediatric-sized 2-milliliter evacuated tubes be used with pediatric-sized tube adapters. All remaining answers are distracters.

References

Kalanick, K. *Phlebotomy Technician Specialist*. Clifton Park, N.Y.: Thomson Delmar Learning, 2004, p. 397.

Hoeltke, L. *The Complete Textbook of Phlebotomy*, 3rd ed. Clifton Park, N.Y.: Thomson Delmar Learning, 2006, p. 132.

151. *ANS:* C

There are other sites where arterial punctures can be performed, such as the umbilicus of the newborn and the dorsalis pedis arteries of an adult patient. All remaining answers are nonsense distracters.

References

Kalanick, K. *Phlebotomy Technician Specialist*. Clifton Park, N.Y.: Thomson Delmar Learning, 2004, p. 445.

Hoeltke, L. *The Complete Textbook of Phlebotomy*, 3rd ed. Clifton Park, N.Y.: Thomson Delmar Learning, 2006, p. 215.

152. *ANS:* D

ABGs are collected in 1- to 5-milliliter syringes depending on the amount of blood required. All remaining answers are distracters.

References

Kalanick, K. *Phlebotomy Technician Specialist*. Clifton Park, N.Y.: Thomson Delmar Learning, 2004, p. 445.

Hoeltke, L. *The Complete Textbook of Phlebotomy*, 3rd ed. Clifton Park, N.Y.: Thomson Delmar Learning, 2006, p. 215.

153. *ANS:* A

The 14th step in the collection of an ABG is the cleansing of the site with povidone-iodine. All remaining answers are distracters.

References

Kalanick, K. *Phlebotomy Technician Specialist*. Clifton Park, N.Y.: Thomson Delmar Learning, 2004, p. 450.

Hoeltke, L. *The Complete Textbook of Phlebotomy*, 3rd ed. Clifton Park, N.Y.: Thomson Delmar Learning, 2006, p. 215.

154. *ANS:* C

PT tests are drawn on a light blue tube. Serology, routine chemistries, blood banking, and therapeutic drug levels are drawn in a red top evacuated tube. Trace element and nutrient studies and toxicology profiles are drawn in a royal blue top evacuated tube.

References

Kalanick, K. *Phlebotomy Technician Specialist*. Clifton Park, N.Y.: Thomson Delmar Learning, 2004, p. 341.

Hoeltke, L. *The Complete Textbook of Phlebotomy*, 3rd ed. Clifton Park, N.Y.: Thomson Delmar Learning, 2006, p. 191.

155. *ANS:* D

A gray tube is required for a plasma specimen. All remaining answers are distracters.

References

Kalanick, K. *Phlebotomy Technician Specialist*. Clifton Park, N.Y.: Thomson Delmar Learning, 2004, p. 341.

Hoeltke, L. *The Complete Textbook of Phlebotomy*, 3rd ed. Clifton Park, N.Y.: Thomson Delmar Learning, 2006, p. 191.

156. *ANS:* D

A yellow sterile tube is drawn *before* any other tubes in the order of draw. All remaining answers are distracters.

References

Kalanick, K. *Phlebotomy Technician Specialist*. Clifton Park, N.Y.: Thomson Delmar Learning, 2004, p. 341.

Hoeltke, L. *The Complete Textbook of Phlebotomy*, 3rd ed. Clifton Park, N.Y.: Thomson Delmar Learning, 2006, p. 191.

157. *ANS:* B

A quick, deep stick is no more painful than a slow superficial stick, but you get a better flow of blood and spare the patient from a second puncture when you stick quickly and deeply only once. All remaining answers are distracters.

References

Kalanick, K. *Phlebotomy Technician Specialist*. Clifton Park, N.Y.: Thomson Delmar Learning, 2004, p. 360.

Hoeltke, L. *The Complete Textbook of Phlebotomy*, 3rd ed. Clifton Park, N.Y.: Thomson Delmar Learning, 2006, p. 187.

158. *ANS:* D

Veins that are located beneath scar tissue, burns, tattoos, or moles should not be used; select another site.

References

Kalanick, K. *Phlebotomy Technician Specialist*. Clifton Park, N.Y.: Thomson Delmar Learning, 2004, p. 384.

Hoeltke, L. *The Complete Textbook of Phlebotomy*, 3rd ed. Clifton Park, N.Y.: Thomson Delmar Learning, 2006, p. 247.

159. *ANS:* A

The Allen test is used to determine collateral circulation prior to performing arterial puncture. All remaining answers are distracters.

References

Kalanick, K. *Phlebotomy Technician Specialist*. Clifton Park, N.Y.: Thomson Delmar Learning, 2004, p. 444.

Hoeltke, L. *The Complete Textbook of Phlebotomy*, 3rd ed. Clifton Park, N.Y.: Thomson Delmar Learning, 2006, p. 216.

160. *ANS:* C

Instruct patients not to carry or lift any heavy objects with the arm the venipuncture occurred on for approximately 1 hour. All remaining answers are distracters.

References

Kalanick, K. *Phlebotomy Technician Specialist*. Clifton Park, N.Y.: Thomson Delmar Learning, 2004, p. 392.

161. *ANS:* C

After a venipuncture is performed, the bleeding should stop within 5 minutes or the nurse and/or physician must be notified. All remaining answers are distracters.

References

Kalanick, K. *Phlebotomy Technician Specialist*. Clifton Park, N.Y.: Thomson Delmar Learning, 2004, p. 427.

Hoeltke, L. *The Complete Textbook of Phlebotomy*, 3rd ed. Clifton Park, N.Y.: Thomson Delmar Learning, 2006, p. 187.

162. *ANS:* B

The most commonly used needle is a 22-gauge, 1-inch for radial and brachial punctures. All remaining answers are distracters.

References

Kalanick, K. *Phlebotomy Technician Specialist*. Clifton Park, N.Y.: Thomson Delmar Learning, 2004, p. 445.

Hoeltke, L. *The Complete Textbook of Phlebotomy*, 3rd ed. Clifton Park, N.Y.: Thomson Delmar Learning, 2006, p. 129.

163. *ANS:* B

The chance of a hematoma is increased in arterial puncture because the blood in the arteries is under great pressure. All remaining answers are nonsense distracters.

References

Kalanick, K. *Phlebotomy Technician Specialist*. Clifton Park, N.Y.: Thomson Delmar Learning, 2004, p. 447.

Hoeltke, L. *The Complete Textbook of Phlebotomy*, 3rd ed. Clifton Park, N.Y.: Thomson Delmar Learning, 2006, p. 207.

164. *ANS:* D

In the collection of an ABG, assess collateral circulation using the Allen test or a Doppler ultrasonic flow indicator. All remaining answers are distracters.

References

Kalanick, K. *Phlebotomy Technician Specialist*. Clifton Park, N.Y.: Thomson Delmar Learning, 2004, p. 449.

Hoeltke, L. *The Complete Textbook of Phlebotomy*, 3rd ed. Clifton Park, N.Y.: Thomson Delmar Learning, 2006, p. 215.

165. *ANS:* D

Clot activators and polymer gels are a special requirement for red-gray, yellow-black, red-green, and green-black tubes.

References

Kalanick, K. *Phlebotomy Technician Specialist*. Clifton Park, N.Y.: Thomson Delmar Learning, 2004, p. 342.

Hoeltke, L. *The Complete Textbook of Phlebotomy*, 3rd ed. Clifton Park, N.Y.: Thomson Delmar Learning, 2006, p. 132.

166. *ANS:* C

The green-gray tube is affected by volume requirements. Red, yellow-black, and red-green evacuated tubes are not affected by volume requirements.

References

Kalanick, K. *Phlebotomy Technician Specialist*. Clifton Park, N.Y.: Thomson Delmar Learning, 2004, p. 342.

Hoeltke, L. *The Complete Textbook of Phlebotomy*, 3rd ed. Clifton Park, N.Y.: Thomson Delmar Learning, 2006, p. 132.

167. *ANS:* C

When collecting a capillary specimen on an infant, label the specimens with the appropriate information. All remaining answers are distracters.

References

Kalanick, K. *Phlebotomy Technician Specialist*. Clifton Park, N.Y.: Thomson Delmar Learning, 2004, p. 362.

Hoeltke, L. *The Complete Textbook of Phlebotomy*, 3rd ed. Clifton Park, N.Y.: Thomson Delmar Learning, 2006, p. 236.

168. *ANS:* A

In the order of draw, a gray top tube is drawn before a brown top tube. All remaining answers are distracters.

References

Kalanick, K. *Phlebotomy Technician Specialist*. Clifton Park, N.Y.: Thomson Delmar Learning, 2004, p. 341.

Hoeltke, L. *The Complete Textbook of Phlebotomy*, 3rd ed. Clifton Park, N.Y.: Thomson Delmar Learning, 2006, p. 191.

169. *ANS:* B

When applying a tourniquet to a patient with fragile skin that tears or bruises easily, apply the tourniquet on top of the patient's shirt or blouse; this reduces the friction applied directly to the skin. You may also wrap gauze around the area prior to application of the tourniquet. All remaining answers are distracters.

References

Kalanick, K. *Phlebotomy Technician Specialist*. Clifton Park, N.Y.: Thomson Delmar Learning, 2004, p. 383.

Hoeltke, L. *The Complete Textbook of Phlebotomy*, 3rd ed. Clifton Park, N.Y.: Thomson Delmar Learning, 2006, p. 149.

170. *ANS:* B

The dorsal hand veins are excellent sites for drawing labs on neonates and children under the age of 2. All remaining answers are distracters.

References

Kalanick, K. *Phlebotomy Technician Specialist*. Clifton Park, N.Y.: Thomson Delmar Learning, 2004, p. 441.

Hoeltke, L. *The Complete Textbook of Phlebotomy*, 3rd ed. Clifton Park, N.Y.: Thomson Delmar Learning, 2006, p. 179.

171. *ANS:* A

The needle is generally inserted so that the entire bevel is in the vein. All remaining answers are distracters.

References

Kalanick, K. *Phlebotomy Technician Specialist*. Clifton Park, N.Y.: Thomson Delmar Learning, 2004, p. 387.

Hoeltke, L. *The Complete Textbook of Phlebotomy*, 3rd ed. Clifton Park, N.Y.: Thomson Delmar Learning, 2006, p. 187.

172. *ANS:* A

If the needle has been inserted through the vein, blood seeps into the tissues, causing a hematoma. All remaining answers are distracters.

References

Kalanick, K. *Phlebotomy Technician Specialist*. Clifton Park, N.Y.: Thomson Delmar Learning, 2004, p. 403.

Hoeltke, L. *The Complete Textbook of Phlebotomy*, 3rd ed. Clifton Park, N.Y.: Thomson Delmar Learning, 2006, p. 207.

173. *ANS:* C

When performing an ABG, a local anesthetic solution of 0.5–1 percent lidocaine is used to numb the site. All remaining answers are distracters.

References

Kalanick, K. *Phlebotomy Technician Specialist*. Clifton Park, N.Y.: Thomson Delmar Learning, 2004, p. 445.

Hoeltke, L. *The Complete Textbook of Phlebotomy*, 3rd ed. Clifton Park, N.Y.: Thomson Delmar Learning, 2006, p. 215.

174. *ANS:* B

A lithium heparin solution of 1,000 units/milliliter is used to prevent the specimen needed for an ABG from clotting. All remaining answers are distracters.

References

Kalanick, K. *Phlebotomy Technician Specialist*. Clifton Park, N.Y.: Thomson Delmar Learning, 2004, p. 446.

Hoeltke, L. *The Complete Textbook of Phlebotomy*, 3rd ed. Clifton Park, N.Y.: Thomson Delmar Learning, 2006, p. 215.

175. *ANS:* B

Lithium iodoacetate is an additive found in a gray top tube. Lithium heparin, ammonium heparin, and sodium heparin are found in a green top evacuated tube. Lithium heparin and polymer gel are found in a green-gray top evacuated tube. Sodium citrate is found in a light blue top evacuated tube.

References

Kalanick, K. *Phlebotomy Technician Specialist.* Clifton Park, N.Y.: Thomson Delmar Learning, 2004, p. 341.

Hoeltke, L. *The Complete Textbook of Phlebotomy,* 3rd ed. Clifton Park, N.Y.: Thomson Delmar Learning, 2006, p. 191.

176. *ANS:* A

Blood cultures are often ordered in sets that may be performed at the same time from two different sites or can be collected 30 minutes apart. All remaining answers are distracters.

References

Kalanick, K. *Phlebotomy Technician Specialist.* Clifton Park, N.Y.: Thomson Delmar Learning, 2004, p. 453.

Hoeltke, L. *The Complete Textbook of Phlebotomy,* 3rd ed. Clifton Park, N.Y.: Thomson Delmar Learning, 2006, p. 286.

177. *ANS:* B

The total volume of blood drawn per day is based on the patient's weight. All remaining answers are distracters.

References

Kalanick, K. *Phlebotomy Technician Specialist.* Clifton Park, N.Y.: Thomson Delmar Learning, 2004, p. 404.

178. *ANS:* D

When warming an area for a capillary blood collection, a warm moist towel must be no hotter than 108 degrees Fahrenheit (42 degrees Celsius). All remaining answers are distracters.

References

Kalanick, K. *Phlebotomy Technician Specialist.* Clifton Park, N.Y.: Thomson Delmar Learning, 2004, p. 359.

Hoeltke, L. *The Complete Textbook of Phlebotomy,* 3rd ed. Clifton Park, N.Y.: Thomson Delmar Learning, 2006, p. 236.

179. *ANS:* B

In sustaining the order of draw, a light blue top evacuated tube must be drawn before a lavender top evacuated tube. All remaining answers are drawn after a lavender top evacuated tube.

References

Kalanick, K. *Phlebotomy Technician Specialist.* Clifton Park, N.Y.: Thomson Delmar Learning, 2004, p. 341.

Hoeltke, L. *The Complete Textbook of Phlebotomy,* 3rd ed. Clifton Park, N.Y.: Thomson Delmar Learning, 2006, p. 191.

180. *ANS:* A

Train yourself to locate veins while wearing gloves because this saves you time in the long run. Do not rub your finger across the patient's arm. All remaining answers are distracters.

References

Kalanick, K. *Phlebotomy Technician Specialist.* Clifton Park, N.Y.: Thomson Delmar Learning, 2004, p. 383.

Hoeltke, L. *The Complete Textbook of Phlebotomy,* 3rd ed. Clifton Park, N.Y.: Thomson Delmar Learning, 2006, p. 179.

181. *ANS:* B

Although the radial artery is smaller than the brachial artery or the femoral artery, the risk of hematoma is considerably less. All remaining answers are distracters.

References

Kalanick, K. *Phlebotomy Technician Specialist.* Clifton Park, N.Y.: Thomson Delmar Learning, 2004, p. 444.

Hoeltke, L. *The Complete Textbook of Phlebotomy,* 3rd ed. Clifton Park, N.Y.: Thomson Delmar Learning, 2006, p. 179.

182. *ANS:* B

Patients that are on anticoagulant therapy or have bleeding disorders must be monitored closely for a minimum of 30 minutes after a blood draw. All remaining answers are distracters.

References

Kalanick, K. *Phlebotomy Technician Specialist.* Clifton Park, N.Y.: Thomson Delmar Learning, 2004, p. 392.

Hoeltke, L. *The Complete Textbook of Phlebotomy,* 3rd ed. Clifton Park, N.Y.: Thomson Delmar Learning, 2006, p. 207.

183. *ANS:* D

Inadvertent contamination can occur by not allowing the antiseptic to dry, using the wrong antiseptic, and by not cleaning the site or blood culture bottles properly.

References

Kalanick, K. *Phlebotomy Technician Specialist.* Clifton Park, N.Y.: Thomson Delmar Learning, 2004, p. 411.

Hoeltke, L. *The Complete Textbook of Phlebotomy,* 3rd ed. Clifton Park, N.Y.: Thomson Delmar Learning, 2006, p. 44.

184. *ANS:* A

Hypodermic needles for an ABG are $5/8$ to $1\frac{1}{2}$ inches in length. All remaining answers are distracters.

References

Kalanick, K. *Phlebotomy Technician Specialist.* Clifton Park, N.Y.: Thomson Delmar Learning, 2004, p. 445.

Hoeltke, L. *The Complete Textbook of Phlebotomy*, 3rd ed. Clifton Park, N.Y.: Thomson Delmar Learning, 2006, p. 215.

185. *ANS:* B

An oxygen concentration is taken prior to the collection of a specimen for an ABG. All remaining answers are distracters.

References

Kalanick, K. *Phlebotomy Technician Specialist*. Clifton Park, N.Y.: Thomson Delmar Learning, 2004, p. 446.

Hoeltke, L. *The Complete Textbook of Phlebotomy*, 3rd ed. Clifton Park, N.Y.: Thomson Delmar Learning, 2006, p. 215.

186. *ANS:* C

Mottled cap colors indicate that the tube has a gel barrier. All remaining answers are distracters.

References

Kalanick, K. *Phlebotomy Technician Specialist*. Clifton Park, N.Y.: Thomson Delmar Learning, 2004, p. 342.

Hoeltke, L. *The Complete Textbook of Phlebotomy*, 3rd ed. Clifton Park, N.Y.: Thomson Delmar Learning, 2006, p. 132.

187. *ANS:* B

To prepare the syringe for an ABG puncture, the phlebotomist needs to draw 0.5 milliliter of heparin in a syringe. All remaining answers are distracters.

References

Kalanick, K. *Phlebotomy Technician Specialist*. Clifton Park, N.Y.: Thomson Delmar Learning, 2004, p. 448.

Hoeltke, L. *The Complete Textbook of Phlebotomy*, 3rd ed. Clifton Park, N.Y.: Thomson Delmar Learning, 2006, p. 215.

188. *ANS:* A

Tubes that contain anticoagulants should be no less than 50 percent full. All remaining answers are distracters.

References

Kalanick, K. *Phlebotomy Technician Specialist*. Clifton Park, N.Y.: Thomson Delmar Learning, 2004, p. 341.

Hoeltke, L. *The Complete Textbook of Phlebotomy*, 3rd ed. Clifton Park, N.Y.: Thomson Delmar Learning, 2006, p. 132.

189. *ANS:* C

The fourth step when collecting a capillary specimen is to explain the procedure. All remaining answers are distracters.

References

Kalanick, K. *Phlebotomy Technician Specialist*. Clifton Park, N.Y.: Thomson Delmar Learning, 2004, p. 361.

Hoeltke, L. *The Complete Textbook of Phlebotomy*, 3rd ed. Clifton Park, N.Y.: Thomson Delmar Learning, 2006, p. 230.

190. *ANS:* B

The most standard ABG kit contains the following items: 1-cc syringe, 25-guage × 1-inch packaged needle, vented tip cap, needle stopper, 2 gauze pads, povidone-iodine prep, alcohol prep, patient identification label, adhesive bandage, and a Ziploc ice bag. A butterfly infusion set and hot packs are not included in a standard ABG kit.

References

Kalanick, K. *Phlebotomy Technician Specialist*. Clifton Park, N.Y.: Thomson Delmar Learning, 2004, p. 346.

Hoeltke, L. *The Complete Textbook of Phlebotomy*, 3rd ed. Clifton Park, N.Y.: Thomson Delmar Learning, 2006, p. 215.

191. *ANS:* A

The improper application or use of tourniquets during a venipuncture can cause hemoconcentration. All remaining answers are distracters.

References

Kalanick, K. *Phlebotomy Technician Specialist*. Clifton Park, N.Y.: Thomson Delmar Learning, 2004, p. 383.

Hoeltke, L. *The Complete Textbook of Phlebotomy*, 3rd ed. Clifton Park, N.Y.: Thomson Delmar Learning, 2006, p. 151.

192. *ANS:* C

An acid-base balance maintains arterial blood at approximately a 7.35 to 7.45 pH level. All remaining answers are distracters.

References

Kalanick, K. *Phlebotomy Technician Specialist*. Clifton Park, N.Y.: Thomson Delmar Learning, 2004, p. 442.

Hoeltke, L. *The Complete Textbook of Phlebotomy*, 3rd ed. Clifton Park, N.Y.: Thomson Delmar Learning, 2006, p. 215.

193. *ANS:* B

For a syringe draw, insert the needle while holding it at a 15- to 30-degree angle. All remaining answers are distracters.

References

Kalanick, K. *Phlebotomy Technician Specialist*. Clifton Park, N.Y.: Thomson Delmar Learning, 2004, p. 387.

Hoeltke, L. *The Complete Textbook of Phlebotomy*, 3rd ed. Clifton Park, N.Y.: Thomson Delmar Learning, 2006, p. 192.

194. *ANS:* B

A blind stick requires approximation of the anatomic location of the vein. With a visual stick, the vein is noticeable to the eye. On a palpated stick, the vein has been located by palpation.

References

Kalanick, K. *Phlebotomy Technician Specialist*. Clifton Park, N.Y.: Thomson Delmar Learning, 2004, p. 401.

195. *ANS:* D

The following are included in the PPE and supplies required for the collection of blood for ABGs: fluid-resistant lab coat, gown, or aprons, gloves, face protection (arterial punctures have an increased risk of splattering blood), and a puncture-resistant sharps container. A 10 percent bleach solution is not included in the PPE and supplies required for an ABG.

References

Kalanick, K. *Phlebotomy Technician Specialist*. Clifton Park, N.Y.: Thomson Delmar Learning, 2004, p. 445.

Hoeltke, L. *The Complete Textbook of Phlebotomy*, 3rd ed. Clifton Park, N.Y.: Thomson Delmar Learning, 2006, p. 215.

196. *ANS:* D

The needle gauge used to administer an anesthetic for an ABG is 25 or 26. All remaining answers are distracters.

References

Kalanick, K. *Phlebotomy Technician Specialist*. Clifton Park, N.Y.: Thomson Delmar Learning, 2004, p. 445.

Hoeltke, L. *The Complete Textbook of Phlebotomy*, 3rd ed. Clifton Park, N.Y.: Thomson Delmar Learning, 2006, p. 215.

197. *ANS:* D

Yellow sterile, black, and lavender top tubes are all required for whole blood specimens.

References

Kalanick, K. *Phlebotomy Technician Specialist*. Clifton Park, N.Y.: Thomson Delmar Learning, 2004, pp. 341–342.

Hoeltke, L. *The Complete Textbook of Phlebotomy*, 3rd ed. Clifton Park, N.Y.: Thomson Delmar Learning, 2006, p. 191.

198. *ANS:* C

Bacteria in the blood is called bacteriemia. Sepsis is a bacterial infection. Septicemia is the presence of pathogenic microorganisms in the blood. Viralemia is a distracter.

References

Kalanick, K. *Phlebotomy Technician Specialist*. Clifton Park, N.Y.: Thomson Delmar Learning, 2004, p. 451.

199. *ANS:* D

If during the venipuncture process the site begins to swell, immediately remove the needle, release the tourniquet, and apply firm pressure with gauze pads on the site for 8–10 minutes. All remaining answers are distracters.

References

Kalanick, K. *Phlebotomy Technician Specialist*. Clifton Park, N.Y.: Thomson Delmar Learning, 2004, p. 405.

Hoeltke, L. *The Complete Textbook of Phlebotomy*, 3rd ed. Clifton Park, N.Y.: Thomson Delmar Learning, 2006, p. 205.

200. *ANS:* C

A green-gray top tube is drawn after a black top tube. Gray, red-green, and red-gray top evacuated tubes are drawn before a black top evacuated tube.

References

Kalanick, K. *Phlebotomy Technician Specialist*. Clifton Park, N.Y.: Thomson Delmar Learning, 2004, p. 342.

Hoeltke, L. *The Complete Textbook of Phlebotomy*, 3rd ed. Clifton Park, N.Y.: Thomson Delmar Learning, 2006, p. 191.

201. *ANS:* B

A phlebotomist should clean the site of a capillary stick with 70 percent isopropyl alcohol pad. All remaining answers are distracters.

References

Kalanick, K. *Phlebotomy Technician Specialist*. Clifton Park, N.Y.: Thomson Delmar Learning, 2004, p. 360.

Hoeltke, L. *The Complete Textbook of Phlebotomy*, 3rd ed. Clifton Park, N.Y.: Thomson Delmar Learning, 2006, p. 231.

202. *ANS:* C

If a plausible vein cannot be found after checking arms, wrists, and back of hands, the phlebotomist should then ask the physician for permission to use the ankle veins. All remaining answers are distracters.

References

Kalanick, K. *Phlebotomy Technician Specialist*. Clifton Park, N.Y.: Thomson Delmar Learning, 2004, p. 384.

Hoeltke, L. *The Complete Textbook of Phlebotomy*, 3rd ed. Clifton Park, N.Y.: Thomson Delmar Learning, 2006, p. 181.

203. *ANS:* D

The brachial artery has sufficient collateral circulation and is the second choice for an arterial draw. The radial artery is the site most commonly selected because it typically has the best collateral circulation. The femoral artery is a third choice, with a physician or specifically trained emergency room personnel performing the procedure. Ulnar is a distracter.

References

Kalanick, K. *Phlebotomy Technician Specialist.* Clifton Park, N.Y.: Thomson Delmar Learning, 2004, p. 444.

Hoeltke, L. *The Complete Textbook of Phlebotomy,* 3rd ed. Clifton Park, N.Y.: Thomson Delmar Learning, 2006, p. 215.

204. *ANS:* D

The 16th step in an evacuated tube system of venipuncture is removing the tourniquet. All remaining answers are distracters.

References

Kalanick, K. *Phlebotomy Technician Specialist.* Clifton Park, N.Y.: Thomson Delmar Learning, 2004, p. 395.

Hoeltke, L. *The Complete Textbook of Phlebotomy,* 3rd ed. Clifton Park, N.Y.: Thomson Delmar Learning, 2006, p. 196.

205. *ANS:* B

If a hematoma develops, release the tourniquet, withdraw the needle immediately, and apply pressure for 5 minutes. All remaining answers are distracters.

References

Kalanick, K. *Phlebotomy Technician Specialist.* Clifton Park, N.Y.: Thomson Delmar Learning, 2004, p. 430.

Hoeltke, L. *The Complete Textbook of Phlebotomy,* 3rd ed. Clifton Park, N.Y.: Thomson Delmar Learning, 2006, p. 207.

206. *ANS:* D

The most common needle size for a femoral arterial draw is a 22 gauge and 1½ inches in length. All remaining answers are distracters.

References

Kalanick, K. *Phlebotomy Technician Specialist.* Clifton Park, N.Y.: Thomson Delmar Learning, 2004, p. 445.

207. *ANS:* C

The 5th step in the collection of an ABG is to obtain and record the patient's temperature, respiratory rate, and breathing mixture on the laboratory slip. The 6th step is opening the ABG kit. The 7th step is to prepare the syringe. The 8th step is to prepare the anesthetic.

References

Kalanick, K. *Phlebotomy Technician Specialist.* Clifton Park, N.Y.: Thomson Delmar Learning, 2004, p. 448.

Hoeltke, L. *The Complete Textbook of Phlebotomy,* 3rd ed. Clifton Park, N.Y.: Thomson Delmar Learning, 2006, p. 215.

208. *ANS:* B

The black top tube contains 3.8 percent buffered sodium citrate. All remaining answers are distracters.

References

Kalanick, K. *Phlebotomy Technician Specialist.* Clifton Park, N.Y.: Thomson Delmar Learning, 2004, p. 342.

Hoeltke, L. *The Complete Textbook of Phlebotomy,* 3rd ed. Clifton Park, N.Y.: Thomson Delmar Learning, 2006, p. 191.

209. *ANS:* A

To anesthetize for an ABG, insert the needle containing anesthesia at a 10-degree angle. All remaining answers are distracters.

References

Kalanick, K. *Phlebotomy Technician Specialist.* Clifton Park, N.Y.: Thomson Delmar Learning, 2004, p. 449.

Hoeltke, L. *The Complete Textbook of Phlebotomy,* 3rd ed. Clifton Park, N.Y.: Thomson Delmar Learning, 2006, p. 215.

210. *ANS:* A

A royal blue top tube has no special requirements. Light blue, black, and brown top evacuated tubes need to be inverted.

References

Kalanick, K. *Phlebotomy Technician Specialist.* Clifton Park, N.Y.: Thomson Delmar Learning, 2004, p. 341.

Hoeltke, L. *The Complete Textbook of Phlebotomy,* 3rd ed. Clifton Park, N.Y.: Thomson Delmar Learning, 2006, p. 191.

211. *ANS:* D

A yellow-black tube must be drawn after a royal blue top tube. Yellow sterile, lavender, and green top evacuated tubes are to be drawn before a yellow-black evacuated tube.

References

Kalanick, K. *Phlebotomy Technician Specialist.* Clifton Park, N.Y.: Thomson Delmar Learning, 2004, pp. 341–342.

Hoeltke, L. *The Complete Textbook of Phlebotomy,* 3rd ed. Clifton Park, N.Y.: Thomson Delmar Learning, 2006, p. 191.

212. *ANS:* A

While performing a venipuncture, do not allow the patient to stand. All remaining answers are distracters.

References

Kalanick, K. *Phlebotomy Technician Specialist*. Clifton Park, N.Y.: Thomson Delmar Learning, 2004, p. 379.

Hoeltke, L. *The Complete Textbook of Phlebotomy*, 3rd ed. Clifton Park, N.Y.: Thomson Delmar Learning, 2006, p. 178.

213. *ANS:* A

Do place the tourniquet 3 to 4 inches above the venipuncture site. Do remove the tourniquet within 1 minute of application. Do remove the tourniquet prior to withdrawing the needle from the patient.

References

Kalanick, K. *Phlebotomy Technician Specialist*. Clifton Park, N.Y.: Thomson Delmar Learning, 2004, p. 383.

Hoeltke, L. *The Complete Textbook of Phlebotomy*, 3rd ed. Clifton Park, N.Y.: Thomson Delmar Learning, 2006, p. 151.

214. *ANS:* C

The radial artery is the site most commonly selected because it typically has the best collateral circulation. The brachial artery is chosen second and the femoral artery is chosen third. Ulnar is a distracter.

References

Kalanick, K. *Phlebotomy Technician Specialist*. Clifton Park, N.Y.: Thomson Delmar Learning, 2004, p. 443.

Hoeltke, L. *The Complete Textbook of Phlebotomy*, 3rd ed. Clifton Park, N.Y.: Thomson Delmar Learning, 2006, p. 179.

215. *ANS:* A

When drawing on an elderly patient, the tourniquet must be in place until just prior to the removal of the needle. All remaining answers are distracters.

References

Kalanick, K. *Phlebotomy Technician Specialist*. Clifton Park, N.Y.: Thomson Delmar Learning, 2004, p. 389.

Hoeltke, L. *The Complete Textbook of Phlebotomy*, 3rd ed. Clifton Park, N.Y.: Thomson Delmar Learning, 2006, p. 151.

216. *ANS:* D

When plasma or serum is required, it must be transferred to an aliquot tube. All remaining answers are distracters.

References

Kalanick, K. *Phlebotomy Technician Specialist*. Clifton Park, N.Y.: Thomson Delmar Learning, 2004, p. 410.

Hoeltke, L. *The Complete Textbook of Phlebotomy*, 3rd ed. Clifton Park, N.Y.: Thomson Delmar Learning, 2006, p. 290.

217. *ANS:* C

Hypodermic needles needed for an ABG are selected from a 20- to 25-gauge range. All remaining answers are distracters.

References

Kalanick, K. *Phlebotomy Technician Specialist*. Clifton Park, N.Y.: Thomson Delmar Learning, 2004, p. 445.

Hoeltke, L. *The Complete Textbook of Phlebotomy*, 3rd ed. Clifton Park, N.Y.: Thomson Delmar Learning, 2006, p. 215.

218. *ANS:* A

The collection syringe for an ABG must be placed in a coolant that can maintain a temperature of 1–5 degrees Celsius (34–41 degrees Fahrenheit). All remaining answers are distracters.

References

Kalanick, K. *Phlebotomy Technician Specialist*. Clifton Park, N.Y.: Thomson Delmar Learning, 2004, p. 446.

Hoeltke, L. *The Complete Textbook of Phlebotomy*, 3rd ed. Clifton Park, N.Y.: Thomson Delmar Learning, 2006, p. 215.

219. *ANS:* C

A green top evacuated tube contains ammonium heparin as an additive. All remaining answers are distracters.

References

Kalanick, K. *Phlebotomy Technician Specialist*. Clifton Park, N.Y.: Thomson Delmar Learning, 2004, p. 341.

Hoeltke, L. *The Complete Textbook of Phlebotomy*, 3rd ed. Clifton Park, N.Y.: Thomson Delmar Learning, 2006, p. 191.

220. *ANS:* B

Glucose determinations are drawn on a gray top evacuated tube. Chemistry determinations and cytogenics are drawn on a green top evacuated tube. Lead determinations are drawn on a brown top evacuated tube.

References

Kalanick, K. *Phlebotomy Technician Specialist*. Clifton Park, N.Y.: Thomson Delmar Learning, 2004, p. 341.

Hoeltke, L. *The Complete Textbook of Phlebotomy*, 3rd ed. Clifton Park, N.Y.: Thomson Delmar Learning, 2006, p. 141.

221. *ANS:* B

Blood cultures drawn for antimicrobial susceptibility testing are drawn in special collection bottles known as ARD (antimicrobial removal devices) bottles. All remaining answers are distracters.

References

Kalanick, K. *Phlebotomy Technician Specialist*. Clifton Park, N.Y.: Thomson Delmar Learning, 2004, p. 452.

222. *ANS:* A

After cleansing, allow the site to dry 30–60 seconds before performing venipuncture. All remaining answers are distracters.

References

Kalanick, K. *Phlebotomy Technician Specialist*. Clifton Park, N.Y.: Thomson Delmar Learning, 2004, p. 385.

Hoeltke, L. *The Complete Textbook of Phlebotomy*, 3rd ed. Clifton Park, N.Y.: Thomson Delmar Learning, 2006, p. 183.

223. *ANS:* B

The femoral artery is used as a last resort and is performed by a physician or specially trained emergency room personnel. The radial artery is chosen first and the brachial artery is the second choice. Ulnar is a distracter.

References

Kalanick, K. *Phlebotomy Technician Specialist*. Clifton Park, N.Y.: Thomson Delmar Learning, 2004, p. 445.

Hoeltke, L. *The Complete Textbook of Phlebotomy*, 3rd ed. Clifton Park, N.Y.: Thomson Delmar Learning, 2006, p. 179.

224. *ANS:* C

The 10th step in an evacuated tube system of venipuncture is allowing the site to air-dry. Assembling the equipment is step 4, applying the tourniquet is step 7, and cleaning the site is step 9.

References

Kalanick, K. *Phlebotomy Technician Specialist*. Clifton Park, N.Y.: Thomson Delmar Learning, 2004, p. 394.

Hoeltke, L. *The Complete Textbook of Phlebotomy*, 3rd ed. Clifton Park, N.Y.: Thomson Delmar Learning, 2006, p. 196.

225. *ANS:* C

"QNS" means quantity not sufficient. All remaining answers are distracters.

References

Kalanick, K. *Phlebotomy Technician Specialist*. Clifton Park, N.Y.: Thomson Delmar Learning, 2004, p. 411.

226. *ANS:* B

To administer an anesthetic for an ABG a 25- to 26-gauge needle is used. All remaining answers are distracters.

References

Kalanick, K. *Phlebotomy Technician Specialist*. Clifton Park, N.Y.: Thomson Delmar Learning, 2004, p. 445.

Hoeltke, L. *The Complete Textbook of Phlebotomy*, 3rd ed. Clifton Park, N.Y.: Thomson Delmar Learning, 2006, p. 215.

227. *ANS:* C

When preparing a syringe for an ABG, check for free movement of the barrel; then attach a 20-gauge needle to draw heparin with. All remaining answers are distracters.

References

Kalanick, K. *Phlebotomy Technician Specialist*. Clifton Park, N.Y.: Thomson Delmar Learning, 2004, p. 448.

Hoeltke, L. *The Complete Textbook of Phlebotomy*, 3rd ed. Clifton Park, N.Y.: Thomson Delmar Learning, 2006, p. 215.

228. *ANS:* C

Serology testing is drawn on a red top tube. Immunodeficiency panels and collection for blood cultures are drawn on a yellow sterile evacuated tube. Coagulations studies, prothrombin time, and activated partial thromboplastin times are drawn on light blue top evacuated tubes. Hematology-Westergren sedimentation rate is drawn on a black top evacuated topped tube.

References

Kalanick, K. *Phlebotomy Technician Specialist*. Clifton Park, N.Y.: Thomson Delmar Learning, 2004, p. 341.

Hoeltke, L. *The Complete Textbook of Phlebotomy*, 3rd ed. Clifton Park, N.Y.: Thomson Delmar Learning, 2006, p. 132.

229. *ANS:* A

A brown top tube contains the additive Na heparin. A gray top tube contains the additives potassium oxalate/sodium fluoride, sodium fluoride, lithium iodoacetate, and lithium iodoacetate/lithium heparin. A green top evacuated tube contains the additives lithium heparin, ammonium heparin, and sodium heparin. A royal blue top evacuated tube contains the additives EDTA and sodium heparin.

References

Kalanick, K. *Phlebotomy Technician Specialist*. Clifton Park, N.Y.: Thomson Delmar Learning, 2004, p. 341.

Hoeltke, L. *The Complete Textbook of Phlebotomy*, 3rd ed. Clifton Park, N.Y.: Thomson Delmar Learning, 2006, p. 132.

230. *ANS:* B

After an ABG has been collected, a patient on anti-coagulation therapy must have pressure applied to the site for 20 minutes. Do not allow the patient to apply the direct pressure. All remaining answers are distracters.

References

Kalanick, K. *Phlebotomy Technician Specialist*. Clifton Park, N.Y.: Thomson Delmar Learning, 2004, p. 450.

Hoeltke, L. *The Complete Textbook of Phlebotomy*, 3rd ed. Clifton Park, N.Y.: Thomson Delmar Learning, 2006, p. 215.

231. *ANS:* B

If the radial artery is damaged during arterial puncture, the ulnar artery supplies blood to the area. All remaining answers are distracters.

References

Kalanick, K. *Phlebotomy Technician Specialist*. Clifton Park, N.Y.: Thomson Delmar Learning, 2004, p. 444.

Hoeltke, L. *The Complete Textbook of Phlebotomy*, 3rd ed. Clifton Park, N.Y.: Thomson Delmar Learning, 2006, p. 215.

232. *ANS:* C

The blood-borne pathogens standard, set by OSHA, prohibits contaminated sharps from being bent, recapped, or removed. All remaining answers are distracters.

References

Kalanick, K. *Phlebotomy Technician Specialist*. Clifton Park, N.Y.: Thomson Delmar Learning, 2004, p. 390.

Hoeltke, L. *The Complete Textbook of Phlebotomy*, 3rd ed. Clifton Park, N.Y.: Thomson Delmar Learning, 2006, p. 62.

233. *ANS:* D

A green-gray top evacuated tube is drawn last in the order of draw sequence. All remaining answers are distracters.

References

Kalanick, K. *Phlebotomy Technician Specialist*. Clifton Park, N.Y.: Thomson Delmar Learning, 2004, p. 342.

Hoeltke, L. *The Complete Textbook of Phlebotomy*, 3rd ed. Clifton Park, N.Y.: Thomson Delmar Learning, 2006, p. 191.

234. *ANS:* B

In the order of draw sequence, a gray top evacuated tube is the 6th tube to be drawn. A royal blue tube is 7th, a lavender tube is 5th, and a brown tube is 8th.

References

Kalanick, K. *Phlebotomy Technician Specialist*. Clifton Park, N.Y.: Thomson Delmar Learning, 2004, p. 341.

Hoeltke, L. *The Complete Textbook of Phlebotomy*, 3rd ed. Clifton Park, N.Y.: Thomson Delmar Learning, 2006, p. 191.

235. *ANS:* C

Fomites are objects such as clothing, towels, and utensils that possibly harbor a disease agent and are capable of transmitting it. A carrier is a person who harbors a specific pathogenic organism; has no discernible symptoms or signs of the disease, condition, or infection; and is potentially capable of spreading the organism to others. A susceptible host is a person who has little resistance to an infectious disease. A pathogen is an organism or substance capable of causing a disease, condition, or infection.

References

Kalanick, K. *Phlebotomy Technician Specialist*. Clifton Park, N.Y.: Thomson Delmar Learning, 2004, p. 173.

Hoeltke, L. *The Complete Textbook of Phlebotomy*, 3rd ed. Clifton Park, N.Y.: Thomson Delmar Learning, 2006, p. 44.

236. *ANS:* A

The phlebotomist most commonly uses a gauze pad that is a 2×2-inch square and is simply referred to as a "two by two." All remaining answers are distracters.

References

Kalanick, K. *Phlebotomy Technician Specialist*. Clifton Park, N.Y.: Thomson Delmar Learning, 2004, p. 329.

Hoeltke, L. *The Complete Textbook of Phlebotomy*, 3rd ed. Clifton Park, N.Y.: Thomson Delmar Learning, 2006, p. 160.

237. *ANS:* C

Microcollection tubes provide for easy measuring, storing, color coding, and centrifugation of the capillary specimen. Microcollection tubes do not provide for chilling.

References

Kalanick, K. *Phlebotomy Technician Specialist*. Clifton Park, N.Y.: Thomson Delmar Learning, 2004, p. 333.

Hoeltke, L. *The Complete Textbook of Phlebotomy*, 3rd ed. Clifton Park, N.Y.: Thomson Delmar Learning, 2006, p. 151.

238. *ANS:* D

Any needle smaller than a 23 gauge causes the red blood cells to lyse. All remaining answers are distracters.

References

Kalanick, K. *Phlebotomy Technician Specialist*. Clifton Park, N.Y.: Thomson Delmar Learning, 2004, p. 335.

Hoeltke, L. *The Complete Textbook of Phlebotomy*, 3rd ed. Clifton Park, N.Y.: Thomson Delmar Learning, 2006, p. 209.

239. *ANS:* B

The point of a needle that has been cut on a slant for ease of entry is called a bevel. A lumen is a passageway or opening to a tubular structure, such as a blood vessel, phlebotomy, or hypodermic needle. The remaining answers are nonsense distracters.

References

Kalanick, K. *Phlebotomy Technician Specialist*. Clifton Park, N.Y.: Thomson Delmar Learning, 2004, p. 336.

Hoeltke, L. *The Complete Textbook of Phlebotomy*, 3rd ed. Clifton Park, N.Y.: Thomson Delmar Learning, 2006, p. 129.

240. *ANS:* B

Tube holders/adapters are disposable, should remain attached to the needle, and should be placed in the sharps container upon completion of the procedure. Tube holders are available in a variety of sizes to accommodate both adult and pediatric evacuated tubes.

References

Kalanick, K. *Phlebotomy Technician Specialist*. Clifton Park, N.Y.: Thomson Delmar Learning, 2004, p. 337.

Hoeltke, L. *The Complete Textbook of Phlebotomy*, 3rd ed. Clifton Park, N.Y.: Thomson Delmar Learning, 2006, p. 138.

241. *ANS:* C

Equipment needed for a finger stick includes the following:
- Lancet
- Latex gloves
- Alcohol prep pads
- 2 × 2-inch gauze pads
- Microcollection container
- Required point-of-care testing equipment
- Biohazardous waste container
- Bandage
- Pen

A tourniquet is not needed to perform a finger stick.

References

Kalanick, K. *Phlebotomy Technician Specialist*. Clifton Park, N.Y.: Thomson Delmar Learning, 2004, p. 359.

Hoeltke, L. *The Complete Textbook of Phlebotomy*, 3rd ed. Clifton Park, N.Y.: Thomson Delmar Learning, 2006, p. 151.

242. *ANS:* B

After the spreader slide has been backed into the drop of blood, it should be lowered to a 30-degree angle in order to quickly push the slide along the length of the stationary glass slide. All remaining answers are distracters.

References

Kalanick, K. *Phlebotomy Technician Specialist*. Clifton Park, N.Y.: Thomson Delmar Learning, 2004, p. 365.

Hoeltke, L. *The Complete Textbook of Phlebotomy*, 3rd ed. Clifton Park, N.Y.: Thomson Delmar Learning, 2006, p. 271.

243. *ANS:* D

The superficial veins of the arm are called basilic, cephalic, median cubital, and median. Radial is an artery.

References

Kalanick, K. *Phlebotomy Technician Specialist*. Clifton Park, N.Y.: Thomson Delmar Learning, 2004, p. 381.

Hoeltke, L. *The Complete Textbook of Phlebotomy*, 3rd ed. Clifton Park, N.Y.: Thomson Delmar Learning, 2006, p. 179.

244. *ANS:* B

Hemoconcentration is a relative increase in the number of red blood cells resulting from a decrease in the volume of plasma. Hemolysis is the destruction of the membrane of red blood cells and the liberation of hemoglobin, which diffuses into the surrounding fluid. Hemostasis is an arrest of bleeding or of circulation, a stagnation of blood. A hematoma is a swelling or mass of blood that is confined to an organ, tissue, or space and that is caused by a break in a blood vessel.

References

Kalanick, K. *Phlebotomy Technician Specialist*. Clifton Park, N.Y.: Thomson Delmar Learning, 2004, p. 383.

245. *ANS:* A

Once a vein is selected, keep a mental picture of its location. Reference the location to an existing landmark, such as a mole or freckle. Temporarily mark the location of a vein with the end of a pen with the writing point retracted by gently pushing it in over the site, leaving a small round indentation over the area where the needle will be inserted. Leave your index finger over the vein and lift it slightly above the vein to allow for cleansing. The corner of a clean alcohol prep pad may also be positioned in direct line with the vein. Ink should not be left on the patient's skin.

References

Kalanick, K. *Phlebotomy Technician Specialist*. Clifton Park, N.Y.: Thomson Delmar Learning, 2004, p. 384.

Hoeltke, L. *The Complete Textbook of Phlebotomy*, 3rd ed. Clifton Park, N.Y.: Thomson Delmar Learning, 2006, p. 181.

246. *ANS:* B

Using the two-finger technique—Thumb and index finger—To pull the skin taut is not recommended. It increases the risk of an accidental needle stick if the patient should suddenly jerk or pull the arm back. The needle may bounce into the phlebotomist's finger. All remaining answers are distracters.

References

Kalanick, K. *Phlebotomy Technician Specialist*. Clifton Park, N.Y.: Thomson Delmar Learning, 2004, p. 387.

Hoeltke, L. *The Complete Textbook of Phlebotomy*, 3rd ed. Clifton Park, N.Y.: Thomson Delmar Learning, 2006, p. 181.

247. *ANS:* D

Evacuated tubes are labeled with the following:
- Patient's name
- Patient or hospital ID number
- Patient's room number (for an inpatient)
- Time and date of collection
- Phlebotomist's initials

Some requisition slips have preprinted numbered tracking labels that are peeled off and placed on the tubes as well.

References

Kalanick, K. *Phlebotomy Technician Specialist*. Clifton Park, N.Y.: Thomson Delmar Learning, 2004, p. 391.

Hoeltke, L. *The Complete Textbook of Phlebotomy*, 3rd ed. Clifton Park, N.Y.: Thomson Delmar Learning, 2006, p. 172.

248. *ANS:* A

Required equipment for an evacuated tube system venipuncture includes a multidraw needle with a 20 to 21 gauge that is 1 to 1½ inches long. All remaining answers are distracters.

References

Kalanick, K. *Phlebotomy Technician Specialist*. Clifton Park, N.Y.: Thomson Delmar Learning, 2004, p. 394.

Hoeltke, L. *The Complete Textbook of Phlebotomy*, 3rd ed. Clifton Park, N.Y.: Thomson Delmar Learning, 2006, p. 132.

249. *ANS:* B

Using a 5-milliliter tube with a 23-gauge needle during a butterfly infusion set draw may cause hemolysis. All remaining answers are distracters.

References

Kalanick, K. *Phlebotomy Technician Specialist*. Clifton Park, N.Y.: Thomson Delmar Learning, 2004, p. 399.

Hoeltke, L. *The Complete Textbook of Phlebotomy*, 3rd ed. Clifton Park, N.Y.: Thomson Delmar Learning, 2006, p. 201.

250. *ANS:* B

On a butterfly infusion set draw, the tourniquet may be left in place until the draw is complete, as long as the draw is accomplished within a 2-minute window. All remaining answers are distracters.

References

Kalanick, K. *Phlebotomy Technician Specialist*. Clifton Park, N.Y.: Thomson Delmar Learning, 2004, p. 399.

Hoeltke, L. *The Complete Textbook of Phlebotomy*, 3rd ed. Clifton Park, N.Y.: Thomson Delmar Learning, 2006, p. 201.

251. *ANS:* C

The patient's full name, identification number, room number (for an inpatient), time and date, and phlebotomist's initials are needed on each tube of blood. All remaining answers are distracters.

References

Kalanick, K. *Phlebotomy Technician Specialist*. Clifton Park, N.Y.: Thomson Delmar Learning, 2004, p. 399.

Hoeltke, L. *The Complete Textbook of Phlebotomy*, 3rd ed. Clifton Park, N.Y.: Thomson Delmar Learning, 2006, p. 171.

252. *ANS:* C

The specimen must be allowed to clot at room temperature for a minimum of 20 minutes and a maximum of 45 minutes. All remaining answers are distracters.

References

Kalanick, K. *Phlebotomy Technician Specialist*. Clifton Park, N.Y.: Thomson Delmar Learning, 2004, p. 408.

Hoeltke, L. *The Complete Textbook of Phlebotomy*, 3rd ed. Clifton Park, N.Y.: Thomson Delmar Learning, 2006, p. 308.

253. *ANS:* B

Bilirubin is the most commonly ordered test that needs to be protected from light. All remaining answers are distracters.

References

Kalanick, K. *Phlebotomy Technician Specialist*. Clifton Park, N.Y.: Thomson Delmar Learning, 2004, p. 406.

Hoeltke, L. *The Complete Textbook of Phlebotomy*, 3rd ed. Clifton Park, N.Y.: Thomson Delmar Learning, 2006, p. 308.

254. *ANS:* C

Specimens that require centrifuging are spun down, and the serum or plasma is pipetted off and transferred into an aliquot tube. All remaining answers are distracters.

References

Kalanick, K. *Phlebotomy Technician Specialist*. Clifton Park, N.Y.: Thomson Delmar Learning, 2004, p. 408.

Hoeltke, L. *The Complete Textbook of Phlebotomy*, 3rd ed. Clifton Park, N.Y.: Thomson Delmar Learning, 2006, p. 308.

255. *ANS:* C

The feathered edge is only one cell thick and is the most important area of the slide. The smear should be at least half the slide's length. If you use frosted slides, you may write the patient's name in pencil on the frosted edge. Do not use ink because it washes off during the staining process. After the slide is made, allow it to air-dry, standing it on end with the drop of blood end down.

References

Kalanick, K. *Phlebotomy Technician Specialist*. Clifton Park, N.Y.: Thomson Delmar Learning, 2004, pp. 365–366.

Hoeltke, L. *The Complete Textbook of Phlebotomy*, 3rd ed. Clifton Park, N.Y.: Thomson Delmar Learning, 2006, p. 271.

256. *ANS:* B

"NPO" means nothing by mouth after midnight. All remaining answers are distracters.

References

Kalanick, K. *Phlebotomy Technician Specialist*. Clifton Park, N.Y.: Thomson Delmar Learning, 2004, p. 378.

257. *ANS:* A

OSHA requires wearing protective apparel during the processing of specimens. All remaining answers are distracters.

References

Kalanick, K. *Phlebotomy Technician Specialist*. Clifton Park, N.Y.: Thomson Delmar Learning, 2004, p. 408.

Hoeltke, L. *The Complete Textbook of Phlebotomy*, 3rd ed. Clifton Park, N.Y.: Thomson Delmar Learning, 2006, p. 62.

258. *ANS:* D

Pull the stopper straight up; do not "pop" it off. All remaining answers are distracters.

References

Kalanick, K. *Phlebotomy Technician Specialist*. Clifton Park, N.Y.: Thomson Delmar Learning, 2004, p. 410.

Hoeltke, L. *The Complete Textbook of Phlebotomy*, 3rd ed. Clifton Park, N.Y.: Thomson Delmar Learning, 2006, p. 196.

259. *ANS:* B

Specimens that require chilling after collection are those for blood gases, ammonia, lactic acid, renin, prothrombin time, partial thromboplastin, and glucagon. Specimens for a thyroid panel, liver enzyme, and CBC do not require chilling.

References

Kalanick, K. *Phlebotomy Technician Specialist*. Clifton Park, N.Y.: Thomson Delmar Learning, 2004, p. 406.

Hoeltke, L. *The Complete Textbook of Phlebotomy*, 3rd ed. Clifton Park, N.Y.: Thomson Delmar Learning, 2006, p. 308.

260. *ANS:* C

Several situations or conditions can cause an arterial blood sample to render inaccurate test results or to be rejected by the laboratory:
- Air bubbles in the specimen
- Inadequate amount of blood collected
- Improperly cooled specimen
- Venous sample instead of arterial sample
- Incorrect anticoagulant used
- Specimen improperly mixed

References

Kalanick, K. *Phlebotomy Technician Specialist*. Clifton Park, N.Y.: Thomson Delmar Learning, 2004, p. 447.

Hoeltke, L. *The Complete Textbook of Phlebotomy*, 3rd ed. Clifton Park, N.Y.: Thomson Delmar Learning, 2006, p. 215.

261. *ANS:* C

Destruction of the membrane of red blood cells and the liberation of hemoglobin, which diffuses into the surrounding fluid, is called hemolysis. All remaining answers are nonsense distracters.

References

Kalanick, K. *Phlebotomy Technician Specialist*. Clifton Park, N.Y.: Thomson Delmar Learning, 2004, p. 335.

Hoeltke, L. *The Complete Textbook of Phlebotomy*, 3rd ed. Clifton Park, N.Y.: Thomson Delmar Learning, 2006, p. 207.

262. *ANS:* B

To minimize the risk of platelets clumping in the collection device, smear slides first, then collect all other samples.

References

Kalanick, K. *Phlebotomy Technician Specialist.* Clifton Park, N.Y.: Thomson Delmar Learning, 2004, p. 363.

Hoeltke, L. *The Complete Textbook of Phlebotomy*, 3rd ed. Clifton Park, N.Y.: Thomson Delmar Learning, 2006, p. 196.

263. *ANS:* D

The following are basic specimen rejection guidelines common to most facilities:
- Discrepancies between requisition forms and labeled tubes
- Unlabeled tubes
- Hemolyzed specimens
- Specimens collected in wrong tube
- Expired tubes
- Insufficient specimen for the test ordered (labeled QNS)
- Specimen collected at the wrong time interval

All remaining answers are distracters.

References

Kalanick, K. *Phlebotomy Technician Specialist.* Clifton Park, N.Y.: Thomson Delmar Learning, 2004, p. 411.

Hoeltke, L. *The Complete Textbook of Phlebotomy*, 3rd ed. Clifton Park, N.Y.: Thomson Delmar Learning, 2006, p. 73.

264. *ANS:* C

Microcollection containers may also contain the same additives as evacuated tubes and are color coded in the same manner. All remaining answers are distracters.

References

Kalanick, K. *Phlebotomy Technician Specialist.* Clifton Park, N.Y.: Thomson Delmar Learning, 2004, p. 363.

Hoeltke, L. *The Complete Textbook of Phlebotomy*, 3rd ed. Clifton Park, N.Y.: Thomson Delmar Learning, 2006, p. 151.

265. *ANS:* D

An incomplete, or short, draw refers to an evacuated tube or syringe that does not contain the required amount of blood to perform the requested tests. All remaining answers are distracters.

References

Kalanick, K. *Phlebotomy Technician Specialist.* Clifton Park, N.Y.: Thomson Delmar Learning, 2004, p. 400.

266. *ANS:* B

It is recommended and accepted practice that the phlebotomist not stick a patient more than twice. If a third attempt is necessary, it is to be preformed by another phlebotomist. All remaining answers are distracters.

References

Kalanick, K. *Phlebotomy Technician Specialist.* Clifton Park, N.Y.: Thomson Delmar Learning, 2004, p. 404.

267. *ANS:* C

A return, or a backward flow, is called reflux. All remaining answers are distracters.

References

Kalanick, K. *Phlebotomy Technician Specialist.* Clifton Park, N.Y.: Thomson Delmar Learning, 2004, p. 388.

268. *ANS:* A

The DIFF-SAFE allows a slide to be prepared from an EDTA tube without removing the stopper. All remaining answers are distracters.

References

Kalanick, K. *Phlebotomy Technician Specialist.* Clifton Park, N.Y.: Thomson Delmar Learning, 2004, p. 366.

269. *ANS:* B

Capillary puncture is an excellent method for collecting blood specimens when only a small amount is needed. Both routine venipucture and butterfly infusion set draws allow for a greater collection of blood over a capillary puncture. IV is a distracter.

References

Kalanick, K. *Phlebotomy Technician Specialist.* Clifton Park, N.Y.: Thomson Delmar Learning, 2004, p. 367.

Hoeltke, L. *The Complete Textbook of Phlebotomy*, 3rd ed. Clifton Park, N.Y.: Thomson Delmar Learning, 2006, p. 236.

270. *ANS:* C

Specimens must be labeled immediately following the collection. All remaining answers are distracters.

References

Kalanick, K. *Phlebotomy Technician Specialist.* Clifton Park, N.Y.: Thomson Delmar Learning, 2004, p. 399.

Hoeltke, L. *The Complete Textbook of Phlebotomy*, 3rd ed. Clifton Park, N.Y.: Thomson Delmar Learning, 2006, p. 171.

271. *ANS:* C

Collection tubes should be transported stopper upward. All remaining answers are distracters.

References

Kalanick, K. *Phlebotomy Technician Specialist.* Clifton Park, N.Y.: Thomson Delmar Learning, 2004, p. 406.

Hoeltke, L. *The Complete Textbook of Phlebotomy,* 3rd ed. Clifton Park, N.Y.: Thomson Delmar Learning, 2006, p. 308.

272. *ANS:* D

Once a specimen is received at the lab, it is logged in, prioritized, and prepared for testing. When a specimen is received at the lab, it is not frozen.

References

Kalanick, K. *Phlebotomy Technician Specialist.* Clifton Park, N.Y.: Thomson Delmar Learning, 2004, p. 407.

Hoeltke, L. *The Complete Textbook of Phlebotomy,* 3rd ed. Clifton Park, N.Y.: Thomson Delmar Learning, 2006, p. 308.

273. *ANS:* C

All are correct except the labeling of the tube. If you send an unlabeled tube to the lab, it will be rejected.

References

Kalanick, K. *Phlebotomy Technician Specialist.* Clifton Park, N.Y.: Thomson Delmar Learning, 2004, p. 411.

Hoeltke, L. *The Complete Textbook of Phlebotomy,* 3rd ed. Clifton Park, N.Y.: Thomson Delmar Learning, 2006, p. 171.

274. *ANS:* C

If a specimen is rejected, the phlebotomist must collect new specimens as quickly as possible. All remaining answers are distracters.

References

Kalanick, K. *Phlebotomy Technician Specialist.* Clifton Park, N.Y.: Thomson Delmar Learning, 2004, p. 411.

Hoeltke, L. *The Complete Textbook of Phlebotomy,* 3rd ed. Clifton Park, N.Y.: Thomson Delmar Learning, 2006, p. 308.

275. *ANS:* D

Powder from gloves can contaminate blood slides and skin punctures. All remaining answers are distracters.

References

Kalanick, K. *Phlebotomy Technician Specialist.* Clifton Park, N.Y.: Thomson Delmar Learning, 2004, p. 411.

276. *ANS:* A

Stat means immediately and indicates that a patient is critical and must be treated or responded to as a medical emergency. Fasting means the patient must fast a certain amount of time before the collection of blood. A timed specimen means that the specimens should be collected at specifically timed intervals. QNS means the quantity is not sufficient.

References

Kalanick, K. *Phlebotomy Technician Specialist.* Clifton Park, N.Y.: Thomson Delmar Learning, 2004, p. 412.

Hoeltke, L. *The Complete Textbook of Phlebotomy,* 3rd ed. Clifton Park, N.Y.: Thomson Delmar Learning, 2006, p. 270.

277. *ANS:* C

The National Accrediting Agency for Clinical Laboratory Sciences (NACCLS) sets the maximum time limit for separating serum and plasma from the cells at 2 hours from time of collection. All remaining answers are distracters.

References

Kalanick, K. *Phlebotomy Technician Specialist.* Clifton Park, N.Y.: Thomson Delmar Learning, 2004, p. 407.

278. *ANS:* B

A type of specimen requiring a near-body temperature (37.5 degrees Celsius, 98.6 degrees Fahrenheit) even during transport is for cold agglutinins. All remaining answers are distracters.

References

Kalanick, K. *Phlebotomy Technician Specialist.* Clifton Park, N.Y.: Thomson Delmar Learning, 2004, p. 407.

Hoeltke, L. *The Complete Textbook of Phlebotomy,* 3rd ed. Clifton Park, N.Y.: Thomson Delmar Learning, 2006, p. 308.

279. *ANS:* B

A centrifuge is a machine used to separate substances of different densities. An autoclave is used for sterilizing instruments. A hemacytometer is an instrument that counts blood cells. An incubator is a chamber that provides determined environmental conditions.

References

Kalanick, K. *Phlebotomy Technician Specialist.* Clifton Park, N.Y.: Thomson Delmar Learning, 2004, p. 332.

Hoeltke, L. *The Complete Textbook of Phlebotomy,* 3rd ed. Clifton Park, N.Y.: Thomson Delmar Learning, 2006, p. 109.

280. *ANS:* A

Blood smears should be free of any holes, lines, or jagged edges, and they must be centered on the slide. All remaining answers are distracters.

References

Kalanick, K. *Phlebotomy Technician Specialist.* Clifton Park, N.Y.: Thomson Delmar Learning, 2004, p. 365.

Hoeltke, L. *The Complete Textbook of Phlebotomy,* 3rd ed. Clifton Park, N.Y.: Thomson Delmar Learning, 2006, p. 271.

281. *ANS:* C

Arterial blood specimens kept at 1–5 degrees Celsius (34–41 degrees Fahrenheit) are accurate for 2–3 hours. All remaining answers are distracters.

References

Kalanick, K. *Phlebotomy Technician Specialist.* Clifton Park, N.Y.: Thomson Delmar Learning, 2004, p. 451.

Hoeltke, L. *The Complete Textbook of Phlebotomy,* 3rd ed. Clifton Park, N.Y.: Thomson Delmar Learning, 2006, p. 215.

282. *ANS:* A

It is important to collect specimens in the correct order to guarantee specimen integrity. To minimize the risk of platelet clumping in the collection device, smear slides first, then collect any hematology samples; then collect all other samples. All remaining answers are distracters.

References

Kalanick, K. *Phlebotomy Technician Specialist.* Clifton Park, N.Y.: Thomson Delmar Learning, 2004, p. 363.

Hoeltke, L. *The Complete Textbook of Phlebotomy,* 3rd ed. Clifton Park, N.Y.: Thomson Delmar Learning, 2006, p. 191.

283. *ANS:* B

The differential is read on the feathered edge of a blood slide. All remaining answers are distracters.

References

Kalanick, K. *Phlebotomy Technician Specialist.* Clifton Park, N.Y.: Thomson Delmar Learning, 2004, p. 365.

Hoeltke, L. *The Complete Textbook of Phlebotomy,* 3rd ed. Clifton Park, N.Y.: Thomson Delmar Learning, 2006, p. 271.

284. *ANS:* C

Routine specimens must arrive at the laboratory within 45 minutes of collection. All remaining answers are distracters.

References

Kalanick, K. *Phlebotomy Technician Specialist.* Clifton Park, N.Y.: Thomson Delmar Learning, 2004, p. 407.

Hoeltke, L. *The Complete Textbook of Phlebotomy,* 3rd ed. Clifton Park, N.Y.: Thomson Delmar Learning, 2006, p. 308.

285. *ANS:* A

Specimens can be centrifuged once. All remaining answers are distracters.

References

Kalanick, K. *Phlebotomy Technician Specialist.* Clifton Park, N.Y.: Thomson Delmar Learning, 2004, p. 409.

Hoeltke, L. *The Complete Textbook of Phlebotomy,* 3rd ed. Clifton Park, N.Y.: Thomson Delmar Learning, 2006, p. 109.

286. *ANS:* D

To clean a centrifuge of a broken evacuated glass tube you should use a wet paper towel, disinfect following the facility's blood spill protocols, and wear heavy-duty utility gloves. You should never sweep the tiny shards of glass into a gloved hand and dispose of them in a sharps container.

References

Kalanick, K. *Phlebotomy Technician Specialist.* Clifton Park, N.Y.: Thomson Delmar Learning, 2004, p. 409.

Hoeltke, L. *The Complete Textbook of Phlebotomy,* 3rd ed. Clifton Park, N.Y.: Thomson Delmar Learning, 2006, p. 109.

287. *ANS:* B

Routine specimens must be centrifuged within 60 minutes of collection. All remaining answers are distracters.

References

Kalanick, K. *Phlebotomy Technician Specialist.* Clifton Park, N.Y.: Thomson Delmar Learning, 2004, p. 407.

Hoeltke, L. *The Complete Textbook of Phlebotomy,* 3rd ed. Clifton Park, N.Y.: Thomson Delmar Learning, 2006, p. 109.

288. *ANS:* D

Lavender top tubes are stable for 24 hours but blood smears must be completed within 1 hour of collection. All remaining answers are distracters.

References

Kalanick, K. *Phlebotomy Technician Specialist.* Clifton Park, N.Y.: Thomson Delmar Learning, 2004, p. 407.

Hoeltke, L. *The Complete Textbook of Phlebotomy,* 3rd ed. Clifton Park, N.Y.: Thomson Delmar Learning, 2006, p. 191.

289. *ANS:* C

Potassium and cortisol specimens must reach the laboratory within a 45-minute window. All remaining answers are distracters.

References

Kalanick, K. *Phlebotomy Technician Specialist*. Clifton Park, N.Y.: Thomson Delmar Learning, 2004, p. 407.

Hoeltke, L. *The Complete Textbook of Phlebotomy*, 3rd ed. Clifton Park, N.Y.: Thomson Delmar Learning, 2006, p. 308.

290. *ANS:* C

Once a specimen drawn in an SST (serum separator tube) is centrifuged, the separator gel prevents glycolysis for up to 24 hours. All remaining answers are distracters.

References

Kalanick, K. *Phlebotomy Technician Specialist*. Clifton Park, N.Y.: Thomson Delmar Learning, 2004, p. 407.

Hoeltke, L. *The Complete Textbook of Phlebotomy*, 3rd ed. Clifton Park, N.Y.: Thomson Delmar Learning, 2006, p. 191.

291. *ANS:* C

A suprapubic specimen is collected for evaluation of microbial analysis or cytology studies. A catheterized specimen is collected when a patient is having trouble voiding, is already catheterized, or when analysis must be done on the urine directly from the bladder. Pediatric specimens present a special challenge. A specially designed plastic urine collection bag with hypoallergenic skin adhesive is used. A midstream collection is used to ensure that the urinary opening is free from contaminates.

References

Kalanick, K. *Phlebotomy Technician Specialist*. Clifton Park, N.Y.: Thomson Delmar Learning, 2004, p. 463.

Hoeltke, L. *The Complete Textbook of Phlebotomy*, 3rd ed. Clifton Park, N.Y.: Thomson Delmar Learning, 2006, p. 270.

292. *ANS:* A

Specimens drawn for glucose determination in tubes containing sodium fluoride, a glycolytic inhibitor, are stable for 24 hours at room temperature and for up to 48 hours when refrigerated. All remaining answers are distracters.

References

Kalanick, K. *Phlebotomy Technician Specialist*. Clifton Park, N.Y.: Thomson Delmar Learning, 2004, p. 407.

Hoeltke, L. *The Complete Textbook of Phlebotomy*, 3rd ed. Clifton Park, N.Y.: Thomson Delmar Learning, 2006, p. 191.

293. *ANS:* B

Chilling a specimen after collection slows down the metabolic processes, which would continue after the draw. All remaining answers are distracters.

References

Kalanick, K. *Phlebotomy Technician Specialist*. Clifton Park, N.Y.: Thomson Delmar Learning, 2004, p. 406.

Hoeltke, L. *The Complete Textbook of Phlebotomy*, 3rd ed. Clifton Park, N.Y.: Thomson Delmar Learning, 2006, p. 308.

294. *ANS:* C

For manually activated clotting times, the tube must be kept warm during as well as before the procedure. All remaining answers are distracters.

References

Kalanick, K. *Phlebotomy Technician Specialist*. Clifton Park, N.Y.: Thomson Delmar Learning, 2004, p. 407.

Hoeltke, L. *The Complete Textbook of Phlebotomy*, 3rd ed. Clifton Park, N.Y.: Thomson Delmar Learning, 2006, p. 281.

295. *ANS:* C

Proper handling of the specimen begins the moment the blood is drawn into the evacuated tube or syringe, and it continues throughout the collection process. All remaining answers are distracters.

References

Kalanick, K. *Phlebotomy Technician Specialist*. Clifton Park, N.Y.: Thomson Delmar Learning, 2004, p. 405.

Hoeltke, L. *The Complete Textbook of Phlebotomy*, 3rd ed. Clifton Park, N.Y.: Thomson Delmar Learning, 2006, p. 308.

296. *ANS:* D

The general guidelines that a phlebotomist must follow in order to maintain specimen integrity contain instructions for handling routine specimens, additive and nonadditive tubes, and transportation; specimens requiring special handling, including, warmth, time, and transportation; and finally exceptions to the general guidelines. Processing the requisition is not part of the general guidelines for maintaining specimen integrity.

References

Kalanick, K. *Phlebotomy Technician Specialist*. Clifton Park, N.Y.: Thomson Delmar Learning, 2004, pp. 405–407.

Hoeltke, L. *The Complete Textbook of Phlebotomy*, 3rd ed. Clifton Park, N.Y.: Thomson Delmar Learning, 2006, p. 308.

297. *ANS:* B

Specimens requiring centrifugation are one of two categories: plasma or serum. All remaining answers are distracters.

References

Kalanick, K. *Phlebotomy Technician Specialist.* Clifton Park, N.Y.: Thomson Delmar Learning, 2004, p. 408.

Hoeltke, L. *The Complete Textbook of Phlebotomy,* 3rd ed. Clifton Park, N.Y.: Thomson Delmar Learning, 2006, p. 109.

298. *ANS:* A

Repeating centrifugation will cause hemolysis and inaccurate test results. All remaining answers are distracters.

References

Kalanick, K. *Phlebotomy Technician Specialist.* Clifton Park, N.Y.: Thomson Delmar Learning, 2004, p. 409.

Hoeltke, L. *The Complete Textbook of Phlebotomy,* 3rd ed. Clifton Park, N.Y.: Thomson Delmar Learning, 2006, p. 109.

299. *ANS:* C

Specially designed amber microcollection containers are available for the collection of bilirubin specimens from infants. All remaining answers are distracters.

References

Kalanick, K. *Phlebotomy Technician Specialist.* Clifton Park, N.Y.: Thomson Delmar Learning, 2004, p. 406.

Hoeltke, L. *The Complete Textbook of Phlebotomy,* 3rd ed. Clifton Park, N.Y.: Thomson Delmar Learning, 2006, p. 151.

300. *ANS:* D

Tests requiring plasma specimens are collected in tubes containing an anticoagulant specific for the requested test. All remaining answers are distracters.

References

Kalanick, K. *Phlebotomy Technician Specialist.* Clifton Park, N.Y.: Thomson Delmar Learning, 2004, p. 408.

Hoeltke, L. *The Complete Textbook of Phlebotomy,* 3rd ed. Clifton Park, N.Y.: Thomson Delmar Learning, 2006, p. 191.

MODULE 7: POINT-OF-CARE TESTING AND NON-BLOOD SPECIMENS

1. *ANS:* C

The reference value range for blood glucose is 75–100 milligrams/deciliter. All other answers are distracters.

References

Kalanick, K. *Phlebotomy Technician Specialist.* Clifton Park, N.Y.: Thomson Delmar Learning, 2004, p. 487.

Hoeltke, L. *The Complete Textbook of Phlebotomy,* 3rd ed. Clifton Park, N.Y.: Thomson Delmar Learning, 2006, p. 276.

2. *ANS:* A

If a GTT (glucose tolerance test) specimen is collected prior to the 2-hour window, an elevated glucose level is recorded and misinterpreted by the physician. All other answers are distracters.

References

Kalanick, K. *Phlebotomy Technician Specialist.* Clifton Park, N.Y.: Thomson Delmar Learning, 2004, p. 488.

Hoeltke, L. *The Complete Textbook of Phlebotomy,* 3rd ed. Clifton Park, N.Y.: Thomson Delmar Learning, 2006, p. 276.

3. *ANS:* B

Coagulation studies must occur at 37 degrees Celsius (98.6 degrees Fahrenheit) to ensure the accuracy of results. All other answers are distracters.

References

Kalanick, K. *Phlebotomy Technician Specialist.* Clifton Park, N.Y.: Thomson Delmar Learning, 2004, p. 491.

Hoeltke, L. *The Complete Textbook of Phlebotomy,* 3rd ed. Clifton Park, N.Y.: Thomson Delmar Learning, 2006, p. 142.

4. *ANS:* D

ACT analyzes the activity of the intrinsic coagulation factors and is used to monitor heparin therapy. All other answers are distracters.

References

Kalanick, K. *Phlebotomy Technician Specialist.* Clifton Park, N.Y.: Thomson Delmar Learning, 2004, p. 492.

Hoeltke, L. *The Complete Textbook of Phlebotomy,* 3rd ed. Clifton Park, N.Y.: Thomson Delmar Learning, 2006, p. 142.

5. *ANS:* D

The prothrombin test (PT) procedure is often performed alone to monitor oral anticoagulation therapy (Coumadin). An activated coagulation time (ACT) is used to monitor heparin therapy. Heat determination and plasma compensation are nonsense distracters.

References

Kalanick, K. *Phlebotomy Technician Specialist.* Clifton Park, N.Y.: Thomson Delmar Learning, 2004, p. 493.

6. *ANS:* C

The PT normal values are 17–22 seconds. All other answers are distracters.

References

Kalanick, K. *Phlebotomy Technician Specialist*. Clifton Park, N.Y.: Thomson Delmar Learning, 2004, p. 493.

7. *ANS:* B

The most common electrolytes measured by POCT (point-of-care testing) are sodium, potassium, chloride, bicarbonate ion, and ionized calcium.

References

Kalanick, K. *Phlebotomy Technician Specialist*. Clifton Park, N.Y.: Thomson Delmar Learning, 2004, p. 497.

8. *ANS:* A

An increase of leukocytes is most commonly present in bacterial urinary tract infections. Red blood cells, platelets, and glucose are not typically increased.

References

Kalanick, K. *Phlebotomy Technician Specialist*. Clifton Park, N.Y.: Thomson Delmar Learning, 2004, p. 518.
Hoeltke, L. *The Complete Textbook of Phlebotomy*, 3rd ed. Clifton Park, N.Y.: Thomson Delmar Learning, 2006, p. 290.

9. *ANS:* A

A blood urea nitrogen (BUN) level is performed to provide a rough estimate of the patient's kidney function. Glucose levels are performed to aid in the diagnosis and management of diabetes mellitus. Prothrombin time is performed to monitor oral anticoagulation therapy. The blood gases test measures pH, partial pressure of carbon dioxide, and partial pressure of oxygen.

References

Kalanick, K. *Phlebotomy Technician Specialist*. Clifton Park, N.Y.: Thomson Delmar Learning, 2004, p. 498.

10. *ANS:* D

The National Institute on Drug Abuse (NIDA) defines the drug testing procedures and requires them to be followed exactly. The other answers are distracters. The CDC is the Centers for Disease Control, CLIA is the Clinical Laboratory Improvement Act, and NCCLS is the National Committee for Clinical Laboratory Standards.

References

Kalanick, K. *Phlebotomy Technician Specialist*. Clifton Park, N.Y.: Thomson Delmar Learning, 2004, p. 499.

11. *ANS:* D

Ordering TDM (therapeutic drug monitoring) allows the physician to establish drug dosage, maintain dosages at beneficial levels, and avoid drug toxicity. A PTT is a partial prothrombin time; P&T and TMD are both nonsense distracters.

References

Kalanick, K. *Phlebotomy Technician Specialist*. Clifton Park, N.Y.: Thomson Delmar Learning, 2004, p. 503.

12. *ANS:* B

Paternity tests are based on ABO and Rh typing, as well as other proteins on the surface of red blood cells. PPD (purified protein derivative) is a skin test used in the determination of tuberculosis. A hematocrit measures the volume of patient's red blood cells as a percentage of whole blood in relationship to the plasma. Tuberculosis is a distracter.

References

Kalanick, K. *Phlebotomy Technician Specialist*. Clifton Park, N.Y.: Thomson Delmar Learning, 2004, pp. 503–504.

13. *ANS:* C

Pregnancy tests determine the levels of human chorionic gonadotrophin (hCG), which is present in increasingly higher levels during pregnancy, in both urine and blood. The remaining answers are distracters. Hct is the abbreviation for hematocrit, Hgb is the abbreviation for hemoglobin, and STD is the abbreviation for sexually transmitted disease.

References

Kalanick, K. *Phlebotomy Technician Specialist*. Clifton Park, N.Y.: Thomson Delmar Learning, 2004, p. 508.

14. *ANS:* B

Cholesterol serves an important function because approximately 80 percent of cholesterol is used to manufacture bile acids that allow the body to digest lipids and fats. Cholesterol located in the skin helps to keep the skin waterproof and aids in the evaporation of water from the body. The remaining answers are distracters.

References

Kalanick, K. *Phlebotomy Technician Specialist*. Clifton Park, N.Y.: Thomson Delmar Learning, 2004, p. 489.

15. *ANS:* A

The desirable cholesterol level is less than 200 milligrams/deciliter. The remaining answers are distracters.

References

Kalanick, K. *Phlebotomy Technician Specialist*. Clifton Park, N.Y.: Thomson Delmar Learning, 2004, p. 491.

16. *ANS:* B

The hematocrit (Hct) measures the volume of the patient's red blood cells as a percentage of whole blood in relationship to the plasma. The remaining answers are distracters. Hgb is the abbreviation for hemoglobin, FBS is the abbreviation for fasting blood sugar, and HDL is the abbreviation for high-density lipoprotein.

References

Kalanick, K. *Phlebotomy Technician Specialist*. Clifton Park, N.Y.: Thomson Delmar Learning, 2004, p. 482.

17. *ANS:* C

The iron-containing protein pigment of the red blood cells, which carries oxygen from the lungs to the tissue, is called hemoglobin (Hgb). The remaining answers are distracters. FSB is the abbreviation for fasting blood sugar, Hct is the abbreviation for hematocrit, LDL is the abbreviation for low-density lipoprotein.

References

Kalanick, K. *Phlebotomy Technician Specialist*. Clifton Park, N.Y.: Thomson Delmar Learning, 2004, p. 485.

18. *ANS:* B

The reference value range for a hematocrit for a female patient is 36–48 percent. The remaining answers are distracters.

References

Kalanick, K. *Phlebotomy Technician Specialist*. Clifton Park, N.Y.: Thomson Delmar Learning, 2004, p. 485.

19. *ANS:* D

The normal values for PTT (partial thromboplastin time) or APTT (activated partial thromboplastin time), when using whole blood, are 93–127 seconds. The remaining answers are distracters.

References

Kalanick, K. *Phlebotomy Technician Specialist*. Clifton Park, N.Y.: Thomson Delmar Learning, 2004, p. 493.

20. *ANS:* D

The drugs most commonly detected in drug screens are alcohol, crack, and marijuana.

References

Kalanick, K. *Phlebotomy Technician Specialist*. Clifton Park, N.Y.: Thomson Delmar Learning, 2004, p. 501.

21. *ANS:* A

Determine whether the patient has taken aspirin or any other salicylate-containing drug in the last 2 weeks. The remaining answers are distracters.

References

Kalanick, K. *Phlebotomy Technician Specialist*. Clifton Park, N.Y.: Thomson Delmar Learning, 2004, p. 495.

22. *ANS:* B

The phlebotomist performs a control "check" daily to ensure that control specimens fall within established range values. The remaining answers are distracters. Performing a control check prior to every test is time-consuming and unnecessary. Control specimens are outdated if they are only checked quarterly or biannually.

References

Kalanick, K. *Phlebotomy Technician Specialist*. Clifton Park, N.Y.: Thomson Delmar Learning, 2004, p. 481.

23. *ANS:* D

Point-of-care testing includes fecal occult blood, coagulation monitoring, and chemistry panels. Immune assay must be performed in the laboratory.

References

Kalanick, K. *Phlebotomy Technician Specialist*. Clifton Park, N.Y.: Thomson Delmar Learning, 2004, p. 480–481.

Hoeltke, L. *The Complete Textbook of Phlebotomy*, 3rd ed. Clifton Park, N.Y.: Thomson Delmar Learning, 2006, p. 9.

24. *ANS:* B

Hyperglycemia pertains to the condition in which the blood sugar (glucose) is increased, as in diabetes mellitus. The remaining answers are distracters. Hyperthyroidism indicates excessive functional activity of the thyroid gland. Hypoglycemia indicates a decreased blood sugar level. Hyperinsulinism indicates the presence of excess insulin in the body, resulting in hypoglycemia.

References

Kalanick, K. *Phlebotomy Technician Specialist*. Clifton Park, N.Y.: Thomson Delmar Learning, 2004, p. 486.

Hoeltke, L. *The Complete Textbook of Phlebotomy*, 3rd ed. Clifton Park, N.Y.: Thomson Delmar Learning, 2006, p. 276.

25. *ANS:* C

Increased cholesterol levels cause fats to deposit in the inner lining of the arteries, creating a condition known as atherosclerosis. Arteriosclerosis is a chronic disease characterized by abnormal thickening and hardening of the arterial walls, with resulting loss of elasticity. Arthrosclerosis and arterisclerosis are nonsense distracters.

References

Kalanick, K. *Phlebotomy Technician Specialist*. Clifton Park, N.Y.: Thomson Delmar Learning, 2004, p. 489.

26. *ANS:* B

Hemoglobin reference value ranges for a newborn are 16.0–23.0 grams/deciliter. The remaining answers are distracters.

References

Kalanick, K. *Phlebotomy Technician Specialist.* Clifton Park, N.Y.: Thomson Delmar Learning, 2004, p. 486.

27. *ANS:* A

Diuretics and corticosteroids may not be taken by a patient scheduled for a GTT. Acetaminophen may be safely taken because it does not affect the results.

References

Kalanick, K. *Phlebotomy Technician Specialist.* Clifton Park, N.Y.: Thomson Delmar Learning, 2004, p. 488.

28. *ANS:* B

The ACT (adrenocorticotropic hormone) analysis is performed by collecting a small volume of blood in a prewarmed special gray top evacuated tube, containing a coagulation activator, such as siliceous earth, silica, or celite. The remaining answers are distracters. Prothrombin time (PT) uses one drop of whole blood or plasma and is typically collected from a capillary puncture. Toxicology profiles depend on the type of specimen being collected (blood, urine, or other body fluid specimens), and a CBC (complete blood count) is collected in a lavender top evacuated tube.

References

Kalanick, K. *Phlebotomy Technician Specialist.* Clifton Park, N.Y.: Thomson Delmar Learning, 2004, p. 492.

29. *ANS:* D

Potassium plays a major role in osmotic pressure, muscle function, nerve conduction, and acid-base.

References

Kalanick, K. *Phlebotomy Technician Specialist.* Clifton Park, N.Y.: Thomson Delmar Learning, 2004, p. 496.

30. *ANS:* C

The normal range for arterial blood pH is 7.35–7.45. The remaining answers are distracters.

References

Kalanick, K. *Phlebotomy Technician Specialist.* Clifton Park, N.Y.: Thomson Delmar Learning, 2004, p. 497.

Hoeltke, L. *The Complete Textbook of Phlebotomy,* 3rd ed. Clifton Park, N.Y.: Thomson Delmar Learning, 2006, p. 215.

31. *ANS:* C

A timed collection test requires a patient to provide urine specimens at specific intervals. In a 24-hour collection, the patient collects all output in a 24-hour period. A random sample can be collected at any time, and a double voided specimen is a distracter.

References

Kalanick, K. *Phlebotomy Technician Specialist.* Clifton Park, N.Y.: Thomson Delmar Learning, 2004, p. 460.

Hoeltke, L. *The Complete Textbook of Phlebotomy,* 3rd ed. Clifton Park, N.Y.: Thomson Delmar Learning, 2006, p. 268.

32. *ANS:* B

A midstream collection method is used to ensure that the urinary opening is free of contaminates, such as genital secretions, pubic hair, and bacteria. A random sample can be collected at any time. A timed collection test requires a patient to provide urine specimens at specific intervals. In a 24-hour collection, the patient collects all output in a 24-hour period.

References

Kalanick, K. *Phlebotomy Technician Specialist.* Clifton Park, N.Y.: Thomson Delmar Learning, 2004, p. 461.

Hoeltke, L. *The Complete Textbook of Phlebotomy,* 3rd ed. Clifton Park, N.Y.: Thomson Delmar Learning, 2006, p. 290.

33. *ANS:* C

Throat cultures are ordered to aid in the diagnosis of streptococcal infections. Semen specimens are collected to determine sperm counts or for forensic testing. Stool samples are collected to determine the presence of occult blood and parasites, and urine specimens are collected to aid in the diagnosis and treatment of urinary tract conditions or disease.

References

Kalanick, K. *Phlebotomy Technician Specialist.* Clifton Park, N.Y.: Thomson Delmar Learning, 2004, p. 453.

Hoeltke, L. *The Complete Textbook of Phlebotomy,* 3rd ed. Clifton Park, N.Y.: Thomson Delmar Learning, 2006, p. 302.

34. *ANS:* A

The first morning specimen is often favored because the urine is at its highest concentration, having been incubating in the bladder while the patient has been sleeping. The remaining answers are distracters.

References

Kalanick, K. *Phlebotomy Technician Specialist.* Clifton Park, N.Y.: Thomson Delmar Learning, 2004, p. 459.

Hoeltke, L. *The Complete Textbook of Phlebotomy*, 3rd ed. Clifton Park, N.Y.: Thomson Delmar Learning, 2006, p. 290.

35. *ANS:* A

A catheterized specimen is collected when a patient is having trouble voiding. The patient is not able to collect a clean catch, random, or 24-hour specimen if he or she is having trouble voiding.

References

Kalanick, K. *Phlebotomy Technician Specialist*. Clifton Park, N.Y.: Thomson Delmar Learning, 2004, p. 463.

Hoeltke, L. *The Complete Textbook of Phlebotomy*, 3rd ed. Clifton Park, N.Y.: Thomson Delmar Learning, 2006, p. 290.

36. *ANS:* A

The Schick test is used to test for diphtheria. The remaining answers are distracters.

References

Kalanick, K. *Phlebotomy Technician Specialist*. Clifton Park, N.Y.: Thomson Delmar Learning, 2004, p. 504.

37. *ANS:* B

The syringe is held at a 15- to 20-degree angle, and the needle is inserted just under the skin, just past the bevel. Remaining answers are distracters.

References

Kalanick, K. *Phlebotomy Technician Specialist*. Clifton Park, N.Y.: Thomson Delmar Learning, 2004, p. 505.

Hoeltke, L. *The Complete Textbook of Phlebotomy*, 3rd ed. Clifton Park, N.Y.: Thomson Delmar Learning, 2006, p. 200.

38. *ANS:* D

Urobilin is one element responsible for the normal color of feces. Bilirubin is a reddish yellow pigment that occurs especially in bile and blood and that causes jaundice if accumulated in excess. A ketone is an organic compound, such as acetone, attached to two carbon atoms. Protein is any of numerous naturally occurring extremely complex substances that consist of amino acid residues joined by peptide bonds and that do not contribute to the color of feces.

References

Kalanick, K. *Phlebotomy Technician Specialist*. Clifton Park, N.Y.: Thomson Delmar Learning, 2004, p. 517.

Hoeltke, L. *The Complete Textbook of Phlebotomy*, 3rd ed. Clifton Park, N.Y.: Thomson Delmar Learning, 2006, p. 304.

39. *ANS:* B

A nitrite test and the leukocyte test are both performed to screen for urinary track infections. A glucose, hemoglobin, or ketones test does not indicate a urinary tract infection.

References

Kalanick, K. *Phlebotomy Technician Specialist*. Clifton Park, N.Y.: Thomson Delmar Learning, 2004, p. 517.

Hoeltke, L. *The Complete Textbook of Phlebotomy*, 3rd ed. Clifton Park, N.Y.: Thomson Delmar Learning, 2006, p. 286.

40. *ANS:* C

A first morning specimen has a heightened concentration of analytes, with a heightened specific gravity.

References

Kalanick, K. *Phlebotomy Technician Specialist*. Clifton Park, N.Y.: Thomson Delmar Learning, 2004, p. 460.

Hoeltke, L. *The Complete Textbook of Phlebotomy*, 3rd ed. Clifton Park, N.Y.: Thomson Delmar Learning, 2006, p. 286.

41. *ANS:* A

Fecal specimens are examined to help evaluate gastrointestinal disorders and conditions. The remaining answers are distracters.

References

Kalanick, K. *Phlebotomy Technician Specialist*. Clifton Park, N.Y.: Thomson Delmar Learning, 2004, p. 456.

Hoeltke, L. *The Complete Textbook of Phlebotomy*, 3rd ed. Clifton Park, N.Y.: Thomson Delmar Learning, 2006, p. 304.

42. *ANS:* C

Semen should be collected in a sterile urine container. Condoms often contain spermicide, which would alter test results. Clean medicine bottles often contain residue from the medication, and a clean baby food jar may contain residue from the baby food, altering the test results.

References

Kalanick, K. *Phlebotomy Technician Specialist*. Clifton Park, N.Y.: Thomson Delmar Learning, 2004, p. 458.

Hoeltke, L. *The Complete Textbook of Phlebotomy*, 3rd ed. Clifton Park, N.Y.: Thomson Delmar Learning, 2006, p. 301.

43. *ANS:* B

The patient must discontinue the use of aspirin and iron intake for at least one week prior to testing. Alcohol consumption, smoking, and eating sugary foods will not alter the test results.

References

Kalanick, K. *Phlebotomy Technician Specialist*. Clifton Park, N.Y.: Thomson Delmar Learning, 2004, p. 504.

44. *ANS:* C

The reaction is read in 24–72 hours, depending on the type of antigen test performed. The remaining answers are distracters.

References

Kalanick, K. *Phlebotomy Technician Specialist*. Clifton Park, N.Y.: Thomson Delmar Learning, 2004, p. 506.

45. *ANS:* B

A strep A test is typically performed when a patient has a sore throat or tonsillitis. Strep A does not cause appendicitis or gastroenteritis, and the test would not be performed given the symptoms that accompany these two conditions.

References

Kalanick, K. *Phlebotomy Technician Specialist*. Clifton Park, N.Y.: Thomson Delmar Learning, 2004, p. 509.

Hoeltke, L. *The Complete Textbook of Phlebotomy*, 3rd ed. Clifton Park, N.Y.: Thomson Delmar Learning, 2006, p. 304.

46. *ANS:* B

A freshly voided specimen should have an aromatic odor. The remaining answers are distracters. An ammonia odor occurs especially during the decomposition of urine when it is standing or retained in the urinary bladder; the odor may be related to some bacterial infections. A fruity or sweet smelling urine may be caused by diabetic acidosis, starvation, or dieting. A foul or putrid odor suggests that the urine is not freshly voided.

References

Kalanick, K. *Phlebotomy Technician Specialist*. Clifton Park, N.Y.: Thomson Delmar Learning, 2004, p. 514.

Hoeltke, L. *The Complete Textbook of Phlebotomy*, 3rd ed. Clifton Park, N.Y.: Thomson Delmar Learning, 2006, p. 286.

47. *ANS:* B

Urinary pH varies from 5 to 9, with 7 being considered neutral. The remaining answers are distracters.

References

Kalanick, K. *Phlebotomy Technician Specialist*. Clifton Park, N.Y.: Thomson Delmar Learning, 2004, p. 516.

Hoeltke, L. *The Complete Textbook of Phlebotomy*, 3rd ed. Clifton Park, N.Y.: Thomson Delmar Learning, 2006, p. 286.

48. *ANS:* A

A fractional or double void specimen requires a patient to drink approximately 200 milliliters of water. The patient waits a required amount of time (typically a half hour), while the urine has time to accumulate in the bladder. A 24-hour collection measures intake and output over a 24-hour period. A 2-hour collection measures intake and output over a 2-hour period. A midstream collection is required to avoid contamination of the specimen.

References

Kalanick, K. *Phlebotomy Technician Specialist*. Clifton Park, N.Y.: Thomson Delmar Learning, 2004, p. 461.

Hoeltke, L. *The Complete Textbook of Phlebotomy*, 3rd ed. Clifton Park, N.Y.: Thomson Delmar Learning, 2006, p. 286.

49. *ANS:* D

The clean catch collection procedure requires a female patient to stand in a squatting position over the toilet. She must open three prepackaged towelettes or prepare three sterile 2 × 2-inch gauze pads with soapy water; use the first towelette or pad to cleanse from front to back, wiping once on the right side of the urinary opening; use the second to wipe once from front to back on the left side of urinary opening; and then use the third to wipe from front to back down the center of urinary opening. Finally, the patient voids the first portion of urine into the toilet (midstream).

References

Kalanick, K. *Phlebotomy Technician Specialist*. Clifton Park, N.Y.: Thomson Delmar Learning, 2004, p. 462.

Hoeltke, L. *The Complete Textbook of Phlebotomy*, 3rd ed. Clifton Park, N.Y.: Thomson Delmar Learning, 2006, p. 290.

50. *ANS:* D

Normal urine color is described as yellow, gold, amber, or straw, and it may be further clarified by pale, light, or dark (i.e., pale yellow or dark amber).

References

Kalanick, K. *Phlebotomy Technician Specialist*. Clifton Park, N.Y.: Thomson Delmar Learning, 2004, p. 510.

Hoeltke, L. *The Complete Textbook of Phlebotomy*, 3rd ed. Clifton Park, N.Y.: Thomson Delmar Learning, 2006, p. 286.

MODULE 8: LEGAL, ETHICAL, PROFESSIONAL COMMUNICATIONS AND CLERICAL SKILLS AND DUTIES

1. *ANS:* D

   Eye contact is not a barrier to effective communication. Non-English–speaking patients and those for whom English is their second language have special concerns. Often non-English–speaking patients understand basic directions through the use of hand signals or sign language. A patient with a hearing impairment requires a different style of communication. Enunciate terms loudly and clearly. A patient's state of health and level of consciousness play an important role in the communication process. Often, patients are heavily medicated or have altered levels of consciousness.

   ## References

   Kalanick, K. *Phlebotomy Technician Specialist.* Clifton Park, N.Y.: Thomson Delmar Learning, 2004, pp. 537–538.

   Hoeltke, L. *The Complete Textbook of Phlebotomy,* 3rd ed. Clifton Park, N.Y.: Thomson Delmar Learning, 2006, p. 326.

2. *ANS:* C

   Approximately 80 percent of all communication is nonverbal. All remaining answers are distracters.

   ## References

   Kalanick, K. *Phlebotomy Technician Specialist.* Clifton Park, N.Y.: Thomson Delmar Learning, 2004, p. 534.

   Hoeltke, L. *The Complete Textbook of Phlebotomy,* 3rd ed. Clifton Park, N.Y.: Thomson Delmar Learning, 2006, p. 326.

3. *ANS:* D

   Comfort zones are based on gender, individual preference, and culture. Comfort zones are not typically based on education.

   ## References

   Kalanick, K. *Phlebotomy Technician Specialist.* Clifton Park, N.Y.: Thomson Delmar Learning, 2004, p. 538.

4. *ANS:* A

   The time of the call, the phone number needed for a return call, and the caller's name should be on the message. There isn't any need for the caller's date of birth (DOB).

   ## References

   Kalanick, K. *Phlebotomy Technician Specialist.* Clifton Park, N.Y.: Thomson Delmar Learning, 2004, p. 540.

5. *ANS:* A

   The use of cologne and perfume is discouraged. The phlebotomist is to be neat, clean, and well-groomed, and he or she is to have good posture. Particular attention is always paid to personal hygiene. Bathing, clean teeth, fresh breath, and the use of antiperspirant/deodorant must be part of the phlebotomist's daily routine.

   ## References

   Kalanick, K. *Phlebotomy Technician Specialist.* Clifton Park, N.Y.: Thomson Delmar Learning, 2004, p. 534.

   Hoeltke, L. *The Complete Textbook of Phlebotomy,* 3rd ed. Clifton Park, N.Y.: Thomson Delmar Learning, 2006, p. 28.

6. *ANS:* B

   The average speaking rate is 120–150 words per minute. All remaining answers are distracters.

   ## References

   Kalanick, K. *Phlebotomy Technician Specialist.* Clifton Park, N.Y.: Thomson Delmar Learning, 2004, p. 535.

7. *ANS:* B

   Ethics is the area of philosophical study that examines society's values, actions, and choices to determine right and wrong. The medical professional's rules of right and wrong are called the medical code of ethics. Duty of care is the responsibility not to infringe on another's rights by either intentionally or carelessly causing him or her harm. Laws hold every health care practitioner to the same legal and ethical standards. "Conditions" is a distracter.

   ## References

   Kalanick, K. *Phlebotomy Technician Specialist.* Clifton Park, N.Y.: Thomson Delmar Learning, 2004, p. 21.

   Hoeltke, L. *The Complete Textbook of Phlebotomy,* 3rd ed. Clifton Park, N.Y.: Thomson Delmar Learning, 2006, p. 21.

8. *ANS:* C

   Malpractice is a claim of improper treatment brought against a professional and/or institution by means of a civil lawsuit. Duty of care is the responsibility not to infringe on another's rights by either intentionally of carelessly causing him or her harm. Libel is a written statement, falsifying facts about someone such that it causes harm to the person's reputation. Battery is the act of intentionally touching someone in a harmful or offensive manner without the person's consent.

   ## References

   Kalanick, K. *Phlebotomy Technician Specialist.* Clifton Park, N.Y.: Thomson Delmar Learning, 2004, p. 19.

9. *ANS:* D

Negligence does not require intent. Fraud, libel, and malpractice require intent.

References

Kalanick, K. *Phlebotomy Technician Specialist*. Clifton Park, N.Y.: Thomson Delmar Learning, 2004, p. 18.

10. *ANS:* B

Battery is the act of intentionally touching someone in a harmful or offensive manner without the person's consent. Assault is the act of intentionally causing someone to fear that he or she is about to become the victim of battery. The intentional infliction of emotional distress is the willful infliction of emotions so as to cause the patient to suffer duress. Malpractice is the misconduct or unprofessional treatment by someone in a professional or official position.

References

Kalanick, K. *Phlebotomy Technician Specialist*. Clifton Park, N.Y.: Thomson Delmar Learning, 2004, p. 18.

11. *ANS:* A

A claim is a billing sent to an insurance carrier. An EOB is an explanation of benefits or services, periodically issued to recipients or providers on whose behalf claims have been paid. A premium is a monthly fee that enrollees pay for medical insurance. A ledger is a distracter.

References

Kalanick, K. *Phlebotomy Technician Specialist*. Clifton Park, N.Y.: Thomson Delmar Learning, 2004, p. 209.

12. *ANS:* D

Active listening does not require physical contact. To actively listen, the phlebotomist gives the patient his or her undivided attention, acknowledges the message sent, and offers an appropriate answer. Active listening also requires concentration and skill, and, when these skills are applied, the phlebotomist can increase the comprehension and retention of information.

References

Kalanick, K. *Phlebotomy Technician Specialist*. Clifton Park, N.Y.: Thomson Delmar Learning, 2004, p. 536.

Hoeltke, L. *The Complete Textbook of Phlebotomy*, 3rd ed. Clifton Park, N.Y.: Thomson Delmar Learning, 2006, p. 326.

13. *ANS:* C

Personal integrity is the ability to do what is right when no one is watching. All remaining answers are distracters.

References

Kalanick, K. *Phlebotomy Technician Specialist*. Clifton Park, N.Y.: Thomson Delmar Learning, 2004, p. 532.

Hoeltke, L. *The Complete Textbook of Phlebotomy*, 3rd ed. Clifton Park, N.Y.: Thomson Delmar Learning, 2006, p. 27.

14. *ANS:* C

Manual requisition forms are generally 3¼ inches wide and 7½ inches long. All of the remaining answers are distracters.

References

Kalanick, K. *Phlebotomy Technician Specialist*. Clifton Park, N.Y.: Thomson Delmar Learning, 2004, p. 203.

15. *ANS:* A

The ICD-9-CM is the reference used to code diagnoses. CPT is the reference used to code procedures. HCPCs and BBP are nonsense distracters.

References

Phlebotomy Kalanick, K. *Phlebotomy Technician Specialist*. Clifton Park, N.Y.: Thomson Delmar Learning, 2004, p. 213.

16. *ANS:* B

Log-on is signing on to a computer system by entering a username and a password. "Online" describes an operational system or being on the Internet. Interface is the hardware and software that enable individual computers and components to interact. Hard copy is the readable paper copy or printout of information.

References

Kalanick, K. *Phlebotomy Technician Specialist*. Clifton Park, N.Y.: Thomson Delmar Learning, 2004, p. 219.

17. *ANS:* A

Ethics is the area of philosophical study that examines society's values, actions, and choices to determine right and wrong. Fraud is an intentional misrepresentation, a deliberate deception intended to produce unlawful gain. Morals and values are distracters.

References

Kalanick, K. *Phlebotomy Technician Specialist*. Clifton Park, N.Y.: Thomson Delmar Learning, 2004, p. 21.

Hoeltke, L. *The Complete Textbook of Phlebotomy*, 3rd ed. Clifton Park, N.Y.: Thomson Delmar Learning, 2006, p. 21.

18. *ANS:* D

Negligence torts occur when a duty of care is breached unintentionally, causing harm. Fraud and libel are intentional torts. Malpractice is a claim of improper treatment or negligence brought against a professional person and/or institution by means of a civil lawsuit.

References

Kalanick, K. *Phlebotomy Technician Specialist.* Clifton Park, N.Y.: Thomson Delmar Learning, 2004, p. 18.

19. *ANS:* A

Due care is the responsibility of health care providers to protect others from harm. A tort is a private wrong or injury, other than a breach of contract, for which the court provides a remedy. "Respondeat superior" is a Latin phrase that means, "Let the master answer." Ethics is the area of philosophical study that examines society's values, actions, and choices to determine right and wrong.

References

Kalanick, K. *Phlebotomy Technician Specialist.* Clifton Park, N.Y.: Thomson Delmar Learning, 2004, p. 19.

20. *ANS:* C

An agreement by the patient to a medical procedure or treatment after reasonable explanation is called informed consent. Chain of custody is the procedure for ensuring that material obtained for diagnosis has been taken from the named patient, is properly labeled, and has not been tampered with en route to the laboratory. Burden of proof is a legal term used in conjunction with the terms "malpractice" and "negligence." Assumed consent is a distracter.

References

Kalanick, K. *Phlebotomy Technician Specialist.* Clifton Park, N.Y.: Thomson Delmar Learning, 2004, p. 20.

21. *ANS:* B

To prove negligence, four conditions must exist. (1) A standard of care must exist. (2) The standard of care must be breached. (3) An injury must be sustained. (4) The injury must be proven to be caused by the acts that resulted from the breach of the standard of care.

References

Kalanick, K. *Phlebotomy Technician Specialist.* Clifton Park, N.Y.: Thomson Delmar Learning, 2004, p. 21.

22. *ANS:* D

A fee for a specific procedure or test is based on the usual and customary fee within the community. All remaining answers are distracters.

References

Kalanick, K. *Phlebotomy Technician Specialist.* Clifton Park, N.Y.: Thomson Delmar Learning, 2004, p. 208.

23. *ANS:* B

An individual or organization covered for protection and loss under the specific terms of an insurance policy is called the insured. The coinsured is covered by coinsurance, which is a cost-sharing requirement specified in a health insurance policy providing that the insured assumes a percentage of the costs for covered services. A guarantor is a person responsible for a payment of services. A PPO (preferred provider organization) is a type of health benefit program in which enrollees receive the highest level of benefits when they obtain services from a physician, hospital, or other health provider designated by their program as a "preferred provider."

References

Kalanick, K. *Phlebotomy Technician Specialist.* Clifton Park, N.Y.: Thomson Delmar Learning, 2004, p. 209.

24. *ANS:* D

The universal health insurance claim form (CMS-1500) is a standard form accepted by most insurance companies. All other answers are distracters.

References

Kalanick, K. *Phlebotomy Technician Specialist.* Clifton Park, N.Y.: Thomson Delmar Learning, 2004, p. 213.

25. *ANS:* D

Nonverbal communication involves body movements, gestures, facial expression, eye contact, touch, use of space, and appearance. Articulation is distinctly and clearly enunciating words, phrases, and sentences. Verbal communication is the spoken word, and the sender must be articulate. Kinesics is a systematic study of the body and the use of its static and dynamic positions as a means of communication.

References

Kalanick, K. *Phlebotomy Technician Specialist.* Clifton Park, N.Y.: Thomson Delmar Learning, 2004, p. 534.

Hoeltke, L. *The Complete Textbook of Phlebotomy,* 3rd ed. Clifton Park, N.Y.: Thomson Delmar Learning, 2006, p. 326.

26. *ANS:* D

A tort is a private wrong or injury, other than a breach of contract, for which the court provides a remedy. Malpractice is the misconduct or unprofessional treatment by someone in a professional or official position. Negligence is the failure to act with reasonable care, resulting in the harming or others. Battery is the act of intentionally touching someone in a harmful or offensive manner without the person's consent.

References

Kalanick, K. *Phlebotomy Technician Specialist*. Clifton Park, N.Y.: Thomson Delmar Learning, 2004, p. 15.

27. *ANS:* A

The Patient Care Partnership is not legally binding; however, this document is accepted throughout the medical health care industry as the standard to which all patients have the right to be treated. All remaining answers are distracters.

References

Kalanick, K. *Phlebotomy Technician Specialist*. Clifton Park, N.Y.: Thomson Delmar Learning, 2004, p. 15.
Hoeltke, L. *The Complete Textbook of Phlebotomy*, 3rd ed. Clifton Park, N.Y.: Thomson Delmar Learning, 2006, p. 22.

28. *ANS:* C

According to the Patient Care Partnership, the patient can expect high-quality hospital care, a clean and safe environment, involvement in care, protection of privacy, preparation for release, and help with billing and the filing of insurance claims. All remaining answers are distracters.

References

Kalanick, K. *Phlebotomy Technician Specialist*. Clifton Park, N.Y.: Thomson Delmar Learning, 2004, pp. 16–17.
Hoeltke, L. *The Complete Textbook of Phlebotomy*, 3rd ed. Clifton Park, N.Y.: Thomson Delmar Learning, 2006, p. 22.

29. *ANS:* B

"Burden of proof" is a legal term used in conjunction with the terms "malpractice" and "negligence." Chain of custody is the procedure for ensuring that material obtained for diagnosis has been taken from the named patient, is properly labeled, and has not been tampered with en route to the laboratory. Informed consent is an agreement by the patient to a medical procedure or treatment after receiving adequate information about the procedure or treatment, its risks, and/or its consequences. Duty of care is the responsibility not to infringe on another's rights by either intentionally or carelessly causing him or her harm.

References

Kalanick, K. *Phlebotomy Technician Specialist*. Clifton Park, N.Y.: Thomson Delmar Learning, 2004, p. 21.

30. *ANS:* B

The most important skill that a successful health care provider can possess is the ability to interact compassionately with patients and their families. Integrity requires adherence to a strict ethical code, to be in an undiminished or unimpaired state. Professionalism is the conduct, behavior, and qualities that characterize a professional person. Communication is the transmission of a message from a sender to a receiver.

References

Kalanick, K. *Phlebotomy Technician Specialist*. Clifton Park, N.Y.: Thomson Delmar Learning, 2004, p. 532.
Hoeltke, L. *The Complete Textbook of Phlebotomy*, 3rd ed. Clifton Park, N.Y.: Thomson Delmar Learning, 2006, p. 27.

31. *ANS:* D

To enunciate words, phrases, and sentences distinctly and clearly is to articulate. To communicate is to transmit a message from a sender to a receiver. To verbalize is to communicate by means of words. To vocalize is to communicate with voice.

References

Kalanick, K. *Phlebotomy Technician Specialist*. Clifton Park, N.Y.: Thomson Delmar Learning, 2004, p. 533.
Hoeltke, L. *The Complete Textbook of Phlebotomy*, 3rd ed. Clifton Park, N.Y.: Thomson Delmar Learning, 2006, p. 326.

32. *ANS:* B

Empathy is defined as an objective awareness of and insight into the feelings, emotions, and behaviors of another person. Sympathy is when one person shares feelings with another. Compassion is knowing and wanting to help when another suffers. Commiseration is feeling sad or sorrowful with someone.

References

Kalanick, K. *Phlebotomy Technician Specialist*. Clifton Park, N.Y.: Thomson Delmar Learning, 2004, p. 537.

33. *ANS:* A

DRGs are a classification system categorizing patient procedures using like diagnoses and treatments. A PPO is a type of health benefit program in which enrollees receive the highest level of benefits when they obtain services from a physician, hospital, or other health provider designated by their program as a "preferred provider." An HMO (health maintenance organization) is a type of health care program in which enrollees receive benefits for services from authorized and preselected providers, usually a primary care physician. Generally, enrollees do not receive coverage for the services of providers who are not in the HMO network, except for emergency services. CDL is a distracter.

References

Kalanick, K. *Phlebotomy Technician Specialist*. Clifton Park, N.Y.: Thomson Delmar Learning, 2004, p. 212.

34. *ANS:* C

Decoding lab tests is not a function of a laboratory computer. The computer has the capability to perform many functions. Based on the specific program the facility is using, the computer can be used to perform one or all of the following: data entry; test requisitions; printing of test request forms, labels, and accession numbers; printing schedules and collection lists; entering test results; maintenance of medical records; and transferring information.

References

Kalanick, K. *Phlebotomy Technician Specialist*. Clifton Park, N.Y.: Thomson Delmar Learning, 2004, pp. 214–215.

35. *ANS:* B

Tricare is a managed health care program offered to spouses and dependents of military service personnel. Champus was replaced by Tricare. Medicare and Medicaid are government agencies that offer support to the general public depending on need, income, and age.

References

Kalanick, K. *Phlebotomy Technician Specialist*. Clifton Park, N.Y.: Thomson Delmar Learning, 2004, p. 208.

36. *ANS:* B

To prevent a lawsuit, the phlebotomist:
- Accurately and legibly documents all information.
- Acquires informed consent prior to specimen collection.
- Documents all incidents immediately.
- Participates in continuing education.
- Performs at the accepted standard of care.
- Strictly adheres to all laboratory policies and procedures.
- Uses proper safety measures.

Having a clean professional background is what a phlebotomist should maintain and what would help in the event of a lawsuit; however, it is not part of the basic guidelines for the prevention of a lawsuit.

References

Kalanick, K. *Phlebotomy Technician Specialist*. Clifton Park, N.Y.: Thomson Delmar Learning, 2004, p. 20.

37. *ANS:* B

Civil law actions comprise the majority of all health care cases. Tort is a private wrong or injury, other than breach or contract, for which the court provides a remedy. Government law and federal law are distracters.

References

Kalanick, K. *Phlebotomy Technician Specialist*. Clifton Park, N.Y.: Thomson Delmar Learning, 2004, p. 15.

38. *ANS:* C

Negligence is the failure to act with reasonable care, resulting in the harming of others. Malpractice is misconduct or unprofessional treatment by someone in a professional or official position. Assault is the act of intentionally causing someone to fear that he or she is about to become the victim of battery, or incomplete battery. Battery is the act of intentionally touching someone in a harmful or offensive manner without the person's consent.

References

Kalanick, K. *Phlebotomy Technician Specialist*. Clifton Park, N.Y.: Thomson Delmar Learning, 2004, p. 19.

39. *ANS:* A

The explanation of benefits (EOB) explains to health care providers that the insurance is not responsible to pay the provider full amount. A deductible is a specific dollar amount that must be paid by the insured before a medical insurance plan or government program begins covering health care costs. A preexisting condition is any illness that began before the insurance policy was written. A copayment (also called copay) is a specific dollar amount that the patient must pay the provider for each encounter.

References

Kalanick, K. *Phlebotomy Technician Specialist*. Clifton Park, N.Y.: Thomson Delmar Learning, 2004, p. 209.

40. *ANS:* D

Most cases against phlebotomists involve malpractice or negligence for practices such as mislabeling specimens; failure to properly identify the patient; failure to use sterile techniques, causing infection; reuse of needles; failure to properly perform a test, resulting in misdiagnosis; injury to a vein, injury to a nerve, and/or scarring; failure to properly inform a patient of the risks, such as fainting; drawing blood without the patient's consent; breech of confidentiality; breakage of equipment, causing injury to the patient; and failure to control the chain of custody.

References

Kalanick, K. *Phlebotomy Technician Specialist*. Clifton Park, N.Y.: Thomson Delmar Learning, 2004, p. 21.

41. *ANS:* D

Patients have the right and responsibility to discuss their medical condition and information about medically appropriate treatment choices, to discuss their treatment plan, to submit information about their medical history, to explain their health care goals and values, and to inform providers as to who will make the decisions when they are unable to do so. It is not the patient's responsibility to diagnose and order lab tests.

References

Kalanick, K. *Phlebotomy Technician Specialist*. Clifton Park, N.Y.: Thomson Delmar Learning, 2004, p. 17.
Hoeltke, L. *The Complete Textbook of Phlebotomy*, 3rd ed. Clifton Park, N.Y.: Thomson Delmar Learning, 2006, p. 22.

42. *ANS:* C

A preferred provider organization (PPO) is a type of health benefit program in which enrollees receive the highest level of benefits when they obtain services from a physician, hospital, or other health provider designated by their program as a "preferred provider." Medicare and Medicaid are government-funded programs that provide services for the insured from authorized providers. An HMO is a type of health care program in which enrollees receive benefits for services from authorized and preselected providers employed by the HMO.

References

Kalanick, K. *Phlebotomy Technician Specialist*. Clifton Park, N.Y.: Thomson Delmar Learning, 2004, p. 212.

43. *ANS:* C

To make informed decisions with the doctor, the patient needs to understand:
- The benefits and risks of each treatment.
- Whether it is experimental or part of a research study.
- What may reasonably be expected from the treatment and any long-term effects it might have on the quality or life.
- What the patient and the family need to do after the patient leaves the hospital.

- The financial consequences of using uncovered services or out-of-network providers.

References

Kalanick, K. *Phlebotomy Technician Specialist*. Clifton Park, N.Y.: Thomson Delmar Learning, 2004, p. 16.

44. *ANS:* D

Caregivers need complete and correct information about a patient's health coverage so that they can make good decisions about care. That includes:
- Past illnesses, surgeries, or hospital stays.
- Past allergic reactions.
- Any medicines or diet supplements the patient is taking.
- Any network or admission requirements under the patient's health plan.

Also, the physician, the family, and the care team all need to know the patient's wishes about health care goals, values, and spiritual beliefs.

References

Kalanick, K. *Phlebotomy Technician Specialist*. Clifton Park, N.Y.: Thomson Delmar Learning, 2004, p. 17.

45. *ANS:* B

Slander is the act of falsifying facts that causes harm to a person's reputation. Slander is spoken; libel is written. Libel is a written statement falsifying facts about someone that causes harm to that person's reputation. Fraud is an intentional misrepresentation, a deliberate deception intended to produce unlawful gain. Duty of care is the responsibility not to infringe on another's rights by either intentionally or carelessly causing him or her harm.

References

Kalanick, K. *Phlebotomy Technician Specialist*. Clifton Park, N.Y.: Thomson Delmar Learning, 2004, p. 19.

46. *ANS:* A

In 1990, the federal government issued the Safe Medical Devices Act. This law was enacted to protect health care workers and patients from injuries caused by health care devices. All remaining answers are distracters.

References

Kalanick, K. *Phlebotomy Technician Specialist*. Clifton Park, N.Y.: Thomson Delmar Learning, 2004, p. 20.

47. *ANS:* D

Duty of care is the responsibility not to infringe on another's rights by either intentionally or carelessly causing him or her harm. Libel is a written statement falsifying facts about someone that causes harm to that person's reputation. Slander is the spoken act of falsifying facts that causes harm to a person's reputation. Invasion of privacy is a tort involving one or more of the following categories: the illegal appropriation of another's name for commercial use, intrusion into a person's privacy, placing a person in false light, or the disclosure of private facts.

References

Kalanick, K. *Phlebotomy Technician Specialist*. Clifton Park, N.Y.: Thomson Delmar Learning, 2004, p. 18.

48. *ANS:* A

A standard is a mode or rule for comparison of measurement that is established by custom or authority. Professionalism is the conduct, behavior, and qualities that characterize a professional person. Ethics is a system of principles governing medical conduct. It deals with the relationship of the health care professional to the patient, the patient's family, associates, and society at large. Integrity requires adherence to a strict ethical code, to be in an undiminished or unimpaired state.

References

Kalanick, K. *Phlebotomy Technician Specialist*. Clifton Park, N.Y.: Thomson Delmar Learning, 2004, p. 532.

Hoeltke, L. *The Complete Textbook of Phlebotomy*, 3rd ed. Clifton Park, N.Y.: Thomson Delmar Learning, 2006, p. 29.

49. *ANS:* D

When verbally communicating with a patient, do not use medical terms that may not be understood. Use terms that are appropriate for the age of your patient. Slang terms and abbreviations should be avoided altogether. Be brief, concise, and accurate when presenting information and answering questions.

References

Kalanick, K. *Phlebotomy Technician Specialist*. Clifton Park, N.Y.: Thomson Delmar Learning, 2004, p. 533.

Hoeltke, L. *The Complete Textbook of Phlebotomy*, 3rd ed. Clifton Park, N.Y.: Thomson Delmar Learning, 2006, p. 326.

50. *ANS:* A

Answer the phone within a maximum of three rings. All remaining answers are distracters.

References

Kalanick, K. *Phlebotomy Technician Specialist*. Clifton Park, N.Y.: Thomson Delmar Learning, 2004, p. 539.

MODULE 9: REGULATORY AGENCIES, SAFETY STANDARDS, AND INFECTION CONTROL

1. *ANS:* B

A microbe that is nondisease producing is called nonpathogenic. All other answers are distracters.

References

Kalanick, K. *Phlebotomy Technician Specialist*. Clifton Park, N.Y.: Thomson Delmar Learning, 2004, p. 162.

Hoeltke, L. *The Complete Textbook of Phlebotomy*, 3rd ed. Clifton Park, N.Y.: Thomson Delmar Learning, 2006, p. 44.

2. *ANS:* B

HIV (human immunodeficiency virus) is a retrovirus that causes AIDS.

References

Kalanick, K. *Phlebotomy Technician Specialist*. Clifton Park, N.Y.: Thomson Delmar Learning, 2004, p. 169.

3. *ANS:* D

The phlebotomist should be tested for HIV antibody as soon as possible after exposure for a baseline and periodically for at least 6 months. All other answers are distracters.

References

Kalanick, K. *Phlebotomy Technician Specialist*. Clifton Park, N.Y.: Thomson Delmar Learning, 2004, p. 192.

4. *ANS:* C

AFB (acid-fast-bacilli) isolation is required for patients with infectious tuberculosis. Strict isolation is complete isolation that is required for all patients with highly contagious diseases. Contact isolation is designed for highly transmittable disease spread primarily by direct contact. Drainage isolation is required for patient with skin infections, open wounds, or burns and sometimes following surgery.

References

Kalanick, K. *Phlebotomy Technician Specialist*. Clifton Park, N.Y.: Thomson Delmar Learning, 2004, p. 168.

Hoeltke, L. *The Complete Textbook of Phlebotomy*, 3rd ed. Clifton Park, N.Y.: Thomson Delmar Learning, 2006, p. 53.

5. *ANS:* D

Enteric isolation procedures are used for patients with intestinal infections that may be transmitted by ingestion.

References

Kalanick, K. *Phlebotomy Technician Specialist*. Clifton Park, N.Y.: Thomson Delmar Learning, 2004, p. 168.

Hoeltke, L. *The Complete Textbook of Phlebotomy*, 3rd ed. Clifton Park, N.Y.: Thomson Delmar Learning, 2006, p. 52.

6. *ANS:* B

HBV (hepatitis B virus) is a blood-borne pathogen that causes a severe acute infection and may progress to chronic infection and permanent liver damage.

References

Kalanick, K. *Phlebotomy Technician Specialist*. Clifton Park, N.Y.: Thomson Delmar Learning, 2004, p. 169.

Hoeltke, L. *The Complete Textbook of Phlebotomy*, 3rd ed. Clifton Park, N.Y.: Thomson Delmar Learning, 2006, p. 51.

7. *ANS:* B

"Blood-borne pathogen" is the term describing any infectious microorganism present in the blood and/or other body fluids and tissue.

References

Kalanick, K. *Phlebotomy Technician Specialist*. Clifton Park, N.Y.: Thomson Delmar Learning, 2004, p. 169.

Hoeltke, L. *The Complete Textbook of Phlebotomy*, 3rd ed. Clifton Park, N.Y.: Thomson Delmar Learning, 2006, p. 44.

8. *ANS:* B

When transmitted by infected patients by means of coughing or sneezing at close range, large-particle droplets generally travel up to only 3 feet.

References

Kalanick, K. *Phlebotomy Technician Specialist*. Clifton Park, N.Y.: Thomson Delmar Learning, 2004, p. 175.

Hoeltke, L. *The Complete Textbook of Phlebotomy*, 3rd ed. Clifton Park, N.Y.: Thomson Delmar Learning, 2006, p. 53.

9. *ANS:* A

Biological hazards, or biohazards, are any materials containing blood or body fluids that are dangerous to health. Chemical hazards are dangerous, especially when they result from mixing wrong chemicals, but they do not contain blood or body fluids. Electrical hazards can occur when using electrical equipment. Radioactive hazards are dangerous based on the level of exposure and the source of the radiation.

References

Kalanick, K. *Phlebotomy Technician Specialist*. Clifton Park, N.Y.: Thomson Delmar Learning, 2004, p. 184.

Hoeltke, L. *The Complete Textbook of Phlebotomy*, 3rd ed. Clifton Park, N.Y.: Thomson Delmar Learning, 2006, p. 67.

10. *ANS:* C

Indirect contact involves exposing a susceptible host to a pathogen by means of an inanimate object.

References

Kalanick, K. *Phlebotomy Technician Specialist*. Clifton Park, N.Y.: Thomson Delmar Learning, 2004, p. 163.

Hoeltke, L. *The Complete Textbook of Phlebotomy*, 3rd ed. Clifton Park, N.Y.: Thomson Delmar Learning, 2006, p. 53.

11. *ANS:* D

Disposable gloves, a lab coat or apron, and/or protective face gear, such as masks and goggles with side shields, are required by OSHA as personal protective equipment (PPE).

References

Kalanick, K. *Phlebotomy Technician Specialist*. Clifton Park, N.Y.: Thomson Delmar Learning, 2004, p. 164.

Hoeltke, L. *The Complete Textbook of Phlebotomy*, 3rd ed. Clifton Park, N.Y.: Thomson Delmar Learning, 2006, p. 57.

12. *ANS:* B

Hand washing is the first line of defense in the fight against the spread of infection. Gloves, lab coats, and face shields are all part of personal protective equipment but are not considered the first line of defense in the fight against the spread of infection.

References

Kalanick, K. *Phlebotomy Technician Specialist*. Clifton Park, N.Y.: Thomson Delmar Learning, 2004, p. 176.

Hoeltke, L. *The Complete Textbook of Phlebotomy*, 3rd ed. Clifton Park, N.Y.: Thomson Delmar Learning, 2006, p. 54.

13. *ANS:* B

Chemical spills require special cleanup kits containing absorbent and neutralizer materials, which are used depending on the type of chemical spill.

References

Kalanick, K. *Phlebotomy Technician Specialist*. Clifton Park, N.Y.: Thomson Delmar Learning, 2004, p. 186.

Hoeltke, L. *The Complete Textbook of Phlebotomy*, 3rd ed. Clifton Park, N.Y.: Thomson Delmar Learning, 2006, p. 70.

14. *ANS:* B

The disposal of chemicals is regulated by the EPA (Environmental Protection Agency). The DEA is the Drug Enforcement Agency, OSHA is the Occupational

Safety and Health Administration, and the CDC is the Center for Disease Control. These agencies do not specifically regulate the disposal of chemicals.

References

Kalanick, K. *Phlebotomy Technician Specialist*. Clifton Park, N.Y.: Thomson Delmar Learning, 2004, p. 186.

Hoeltke, L. *The Complete Textbook of Phlebotomy*, 3rd ed. Clifton Park, N.Y.: Thomson Delmar Learning, 2006, p. 70.

15. *ANS:* A

The Environment Protection Agency recommends the use of a 1:10 bleach solution or other EPA-approved disinfectant.

References

Kalanick, K. *Phlebotomy Technician Specialist*. Clifton Park, N.Y.: Thomson Delmar Learning, 2004, p. 190.

Hoeltke, L. *The Complete Textbook of Phlebotomy*, 3rd ed. Clifton Park, N.Y.: Thomson Delmar Learning, 2006, p. 50.

16. *ANS:* C

Electrical equipment fires require a Class C fire extinguisher, which is designed for ordinary combustibles, such as wood, paper, or clothing. A Class B extinguisher is designed for flammable liquids and vapors, such as paint, oil, grease, or gasoline. Class D extinguishers are designed for combustible or reactive metals, such as sodium, potassium, magnesium, and the like.

References

Kalanick, K. *Phlebotomy Technician Specialist*. Clifton Park, N.Y.: Thomson Delmar Learning, 2004, p. 188.

Hoeltke, L. *The Complete Textbook of Phlebotomy*, 3rd ed. Clifton Park, N.Y.: Thomson Delmar Learning, 2006, p. 71.

17. *ANS:* B

A material safety data sheet provides detailed information for each hazardous chemical manufactured or imported.

References

Kalanick, K. *Phlebotomy Technician Specialist*. Clifton Park, N.Y.: Thomson Delmar Learning, 2004, p. 186.

Hoeltke, L. *The Complete Textbook of Phlebotomy*, 3rd ed. Clifton Park, N.Y.: Thomson Delmar Learning, 2006, p. 69.

18. *ANS:* C

Disposable instruments would be discarded in a biohazards sharps container and not in a biohazards waste container. Gowns may be disposable and discarded in a biohazards container. Disposable gloves are never washed and reused. They should be appropriately removed and disposed of in a biohazards waste container. Lab coats can either remain at the laboratory and be laundered or disposed of in the biohazards container.

References

Kalanick, K. *Phlebotomy Technician Specialist*. Clifton Park, N.Y.: Thomson Delmar Learning, 2004, pp. 174, 175, 176.

Hoeltke, L. *The Complete Textbook of Phlebotomy*, 3rd ed. Clifton Park, N.Y.: Thomson Delmar Learning, 2006, p. 57.

19. *ANS:* B

To maintain medical asepsis, hands and wrists are washed for a minimum of 2 minutes with antimicrobial or antibacterial soap.

References

Kalanick, K. *Phlebotomy Technician Specialist*. Clifton Park, N.Y.: Thomson Delmar Learning, 2004, p. 177.

20. *ANS:* D

If an electrical accident occurs, you must shut off the source of electricity immediately.

References

Kalanick, K. *Phlebotomy Technician Specialist*. Clifton Park, N.Y.: Thomson Delmar Learning, 2004, p. 187.

Hoeltke, L. *The Complete Textbook of Phlebotomy*, 3rd ed. Clifton Park, N.Y.: Thomson Delmar Learning, 2006, p. 71.

21. *ANS:* C

Quality assurance is a group of activities and programs designed to guarantee the highest level of quality patient care.

References

Kalanick, K. *Phlebotomy Technician Specialist*. Clifton Park, N.Y.: Thomson Delmar Learning, 2004, p. 25.

Hoeltke, L. *The Complete Textbook of Phlebotomy*, 3rd ed. Clifton Park, N.Y.: Thomson Delmar Learning, 2006, p. 34.

22. *ANS:* C

Risk management is a program, used in conjunction with QA/QC (quality assurance/quality control), designed to minimize the risk of loss or injury for both the health care provider and the patient.

References

Kalanick, K. *Phlebotomy Technician Specialist*. Clifton Park, N.Y.: Thomson Delmar Learning, 2004, p. 26.

Hoeltke, L. *The Complete Textbook of Phlebotomy*, 3rd ed. Clifton Park, N.Y.: Thomson Delmar Learning, 2006, p. 34.

23. *ANS:* D

OSHA regulates standards for blood-borne pathogens, personal protective equipment, formaldehyde (standard), eye wash protection, respirator (standard), maintenance of the log for injuries and illnesses, electrical systems, and disposal of biohazardous wastes.

References

Kalanick, K. *Phlebotomy Technician Specialist*. Clifton Park, N.Y.: Thomson Delmar Learning, 2004, p. 22.
Hoeltke, L. *The Complete Textbook of Phlebotomy*, 3rd ed. Clifton Park, N.Y.: Thomson Delmar Learning, 2006, p. 62.

24. *ANS:* A

Moderate-complexity tests are more complicated to perform than waived tests; they require an understanding of methodology, quality control, reagent stability, and instrument calibration. High-complexity tests include sophisticated testing methodology and often require independent judgment for interpretation. Waived tests are simple to perform, require a minimum of quality control, and have insignificant risk of harm to the patient. Low-complexity tests is a distracter.

References

Kalanick, K. *Phlebotomy Technician Specialist*. Clifton Park, N.Y.: Thomson Delmar Learning, 2004, p. 24.

25. *ANS:* A

The Joint Commission of Accreditation of Healthcare Organizations (JCAHO) is the leading national accreditation body for hospitals. CLSI is the Clinical Laboratory Standard Institute, NACCLS is the National Accrediting Agency for Clinical Laboratory Sciences, and HIPAA is the Health Insurance Portability and Accountability Act.

References

Kalanick, K. *Phlebotomy Technician Specialist*. Clifton Park, N.Y.: Thomson Delmar Learning, 2004, p. 25.

26. *ANS:* B

In essence, a reservoir host is the breeding ground for the transmission of pathogens to others.

References

Kalanick, K. *Phlebotomy Technician Specialist*. Clifton Park, N.Y.: Thomson Delmar Learning, 2004, p. 162.

Hoeltke, L. *The Complete Textbook of Phlebotomy*, 3rd ed. Clifton Park, N.Y.: Thomson Delmar Learning, 2006, p. 44.

27. *ANS:* B

A pathogen is an organism or substance capable of causing a disease, condition, or infection. A nonpathogenic organism is a microbe that is nondisease producing. Curative and corroborative are nonsense distracters.

References

Kalanick, K. *Phlebotomy Technician Specialist*. Clifton Park, N.Y.: Thomson Delmar Learning, 2004, p. 162.
Hoeltke, L. *The Complete Textbook of Phlebotomy*, 3rd ed. Clifton Park, N.Y.: Thomson Delmar Learning, 2006, p. 44.

28. *ANS:* B

The Centers for Disease Control (CDC), Occupational Safety and Health Administration (OSHA), Joint Committee for Accrediting Healthcare Organizations (JCAHO), and Hospital Infection Control Practices Advisory Committee (HICPAC) all assist hospitals, clinics, and laboratories to maintain up-to-date isolation practices, establish guidelines, and enforce regulations governing infection control. HIPAA is the Health Insurance Portability and Accountability Act and is not involved in isolation practices.

References

Kalanick, K. *Phlebotomy Technician Specialist*. Clifton Park, N.Y.: Thomson Delmar Learning, 2004, p. 164.

29. *ANS:* A

Contact isolation was designed for highly transmittable diseases that are spread primarily by direct contact and that do not warrant strict isolation. Examples of these conditions are antibiotic-resistant pathogens and respiratory disorders, such as bronchitis, croup, epiglottitis, and pneumonia.

References

Kalanick, K. *Phlebotomy Technician Specialist*. Clifton Park, N.Y.: Thomson Delmar Learning, 2004, p. 167.
Hoeltke, L. *The Complete Textbook of Phlebotomy*, 3rd ed. Clifton Park, N.Y.: Thomson Delmar Learning, 2006, p. 53.

30. *ANS:* C

In 1970, the CDC published a detailed manual entitled *Isolation Techniques for Use in Hospitals* to assist general hospitals with isolation precautions.

References

Kalanick, K. *Phlebotomy Technician Specialist*. Clifton Park, N.Y.: Thomson Delmar Learning, 2004, p. 166.

Appendix B

Answers to Critical Thinking

MODULE 4

1. Patient, complains of, lower left quadrant, after eating, level of consciousness, patient, history, hepatitis B virus, complete blood count, calcium, and hemoglobin and hematocrit, liver test, morning, Patient, nothing by mouth, before operation, 4 hours, after operation.

2. Labor and delivery, without, neonatal intensive care unit, immediately, aspartate aminotransferase (also known as SGOT serum glutamic oxaloacetic), creatinine kinase, electrocardiogram.

    Murmurs are defects in the valves of the heart. The valves help to regulate the flow of blood from one chamber to another chamber of the heart. When one or more are not working properly, the blood pools, causing unoxygenated or superoxygenated blood to be in the incorrect chamber, depending on which valve is involved. This causes a lack of oxygenation to the tissues and the skin to appear blue.

3. Jamie was drawing blood from an artery, not a vein. Jamie should have known from the bright red blood spurting into the tube. Venous blood is dark red and typically does not spurt.

    Dr. Smart will remove the tourniquet and apply direct pressure on the puncture site until the bleeding stops. He may also elevate the arm and ask the nurse to apply a pressure dressing.

    Jamie should get the nurse as requested. After the patient has been taken care of, Jamie should help clean up and then must report the incident to her supervisor. An incident report also needs to be completed and filed.

MODULE 5

1. Emergency room, physician, radiology, radiologist, phlebotomist, certified nursing assistant, respiratory therapist, pharmacist, nurse's

2. Oncologist, cytology

3. A PA works under the direct supervision of an M.D. and can provide skills comparable to an M.D. (physical examinations to surgical procedures).

MODULE 6

1. *Autologous blood donation:* Autologous transfusions are transfusions in which the blood donor and transfusion recipient are the same. In other words, a person donates blood for his or her own use. This may be done prior to elective surgeries or when an anticipated transfusion is required. A person may donate one unit of blood each week for up to 6 weeks before surgery. Blood can be stored in its liquid form for up to 42 days. Preoperative autologous donations may not be made within 72 hours of surgery. Using one's own blood for transfusion eliminates numerous risks associated with donor transfusions, such as disease transmission and incompatibilities. If the blood is not required for transfusion, the blood may be used for the general population with the donor's permission.

    She can donate a unit of blood per week, for up to 6 weeks before surgery. Her blood can be stored in liquid form for up to 42 days.

    Blood bank specimens require:
    - The patient's full name, including middle initial.
    - The patient's hospital identification number or, if an outpatient, social security number.
    - The patient's date of birth.
    - The date and time of collection.
    - The phlebotomist's initials.
    - The room number and bed number (optional).

2. Physically support the patient to prevent further injury, loosen any tight clothing, such as collars or ties. Apply a cold compress or washcloth to the forehead and back of the neck, if necessary; use an ammonia inhalant to bring the patient "back around." Alert the nurse and/or physician as quickly as possible. Monitor the patient's vital signs, until he returns to normal or a nurse or physician assumes responsibility for him.

3. First mistake: Never tell a patient that it isn't going to hurt. You may need to enlist the help of Suzie's doctor or one of the medical staff with whom Suzie is more familiar to help calm her down. If this is not

217

effective, the physician may suggest you wait a few minutes, use distractions, or send the patient to the ER where they can restrain or sedate her. What you don't want is to have to stick her more than once or to have her fight you and cause a contaminated needle stick.

MODULE 7

1. The clinician should have:
   - Had the consent form signed and the picture ID before collecting the specimen.
   - Never collected the specimen without the bluing for the water.
   - Contacted the potential employer about the refusal to sign the consent form by the employee candidate.
2. Choose the capillary stick because it is stat. His range should be 42–52 percent.
3. The test will tell the physician nothing because the test results are not valid. Melanie should not have taken her blood pressure medication this morning prior to testing.

MODULE 8

1. Dr. Korn is guilty of a civil offense. He caused a tort called intentional infliction of emotional distress.
2. Mr. Leonard signed a consent form stating he didn't want the insurance billed. Obviously, if he received an EOB, the insurance was billed and the office violated HIPAA. Any test for STD (e.g., HIV, Chlamydia, hepatitis C) is to be kept confidential. Mr. Leonard is upset probably because, if the test were to be positive, his insurance company now knows, which could possibly cause problems for Mr. Leonard's coverage in the future.

3. Jim feels this way about the health clinic because of the staff's effective verbal and nonverbal communication.

MODULE 9

1. Airborne transmission occurs by dissemination of either airborne droplet nuclei or dust particles containing the infectious agent. Microorganisms carried in this manner can be dispersed widely by air currents and may become inhaled by a susceptible host in the same room or over a longer distance from the source patient, depending on environmental factors.

   AFB (acid-fast-bacilli) isolation is the appropriate protocol for Mr. Franklin. AFB isolation is required for patients with infectious tuberculosis. OSHA implemented a new policy, requiring the use of a high-efficiency particulate air (HEPA) respirator as a minimum level of respiratory protection for all health care workers who care for AFB patients. Gowns and gloves are also required as part of the barrier precautions. All supplies must be disposed of inside the patient's room.
2. Phyllis should enlist the help of the nurse to untangle the boy from her earring as Phyllis keeps the needle secure in the boy's arm. Or Phyllis should remove the needle, release the tourniquet, and apply pressure on the venipuncture site (or ask the nurse to apply pressure) as she removes the earring from the ear or the boy's hand from the earring.

   Phyllis should not be wearing loop earrings to begin with; this is one of the first lab safety rules you learn.
3. The answer is level 1—Moderate complexity.

   It is more complicated to perform than waived tests, and it requires an understanding of methodology, quality control, reagent stability, and instrument calibration.

Index

Phlebotomy Technician Specialist: Certification Exam Review

LICENSE AGREEMENT: IMPORTANT! READ CAREFULLY: This End User License Agreement ("Agreement") sets forth the conditions by which Thomson Delmar Learning, a division of Thomson Learning Inc. ("Thomson") will make electronic access to the Thomson Delmar Learning-owned licensed content and associated media, software, documentation, printed materials, and electronic documentation contained in this package and/or made available to you via this product (the "Licensed Content"), available to you (the "End User"). BY CLICKING THE "I ACCEPT" BUTTON AND/OR OPENING THIS PACKAGE, YOU ACKNOWLEDGE THAT YOU HAVE READ ALL OF THE TERMS AND CONDITIONS, AND THAT YOU AGREE TO BE BOUND BY ITS TERMS, CONDITIONS, AND ALL APPLICABLE LAWS AND REGULATIONS GOVERNING THE USE OF THE LICENSED CONTENT.

1.0 SCOPE OF LICENSE

1.1 *Licensed Content.* The Licensed Content may contain portions of modifiable content ("Modifiable Content") and content which may not be modified or otherwise altered by the End User ("Non-Modifiable Content"). For purposes of this Agreement, Modifiable Content and Non-Modifiable Content may be collectively referred to herein as the "Licensed Content." All Licensed Content shall be considered Non-Modifiable Content, unless such Licensed Content is presented to the End User in a modifiable format and it is clearly indicated that modification of the Licensed Content is permitted.

1.2 Subject to the End User's compliance with the terms and conditions of this Agreement, Thomson Delmar Learning hereby grants the End User, a nontransferable, nonexclusive, limited right to access and view a single copy of the Licensed Content on a single personal computer system for noncommercial, internal, personal use only. The End User shall not (i) reproduce, copy, modify (except in the case of Modifiable Content), distribute, display, transfer, sublicense, prepare derivative work(s) based on, sell, exchange, barter or transfer, rent, lease, loan, resell, or in any other manner exploit the Licensed Content; (ii) remove, obscure, or alter any notice of Thomson Delmar Learning's intellectual property rights present on or in the Licensed Content, including, but not limited to, copyright, trademark, and/or patent notices; or (iii) disassemble, decompile, translate, reverse engineer, or otherwise reduce the Licensed Content.

2.0 TERMINATION

2.1 Thomson Delmar Learning may at any time (without prejudice to its other rights or remedies) immediately terminate this Agreement and/or suspend access to some or all of the Licensed Content, in the event that the End User does not comply with any of the terms and conditions of this Agreement. In the event of such termination by Thomson Delmar Learning, the End User shall immediately return any and all copies of the Licensed Content to Thomson Delmar Learning.

3.0 PROPRIETARY RIGHTS

3.1 The End User acknowledges that Thomson Delmar Learning owns all rights, title and interest, including, but not limited to all copyright rights therein, in and to the Licensed Content, and that the End User shall not take any action inconsistent with such ownership. The Licensed Content is protected by U.S., Canadian and other applicable copyright laws and by international treaties, including the Berne Convention and the Universal Copyright Convention. Nothing contained in this Agreement shall be construed as granting the End User any ownership rights in or to the Licensed Content.

3.2 Thomson Delmar Learning reserves the right at any time to withdraw from the Licensed Content any item or part of an item for which it no longer retains the right to publish, or which it has reasonable grounds to believe infringes copyright or is defamatory, unlawful, or otherwise objectionable.

4.0 PROTECTION AND SECURITY

4.1 The End User shall use its best efforts and take all reasonable steps to safeguard its copy of the Licensed Content to ensure that no unauthorized reproduction, publication, disclosure, modification, or distribution of the Licensed Content, in whole or in part, is made. To the extent that the End User becomes aware of any such unauthorized use of the Licensed Content, the End User shall immediately notify Thomson Delmar Learning. Notification of such violations may be made by sending an e-mail to delmarhelp@thomson.com.

5.0 MISUSE OF THE LICENSED PRODUCT

5.1 In the event that the End User uses the Licensed Content in violation of this Agreement, Thomson Delmar Learning shall have the option of electing liquidated damages, which shall include all profits generated by the End User's use of the Licensed Content plus interest computed at the maximum rate permitted by law and all legal fees and other expenses incurred by Thomson Delmar Learning in enforcing its rights, plus penalties.

6.0 FEDERAL GOVERNMENT CLIENTS

6.1 Except as expressly authorized by Thomson Delmar Learning, Federal Government clients obtain only the rights specified in this Agreement and no other rights. The Government acknowledges that (i) all software and related documentation incorporated in the Licensed Content is existing commercial computer software within the meaning of FAR 27.405(b)(2); and (2) all other data delivered in whatever form, is limited rights data within the meaning of FAR 27.401. The restrictions in this section are acceptable as consistent with the Government's need for software and other data under this Agreement.

7.0 DISCLAIMER OF WARRANTIES AND LIABILITIES

7.1 Although Thomson Delmar Learning believes the Licensed Content to be reliable, Thomson Delmar Learning does not guarantee or warrant (i) any information or materials contained in or produced by the Licensed Content, (ii) the accuracy, completeness or reliability of the Licensed Content, or (iii) that the Licensed Content is free from errors or other material defects. THE LICENSED PRODUCT IS PROVIDED "AS IS," WITHOUT ANY WARRANTY OF ANY KIND AND THOMSON DELMAR LEARNING DISCLAIMS ANY AND ALL WARRANTIES, EXPRESSED OR IMPLIED, INCLUDING, WITHOUT LIMITATION, WARRANTIES OF MERCHANTABILITY OR FITNESS OR A PARTICULAR PURPOSE. IN NO EVENT SHALL THOMSON DELMAR LEARNING BE LIABLE FOR: INDIRECT, SPECIAL, PUNITIVE OR CONSEQUENTIAL DAMAGES INCLUDING FOR LOST PROFITS, LOST DATA, OR OTHERWISE. IN NO EVENT SHALL THOMSON DELMAR LEARNING'S AGGREGATE LIABILITY HEREUNDER, WHETHER ARISING IN CONTRACT, TORT, STRICT LIABILITY OR OTHERWISE, EXCEED THE AMOUNT OF FEES PAID BY THE END USER HEREUNDER FOR THE LICENSE OF THE LICENSED CONTENT.

8.0 GENERAL

8.1 *Entire Agreement.* This Agreement shall constitute the entire Agreement between the Parties and supercedes all prior Agreements and understandings oral or written relating to the subject matter hereof.

8.2 *Enhancements/Modifications of Licensed Content.* From time to time, and in Thomson Delmar Learning's sole discretion, Thomson Delmar Learning may advise the End User of updates, upgrades, enhancements and/or improvements to the Licensed Content, and may permit the End User to access and use, subject to the terms and conditions of this Agreement, such modifications, upon payment of prices as may be established by Thomson Delmar Learning.

8.3 *No Export.* The End User shall use the Licensed Content solely in the United States and shall not transfer or export, directly or indirectly, the Licensed Content outside the United States.

8.4 *Severability.* If any provision of this Agreement is invalid, illegal, or unenforceable under any applicable statute or rule of law, the provision shall be deemed omitted to the extent that it is invalid, illegal, or unenforceable. In such a case, the remainder of the Agreement shall be construed in a manner as to give greatest effect to the original intention of the parties hereto.

8.5 *Waiver.* The waiver of any right or failure of either party to exercise in any respect any right provided in this Agreement in any instance shall not be deemed to be a waiver of such right in the future or a waiver of any other right under this Agreement.

8.6 *Choice of Law/Venue.* This Agreement shall be interpreted, construed, and governed by and in accordance with the laws of the State of New York, applicable to contracts executed and to be wholly preformed therein, without regard to its principles governing conflicts of law. Each party agrees that any proceeding arising out of or relating to this Agreement or the breach or threatened breach of this Agreement may be commenced and prosecuted in a court in the State and County of New York. Each party consents and submits to the nonexclusive personal jurisdiction of any court in the State and County of New York in respect of any such proceeding.

8.7 *Acknowledgment.* By opening this package and/or by accessing the Licensed Content on this Web site, THE END USER ACKNOWLEDGES THAT IT HAS READ THIS AGREEMENT, UNDERSTANDS IT, AND AGREES TO BE BOUND BY ITS TERMS AND CONDITIONS. IF YOU DO NOT ACCEPT THESE TERMS AND CONDITIONS, YOU MUST NOT ACCESS THE LICENSED CONTENT AND RETURN THE LICENSED PRODUCT TO DELMAR LEARNING (WITHIN 30 CALENDAR DAYS OF THE END USER'S PURCHASE) WITH PROOF OF PAYMENT ACCEPTABLE TO THOMSON DELMAR LEARNING, FOR A CREDIT OR A REFUND. Should the End User have any questions/comments regarding this Agreement, please contact Thomson Delmar Learning at delmarhelp@thomson.com.

SETUP INSTRUCTIONS:
1. Insert disk into CD-ROM player. The installation program should start momentarily.
2. If the installation program does not start, then choose Run... from the Start menu.
3. In the Open text box, enter d:setup.exe then click the OK button. (Substitute the letter of your CD-ROM drive for d:)
4. Follow the installation prompts from there.

SYSTEM REQUIREMENTS:
- Operating system: Microsoft® Windows™ 98, 2000, Me, XP, or newer
- Processor: Pentium (or newer) CPU
- Memory: 32 MB or more of RAM
- Hard drive space: 10 MB or more
- Monitor: 256 color display or better
- CD-ROM drive

Microsoft® is a registered trademark and Windows™ and Windows NT® are trademarks of Microsoft Coporation.